Musculoskeletal and Sports Injuries

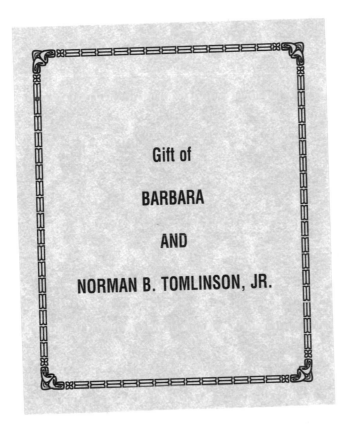

Musculoskeletal and Sports Injuries

Brian Corrigan
MB, BS, FRCP, FRCPE, FRACP, FACRM, DPhysMed
Head, Department of Rheumatology, Concord Hospital, Sydney, Australia

G.D. Maitland
MBE, AUA, FCSP, FACP, FACP (Specialist in Manipulative Physiotherapy), MAPPLSci
Specialist Lecturer, University of South Australia

BUTTERWORTH
HEINEMANN

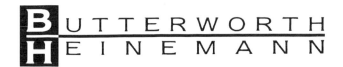

Butterworth-Heinemann Ltd
Linacre House, Jordan Hill, Oxford OX2 8DP

 A member of the Reed Elsevier group

OXFORD   LONDON   BOSTON
MUNICH   NEW DELHI   SINGAPORE   SYDNEY
TOKYO   TORONTO   WELLINGTON

First published 1994   # 28802067

British Library Cataloguing in Publication Data
Corrigan, Brian
  Musculoskeletal and Sports Injuries
  I. Title   II. Maitland, G. D.
  617.3

ISBN 0 7506 1485 4

Library of Congress Cataloguing in Publication Data
Corrigan, Brian
  Musculoskeletal and sports injuries/Brian Corrigan, G. D.
  Maitland.
  p.   cm.
  Includes bibliographical references and index.
  ISBN 0 7506 1485 4
  1. Sports – Accidents and injuries. 2. Musculoskeletal system –
  Wounds and injuries. 3. Sports physical therapy. I. Maitland,
  G. D. (Geoffrey Douglas) II. Title.
  [DNLM: 1. Athletic Injuries – therapy. 2. Sports Medicine. QT
  260 C825m]
  RD97.C67   93–34395
  617.1'027–dc20   CIP

Composition by Scribe Design, Gillingham, Kent
Printed and bound in Great Britain by the Bath Press, Avon

Contents

Preface

This book has evolved from our text *Practical Orthopaedic Medicine*. This has been so very well received and a new edition was needed. During the preparation of the new edition we discarded virtually every reference due to the huge increase in the sports medicine literature and since sports medicine is a major interest for us both, we decided to increase markedly the sports injuries content in this book. Thus the book has a new title *Musculoskeletal and Sports Injuries* to reflect this change, but the original principles of the first book have been retained: a clinical approach based on history and examination of musculoskeletal disorders with an emphasis on function. This increase in content has meant that we can only deal with peripheral, and not spinal, joints.

Musculoskeletal and Sports Injuries deals with soft tissue lesions but stresses mainly sporting injuries. The emphasis in treatment is on conservative management including physiotherapy, especially the role that gentler manual methods and stretching can play.

However, a shoulder lesion such as supraspinatus tendinitis should present the same problem whether or not it is to a sport clinic, physical medicine clinic, rheumatology clinic, physiotherapy clinic or an orthopaedic clinic. Its cause may be different but clinical signs are basically the same in each type of clinic. Our concept was to attempt to weld together all these approaches.

Our thanks for bringing about this book goes to many people but especially to Dr C. Needs, S. Graham, B. Shenstone and M. Brown for useful suggestions and reading the manuscript; Tania Rtshaldze and Deidre Tapscott for not only their typing but also valuable advice; Virginia Staggs and the library staff at Concord Hospital for finding so many references so efficiently; Andrew McArthur and the staff of the Photography Department; Anne Maitland for artwork; and Tania Brinsden our most photogenic model from the Physiotherapy Unit at Concord Hospital. Finally, but not at all least, the staff at Butterworth-Heinemann: John Coxhill, Charles Fry and Caroline Makepeace – not only for their help to us, but also for bearing with us for a few difficult years with troubles not of their making.

Brian Corrigan
G. D. Maitland

1 Pain in the limbs

Musculoskeletal pain in the limb may be classified under four headings: joint pain, soft tissue pain, neurogenic pain, and orthopaedic causes including fractures, dislocations, tumours and infections.

Joint pain

Although the microstructure of peripheral joints is complex, their basic design is relatively simple. The bone ends forming the joint are lined by avascular articular cartilage, nourished by synovial fluid derived from the highly vascular synovial membrane. Two joints, the shoulder and hip, are deepened by a cartilaginous labrum. Five joints – knee, wrist, sternoclavicular, temporomandibular and acromioclavicular – also contain an intra-articular fibrocartilaginous meniscus. These structures reduce joint compressive loads by distributing them uniformly over a large joint surface area protecting the articular cartilage, aiding joint nutrition and helping to stabilize the joints.

Synovial joints are movable joints and normal movement depends on several factors. Each peripheral joint has a normal, physiological range of movement determined to some extent by the configuration of the opposing joint surfaces. On joint movement, these opposing surfaces can slide, roll and spin on one another. This normal range also depends on the integrated action of the surrounding soft tissues, which is under voluntary neurological control, and on a series of involuntary, or accessory, joint movements that vary for each joint.

Joint stability depends on static and dynamic factors. Static factors depend on the shape of the bony joint surfaces with the integrity of surrounding capsular and ligamentous supports. Ligaments function to guide joints through their physiological range of motion and to resist applied tensile and shear forces. The menisci and labra assist in stabilizing joints by deepening them. Dynamic factors are the surrounding muscles with their tendons. Stability is essential for normal movement and the joint must remain within the constraints that hold it together but allow movement to the limit of these constraints.

Joint disorders may be caused by:

1   Inflammation. Inflammatory changes, often on the basis of altered immunity, first involve the synovial membrane. Synovitis produces soft tissue swelling and synovial effusion with pain, stiffness and loss of function.
2   Degeneration. Degenerative changes first involve the articular cartilage with fibrillation, fissuring and erosions, focal at first but then becoming confluent with reactive changes in surrounding articular tissues.
3   Abnormality or alteration in the normal range of joint movements. Thus movement may be:
    (a) Decreased: this is called hypomobility (where there is a loss of physiological and accessory movement).
    (b) Ankylosed with no joint movement.
    (c) Increased because of hypermobility.
    (d) Abnormal as a result of joint instability.
    (e) Blocked owing to an internal derangement of the joint, e.g. a torn intra-articular meniscus or loose foreign body.

Link system

The joints in a limb may be looked on as forming links in a chain, moved by muscles whose action is integrated through this system of links. During activity large internal forces may be generated around a joint, which then acts as fulcrum both for proximal and for distal lever arms. Sporting movements require muscular activity of a ballistic type, that once set in motion tend to remain so because of momentum. The body has been likened to a rocket which has been set in motion with a burst of energy. This propulsive effort is then maintained through an integrated muscle mechanism that propels the moving parts through this linked system of joints. Musculoskeletal pain may develop as the result of an alteration in other parts of the system of links. Accordingly, when examining a patient with joint pain the whole of the limb must be examined to determine whether any abnormality is present in another part of the link. These abnormalities include joint stiffness, muscular weakness or tightness, and postural abnormalities or misalignments, such as knee or foot deformities with excessive subtalar joint pronation or unequal leg lengths. They may not become clinically apparent until strenuous sporting, recreational or occupational loads are placed upon them.

Soft tissue lesions

The soft tissues around the joints are the joint capsule and ligaments, muscles, tendons with their surrounding synovial sheaths or bursae. Pain in the soft tissues may be generalized or localized.

Generalized causes

These include:

1 Viral diseases. Almost every viral disease, e.g. influenza, can have generalized aches and pains as a prodrome.
2 Many drugs, especially antibiotics, antihypertensives, antiepileptics and cardiac drugs. If the diagnosis is in doubt, it is often wise to stop the drug first.
3 The prodromal stages of any connective tissue disease, e.g. rheumatoid arthritis, systemic lupus, polymyalgia rheumatica. Metabolic and endocrine disorders, e.g. hyper- or hypothyroidism.

4 Psychogenic causes should also be considered in any consideration of limb pain. The most common causes are depression and anxiety-tension states. Depressed people often have sleep disturbances but believe this to be due to their pain. In addition, a psychogenic overlay may be present, often associated with a secondary gain, either emotional or financial, or can be related to a fear of becoming crippled, especially if there is a family history of arthritis. Finally, hysteria or malingering, but they are distinctly uncommon causes of such pain.
5 Fibrositis or fibromyalgia syndrome exists in two forms. A localized form is related to spinal hypomobility lesions. A generalized form occurs usually in young people of either sex with variable degrees of generalized non-articular pain, stiffness, fatigue, a disturbance in sleep quality, and localized areas of tenderness in muscles (trigger spots). Its aetiology is unknown but it may be stress related and may represent a state of abnormal peripheral sensorineural activation.

Localized causes

Localized causes in the peripheral joints, or regional pain syndromes, can be classified according to the joint involved (e.g. shoulder, elbow) and the soft tissue involved (e.g. muscle tendon, bursa). Most joints have several typical lesions in the surrounding soft tissues. Their diagnosis is mainly clinical (see Chapter 3) and are described in subsequent chapters.

Neurogenic causes

The musculoskeletal system is intimately related to the peripheral nerves, surrounding neural sheath, and their dural supportive structures, so much so that it can be looked on as a neuromusculoskeletal system.

Neurogenic limb pain may have one of three causes:

1 Nerve root compression due to spine disorders, especially intervertebral disc prolapse with radicular pain.
2 Referred pain may arise from spinal joints with pain referred distally into the limb. Referred pain may also arise in one peripheral joint and

again be referred distally. The common example given is of knee pain referred from the hip.

3 Peripheral nerve entrapments result as a nerve is compressed as it runs through its normal anatomical confines in soft tissues or fibro-osseous canals. The most common site is the median nerve in the carpal tunnel, but nerve entrapment may also complicate soft tissue lesions such as tenosynovitis resulting from overuse, trauma or rheumatoid arthritis.

2 Sports injuries

Soft tissue sporting injuries may be classified into one of three categories according to their mechanism of production: (1) direct injuries, (2) indirect injuries, and (3) overuse injuries.

Direct injuries

Direct injuries are produced, as their name suggests, by a direct blow by an opponent, or a sporting implement such as a stick, ball or a fall. They most commonly occur in body-contact sports resulting in a contusion injury with disruption of blood vessels in either muscles or joints.

Muscles

Muscle is supplied by an extensive capillary network measuring approximately 3000 per mm^2 on cross-section. At rest, most of these are closed. In actively exercising muscles, the rate of blood flow is markedly increased and in the large muscle groups of the leg blood flow may be increased up to eight times the resting rate. During activity, a direct blow to this highly vascular tissue is capable of producing an extensive intramuscular haemorrhage. This injury results in haematoma formation, usually between the muscle fibres themselves, without any particular disruption of muscle fibres, but with a varying degree of reflex muscle spasm. This type of injury is most liable to occur in the thigh and haemorrhage into the quadriceps muscles produces the colloquially termed 'corked thigh'. Direct muscle injuries in body-contact sports may also occur at any other site, most commonly the upper arm.

Pain in the muscle is present and is made worse by movement. Bruising may be found in the skin of the injured area and over the following days it may track down tissue planes to appear more distally. Swelling and tenderness are usually found in the involved area, and following a direct injury to the quadriceps muscle in the thigh, blood may track down the fascial planes to the knee joint irritating the synovial membrane and producing a synovial effusion into the knee. This can cause considerable diagnostic confusion unless an accurate history of a direct injury to the thigh is obtained.

Disturbances of function are dependent on the loss of several muscle characteristics. Flexibility is the ability of muscles to stretch and to relax. This also allows the muscle to achieve its explosive force. The further the joint is stretched, within limits, the more force will it yield. This principle can be readily observed in most sporting actions requiring rapid movement. Muscle strength is the amount of force that a muscle can exert isometrically. Muscle power is the ability to use strength dynamically and is the product of force times the distance through which the force acts over time. It is dependent on torque which produces rotation or torsion.

Loss of muscle function is evidenced by weakness on active contraction and loss of flexibility. Weakness can be tested clinically by maximally resisting muscle action either as an isometric or isotonic contraction. They are best tested and quantified by use of isokinetic machines (see below). To test for flexibility, e.g. in the quadriceps muscles, the patient lies prone and the knee is fully passively flexed. In the unaffected leg, the patient's heel can usually be touched on to the buttock; in the affected leg, this range cannot be attained as the quadriceps cannot be stretched out. The distance of heel from the buttock is measured as an assessment of the degree of injury, and its subsequent progress towards recovery.

Joints

Joints may also be involved by direct injury resulting in local bleeding with haematoma formation. This most commonly occurs over the knee ligaments where haematoma in the medial collateral ligament of the knee joint may subsequently ossify, producing a Pellegrini–Stieda lesion (see p. 153) with a locally painful tender swelling in the proximal attachment of the ligament, evident clinically and on radiographs.

Management of direct injuries

Immediate treatment

The important principles are: (1) to control haemorrhage and so limit haematoma formation, and (2) to avoid any further aggravation of the injury.

The optimum management for moderate to severe degrees of injury consists of rest, ice, compression and elevation. Rest for 24–48 h is necessary to reduce blood flow and allows an accurate assessment of the degree of injury. Ice (see p. 29) is used to reduce blood flow and decrease subsequent oedema and inflammatory response. The ice is best applied crushed, wrapped in a wet towel and applied over the injured area.

Compression to minimize haemorrhage may be applied over the ice. It is also assisted by elevation of the injured limb. This current management regimen should be contrasted with previous immediate treatment regimens which used heat, forceful massage and exercising, and usually resulted in aggravation of the injury and the degree of subsequent swelling.

Subsequent management

After the first 48 h, an active rehabilitation programme is commenced. This approach to management has developed because prolonged rest is neither necessary nor desirable and fails to utilize the patient's motivation for speedy recovery. Immobilization, even for short periods, leads to adverse effects in muscle, ligaments, bone and articular cartilage.

In muscles, disuse atrophy commences immediately and may be significant by 1 week. Muscle biopsy studies show that slow twitch muscle fibres and their associated oxidative enzyme systems deteriorate with immobilization [1,2].

Similarly, immobilization produces a rapid decline in the biomechanical properties of ligaments and bone but exercise can increase the strength and stiffness of ligaments and the ligament–bone unit. Articular cartilage suffers changes in its biochemistry and ultrastructure on immobilization. These can be reversed by activity [3–7]. O'Driscoll *et al* [8] described the beneficial effects of continuous passive movement on the nourishment and healing of cartilage, clearance of hemarthrosis and prevention of intra-articular adhesions.

Management is by active exercises within the limits of pain tolerance; this enhances the local circulation, helps to absorb the haematoma and restores strength and flexibility to the injured muscle. Exercise regimens need to be properly supervised by a physiotherapist, graded according to the degree of pain and disability, and progressed in intensity.

Isometric (static) exercises

In these exercises the joint is not moved when the muscle is tensed; resistance is sufficient to allow no, or actually very little, change in the length of muscle fibres. This allows maximum muscle use without approximation of its attachments and without joint movement or trauma to joint surfaces.

The athlete is taught the correct isometric regimen and a few minutes are spent on each exercise several times throughout the day. They need to be done in a set rhythmical pattern and the patient is taught to contract, hold, relax and then rest the muscle. The contraction is usually held for 6 s and the rest period for 6 s. The exercises are best carried out at a joint angle which permits the highest mechanical output of the muscle, slightly shorter than its resting length. They produce maximal muscle loading but only in one point in the range of joint motion and so they should be performed at multiple joint angles.

ADVANTAGES
They are simple to teach and carry out, require no special apparatus, can be done virtually at any place or time, particularly at home, and require little time to perform. They can be commenced early in the treatment programme before progressing to other forms of exercise as they usually produce little pain or discomfort.

PROBLEMS

Maximum isometric strength is not attained for a few months and there is difficulty with motivation and poor patient compliance. There is no evidence that their use produces an improvement in specific motor skills or isotonic muscle strength and endurance.

Isotonic dynamic exercises

In these, the joint is moved by the athlete against a constant resistance offered either by the therapist or more commonly by some form of apparatus. It is usually applied as a form of progressive resisted exercise, i.e. the resistance is increased as the muscle strength increases or according to a predetermined schedule of increments. Its rationale is overload; a stress sufficient to cause a muscle to fatigue will stimulate the muscle to adapt by increasing in strength and endurance. For increasing muscle power, exercise using a low repetition rate with high resistance is used. Endurance exercises require high repetition with low resistance.

METHODS

First, the ten repetition maximum of a muscle, the maximum weight that can be lifted ten times against gravity through a full range of movement, is calculated. An increasing loading of the muscle during a training session was first used. Retesting followed each week so that the load for each session could then be increased. Different techniques have since been described using either high or low loads and high or low repetitions.

PROBLEMS WITH THEIR USE

These techniques are highly effective at increasing muscle strength but require specialized equipment and expertise for optimal use, and errors may be made in estimating the ten repetition maximum or its progression. In the knee, excess loading of the patello-femoral joint may exacerbate knee pain. These exercises are performed through a range of joint motion with a set resistance. However, neither the forces nor the resistance remain constant during the range and so loading occurs at the weakest point in the system whereas the rest of the system works at less than its full capacity.

Isotonic variable resistance exercises

Isotonic variable resistance exercises are used to overcome the latter problem. The resistance, which may be on a hydraulic or cam-shaped machine, such as Nautilus, is designed to match the angle-specific strength capacity of muscle. One of their advantages is the ability to strengthen muscles both eccentrically and concentrically with a greater capacity to work at a higher maximal rate than with constant resistance isotonic exercises. This also allows for increased joint flexibility.

Isokinetic exercises

Isokinetic exercises have been a significant advance in therapy. Resisted exercise is performed against a machine which provides a defined time and rate of movement of the joint and also a quantifiable evaluation of the patient's progress. Isokinetic strength is the maximum torque that can be exerted against a preset rate-limiting device. The training effect on a muscle depends on the load but also on the relationship of that load to the muscle position during voluntary maximal contraction; a constant load will have a variable effect at different positions within the range.

The Cybex machine allows for changes in the rate of training, using either slower or faster repetitions. It uses an accommodating resistance and involves exercising at a constant velocity of joint motion. The muscle force can be varied by the patient so that the resistance matches the patient's muscular exertion at specific velocities. It also uses a dynamometer to provide a direct measurement of muscle torque, power and endurance under reproducible velocities. As the muscle becomes fatigued its torque output decreases and the machine can accommodate to this decrease with less resistance. The dynamometer produces a graphic analysis of muscle performance throughout the range of joint movement which allows quantification of different test or exercise patterns and is a powerful motivating force. A variant, Kin-Com, also contains a computer which can control and modify the force, velocity and range of movement and so allow isometric, concentric and eccentric contractions that can be monitored on a video display unit.

ADVANTAGES

Isokinetics are superior to isometrics as muscle re-education takes place throughout the full range of its length instead of at one static length. The advantage over isotonic exercise is that muscle force can be varied so that resistance can be applied and increased to weaker regions in the muscle. It is safer to use at an earlier stage in treatment as muscle fibres can be subjected to controlled, gradually increasing loads. Because muscle resistance can be optimized throughout the full range of motion, more work can be performed with each repetition of exercises in comparison to other methods. In retraining athletes for specific muscle skills, other strengthening exercises cannot attain high velocities of joint ranges of motion. Velocities can be achieved with isokinetic exercise machines that match the velocity required for athletic skills.

Passive movements

Exercises are combined with two passive movement techniques. The first passive movement is stretching (see Chapter 4). The exercise programme should be combined with muscle stretching applied by the physiotherapist for approximately 10 s with a 10 s rest. The muscle is taken to the limit of discomfort and released slowly but as large a range of movement as possible should be used. This stretching regimen is carried out slowly and gently for up to 10 min at approximately intervals of 2 h.

Heat, such as ultrasound, may be used before the active exercise and stretching regimen as a type of 'warm-up procedure' to help relieve pain and reduce muscle spasm. Paradoxically, ice may still be used in preference to heat to achieve the same desired results or else use of alternating heat and cold.

The second exercise uses slow and gentle movements performed within the limits of pain but up to as large a range of movement as is possible. These are performed for approximately 5 min every 2 h in the early stage.

Medication

These injuries usually cause a considerable degree of pain and non-narcotic analgesics may be used. The use of non-steroidal anti-inflammatory drugs is controversial although they do allow for earlier mobilization and rehabilitation. Prostaglandins released in these injuries play a role in the production of pain and the inflammatory response and so the use of anti-inflammatories would appear to be justified. Other pharmacological agents, such as proteolytic enzymes and muscle relaxants, have not been proven to be of sufficient value to justify their use.

Direct muscle injuries can usually be treated without any necessity for aspiration or injection of the haematoma.

Rehabilitation

While the injured muscle steadily increases in strength, power, endurance and flexibility, the athlete is encouraged to continue to exercise other non-injured muscle groups. As muscle function is being retrained, attention must also be given to exercises to maintain general fitness, aerobic capacity and prevent any increase in body-weight. Cycling, which can be on a stationary bike, swimming and walking in water, perhaps with a flotation device, are ideal. With leg injuries jogging can be commenced, gradually increasing in pace and distance. Functional activities aimed at restoring motor skills should be instituted and graduated. With ankle injuries, tilt or wobble boards can be used to increase strength through increased proprioceptive feedback.

Complications

Complications of direct muscle injuries may occur especially in patients who have been improperly managed and include fibrosis, rupture, cyst formation, calcification and myositis ossificans.

Haematoma formation results in fibrin deposition within the muscle fibres which may produce fibrosis with adhesion formation and resultant loss of normal muscle extensibility. Activity may then cause pain and stiffness or result in rupture of the muscle fibres. A cystic swelling filled with a serous exudate may become walled off and is unlikely to resorb spontaneously. These are to be found particularly in the lax tissues around the lower lumbar spine.

In myositis ossificans, bone forms in the muscle haematoma and produces considerable disability (Figure 2.1). This condition should not be confused with the calcification which may occur as a rare and late complication in a localized area of haematoma. The pathogenesis is presumably osteoblastic invasion from the periosteum into the overlying muscle haematoma [9]. Subsequently, a large bony mass is formed with trabeculae and even marrow spaces. This is invariably attached to the underlying bone, usually the femur and less commonly the humerus. Any procedure that 'irritates' the bone, such as massage or perhaps excessive muscular action, may result in this condition.

The athlete presents with increasing pain and loss of function in the involved muscle. Pain is usually intense, is made worse with most activities, and disturbs sleep at night. The activity of the bone lesion may be gauged by the degree of pain. Clinical findings include muscle weakness, atrophy, loss of extensibility and a palpable tender mass in the involved muscle. Radiography, bone scan or computed tomography (CT) reveals the presence of fluffy bone, indistinct at first but later more solidified, growing out into the involved muscle.

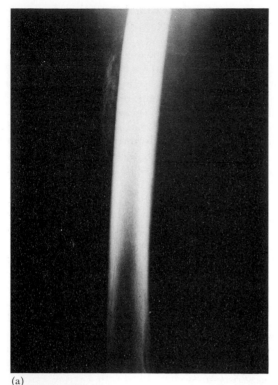

(a)

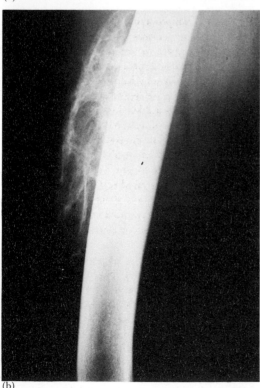

(b)

Figure 2.1 Myositis ossificans: (a) early; (b) late

MANAGEMENT OF MYOSITIS OSSIFICANS

In severe cases, all activities and physical methods of treatment must cease; at first the patient may even need to be kept at rest in bed for a few days. Analgesics and anti-inflammatory agents are given in sufficient dosage to ease pain. As pain and tenderness settle, treatment to include a gradual active and passive stretching and strengthening of the involved muscle group is commenced. This combination may also be achieved by the use of proprioceptive neuromuscular facilitation techniques. The bony mass usually regresses slowly and after a period of some months the patient can return to active sports. Surgery is never indicated.

Because myositis ossificans is a potential complication of any direct muscle injury, too early or overvigorous activity and the use of massage in treatment must be avoided. The injured area needs to have protection and padding on the return to body contact sports.

Indirect injuries

Indirect injuries result from forces generated within the musculoskeletal structures during activity. When this force is sufficient it may result in a fracture or dislocation, whereas indirect soft tissue injuries commonly involve either muscles or joints. In muscles, overloading results in disruption of muscle fibres, known then as a muscle tear, pull or strain. In the joints, indirect injuries may produce disruption of ligament fibres resulting in a sprain or injury to intra-articular structures, such as a meniscus.

Muscles

A muscle tear from an indirect injury may occur at any site between its origin and its insertion although they tend to occur most commonly in the mid-section of the muscle belly in younger patients. Tears usually involve muscles that span two joints. These muscles have different actions according to the relative position in the limb. The most likely cause is a neuromuscular incoordination which results in a disordered muscle action that leads to a muscle tear. This type of muscle injury tends to occur either in the early stages of a sporting event, when it may be associated with an inadequate stretching or warm-up procedure, or in the late stages of a sporting event when it may be associated with fatigue, lack of muscular fitness, an unguarded movement or an inadequate technique. Other mechanisms that may produce muscle tears are not so common. They may occur if the muscle is suddenly overstretched or alternatively at the height of a muscular contraction especially if its further action is then blocked, e.g. kicking against an inert object or on sudden deceleration.

Sprinting requires an explosive muscular effort over a short period of time and in sprinters the hamstring muscle is most commonly involved. The typical history is that the patient either tries to increase speed or suddenly change direction while running, feels a sudden painful tearing sensation in the posterior thigh and is unable to continue running. Two other muscle groups commonly involved in indirect injury are the quadriceps and the gastrocnemius. The latter occurs commonly in middle-aged runners and the site of the tear is usually either in the medial belly of the muscle or at its musculotendinous junction.

Clinical examination demonstrates a loss of muscle strength and flexibility, with pain reproduced on isometric contraction and by stretching the involved muscle. Palpation reveals a locally tender area over the site of the tear. In a more severe degree of injury, a palpable gap may be felt in the muscle or in the musculotendinous junction above it a rolled-up portion of muscle.

Management

Immediate management for the first 24–48 h is similar to that described above for direct injuries using rest, ice, compression and elevation.

Subsequent management involves an active programme of rehabilitation for muscle strengthening and stretching with gently controlled passive movements. The rate of increase of improvement is usually more gradual than in direct injuries but, nevertheless, should still steadily progress. Active treatment is necessary because prolonged rest will increase the underlying loss of muscle function. Isometric, isotonic and isokinetic exercises are given as above to the injured muscle and to its antagonists. Passive stretching is supervised by the physiotherapist and the patient can be taught how to perform some of the techniques himself.

Aftercare

Principles are the same as discussed above. As lower limb injuries improve the athlete is encouraged to jog or run at half pace, thus both exercising and stretching the muscle. The muscle is actively exercised until it attains full strength and extensibility before the patient is allowed to return to full sporting activity.

Complications

1 Complete rupture of a muscle is uncommon. It may be diagnosed by the presence of a palpable gap in the muscle belly with a proximal rolled-up segment of muscle. It most commonly involves the rectus femoris muscle or the biceps in the upper arm.
2 The surrounding muscle sheath may be torn allowing the muscle to herniate through it. This swelling may become more prominent on contracting the muscle.
3 As a muscle tear heals, a small area of fibrosis may result, palpable as a small, locally tender thickening in the muscle. Treatment (see Chapter 4) is with ultrasound, deep pressures, stretching and injection of local anaesthetics and corticosteroid into the tender area.

Ligaments

Ligaments are composed of dense bundles of suitably orientated collagen fibres containing only a small number of fibrocytes, a limited blood supply and numerous sensory and proprioceptive nerve fibres. Some ligaments form a localized thickening of a joint capsule and in the two most commonly injured joints, the knee and ankle, they form thicker collateral ligaments. Their function is to prevent excessive or abnormal movement in the joint and therefore indirect injuries, which apply excessive force or movement to a joint, may produce ligament sprains. The most commonly injured ligaments are anterior cruciate and medial collateral ligament of the knee and the lateral collateral ligament of the ankle. Sprains can be graded in severity into one of three degrees:

1 A first degree sprain involves a tear of a few ligament fibres only. As much of the ligament is still intact, the joint remains stable.
2 In second degree sprains there is a moderate degree of ligament fibre tearing and some stretching of the remaining ligaments. Ligament function is impaired and some degree of joint laxity may become possible. This injury, when associated with damage to the joint capsule or synovium, may result in a synovial effusion.

3 In third degree sprains, ligament fibres are completely disrupted or the ligament attachments are detached from the bone. The loss of ligamentous function causes the joint to become unstable.

Some degree of overlap exists clinically between these three categories so that repeated examination may be necessary to assess the degree in individual cases.

The history should include the mechanism of injury, whether activity could be continued or how soon after the injury was activity necessarily ceased. The presence and degree of pain and swelling are important. The subsequent history of any limp, ability to run or exercise, any sensation of instability or giving way, and the degree of stiffness are important.

First and second degree sprains are usually quite painful for a time and may be associated with some degree of swelling and muscle spasm. In third degree sprains, blood and fluid may escape from the joint into the extra-articular structures; subsequently, pain may not necessarily be a prominent clinical feature, especially in comparison to the degree of injury, and joint swelling may be absent.

Clinical examination is designed to confirm the presence of a sprained ligament, the exact site of the tear and its degree of damage. It is an advantage to examine the patient as soon as possible after the injury, to know if the patient has had any previous ligamentous laxity and to examine the normal side.

1 Swelling may result from a localized area of oedema, visible and palpable over the site of injury. Discoloration from bruising often appears after several days. The presence of a synovial effusion usually indicates a second degree sprain with damage to the synovial membrane, and a haemarthrosis usually indicates additional injury to intra-articular structures such as the anterior cruciate ligament or menisci. Swelling as a result of haemarthrosis occurs almost immediately whereas a synovial effusion will appear gradually.

2 Stress tests: the ligament should be passively stretched in the direction of the original injury. There are three important findings:
   (a) Whether any pain is produced.
   (b) The degree of any instability or protective muscle spasm present. This technique must be learned for each individual joint.
   (c) The 'end-feel' of the movement. In grade 2 collateral ligament tear with some degree of instability, there is usually a firm springy type of end-feel. In a grade 3 tear, the endpoint usually has a characteristic mushy quality.

3 Palpation may reveal a gap in the ligament, most easily appreciated in cases of rupture of the medial collateral ligament of the knee. Tenderness tends to be localized over the site of the ligament tear and its presence helps to confirm the diagnosis. Tenderness may sometimes be diffuse in recent acute injuries or in ligaments deep to the surface, e.g. the capsular ligaments of the knee.

Management

Diagnosis and management of ligament injuries of the various joints are considered in the following chapters. As with muscle injuries, the emphasis in management is on an active treatment regimen of exercises. The junctional strength of experimental bone–ligament–bone preparations is increased by exercises and is decreased by immobilization. Similarly, the strength of the injured ligament is decreased by immobilization and is increased by exercise training and continued slow passive mobilization.

Overuse injuries

Overuse injuries, in which inflammatory lesions are produced as a result of long continued or repetitive musculoskeletal action, are becoming increasingly more common since the relatively recent introduction of heavy training loads. The basic cause lies in the repetitive type of action and high loads necessary for a particular sport so that inflammatory changes in any part of the motor unit result from overuse. A motor unit consists of a muscle, its tendons and insertions, and surrounding tenosynovium or bursa.

The important principle here is adaptation; when stress or overload is applied to soft tissues, time must be given for them to adapt so that a training effect is produced. Soft tissues can also be so conditioned to the stress without suffering any injury. If sufficient time is not given for recuperation, overuse conditions may result.

The aetiology of overuse injuries may be classified as: (1) training errors, (2) biomechanical abnormalities, and (3) problems with shoes or terrain.

Training errors

These can generally be typified as too much too soon or may result from abuse of the body part, and are the single most important factor in causing overuse injuries. Hard training days should have easy days interposed so that the musculoskeletal system can adapt to the load placed on it. Appropriate adaptation can then allow more stress to be placed gradually on the body. If not then overuse injuries may accumulate.

Causes include: (1) inadequate warm-up, (2) excessive mileage, (3) rapid increase in the distance run, (4) rapid increase in the intensity of running, (5) increased resistance in running, e.g. in water or on sand or up hills, (6) a single severe training or competitive event, and (7) a sudden load applied after injury.

A coach may undertake a training programme without regard to the athlete's own capabilities or background. Extra care must be taken when a player returns to training after injury or alters his techniques ('new-use').

Biomechanical abnormalities

Biomechanical factors in the lower leg are commonly associated with overuse conditions. In general, they are caused by malalignments, joint stiffness or instabilities, and muscle weakness or tightness. These factors may be minor variations of the normal but with the training loads that athletes apply they can result in changes at any site in the linked system of joints. Alterations in one limb may predispose to an overuse condition in the other limb, e.g. an overuse injury such as a stress fracture or an Achilles tendinitis may occur in one leg following a minor degree of injury in the opposite leg that resulted in an alteration of the running action. Overloading of the patellofemoral joint may occur especially in patients with structural abnormalities of the leg, e.g. tight hamstrings, or with overpronation of the subtalar joint.

Biomechanical abnormalities in the lower limb include:

1 Hip: femoral neck anteversion; leg length discrepancy.
2 Knee: muscle weakness or tightness involving quadriceps, hamstrings, genu valgum, varum or recurvatum, excessive Q angle, patella misalignments.
3 Lower leg: tibial varum, tibial torsion, gastrocnemius–soleus weakness or tightness.
4 Ankle: equinus deformity.
5 Foot: subtalar joint stiffness or excess pronation, pes planus or cavus, valgus or varus rear foot deformities; valgus or varus forefoot deformities.

Problems with shoes or terrain

Shoes and surfaces can also contribute to overuse injuries. The shoes may be ill-fitting, excessively worn, too inflexible and, especially, lack adequate cushioning or provide inadequate support and control to the heel. Wearing different shoes can produce differences in the range of subtalar joint motion. Shoes need to provide shock-absorbing qualities.

Difficulties in finding suitable running surfaces are often a problem. Not all surfaces around the world have the soft gentle underfooting to be found in some European forests. The road surface may be too hard, sand may be too soft, the beach may be excessively cambered, grass may be too uneven. The action required to run uphill is quite different from that of running downhill, or sloping surfaces causing supination of the downhill foot and pronation of the uphill foot. Loss of shock absorbing and increased tibial rotation can result.

Grading

The overuse injuries should be graded 1–4 according to severity of symptoms. Obviously, these gradings also indicate the degree of underlying inflammation or soreness, although there is some overlap between them.

Grade 1: Pain or soreness comes on immediately after activity and usually lasts for a varying time up to a few hours. It is always gone by the following morning.

Grade 2: Pain comes on towards the end of the activity and lasts for some time afterwards. It is not always gone by the next morning and the part then feels stiff for an hour or so.

Grade 3: Pain comes on at the beginning or early in activity and limits the degree of activity. Pain and stiffness will be present at times during the day.

Grade 4: Pain may be present at night and severely limits or prevents activity.

Overuse injuries are classified according to the structure in which the motor power unit is most involved. They are divided into injuries of: (1) tendons with their tendon sheath and bursae, (2) tenoperiosteal lesions, (3) joints, (4) bone and (5) neural tissues.

Tendons

Tendons, made up of parallel bundles of collagen fibres and small numbers of fibrocytes, combine great tensile strength with some degree of elasticity.

Tendons form either at the origin of a muscle or blend with muscle fibres at a musculotendinous junction to form its insertion and so concentrate the muscle force into a relatively small area. As they attach to bone, tendons first become cartilaginous, then calcified and finally are cemented into the bone. At both the origin and insertion they form into a network of fibres (Sharpeys fibres) that penetrate deeply into the cortex of the bone to anchor the tendon. This attachment, known as an enthesis, is metabolically active and receives its blood supply from the periosteum. A tendon may be surrounded by a synovial sheath, tenosynovium, or a connective tissue layer, the paratenon, whereas bursae are commonly related to the tendon attachments to bone.

Overuse injuries of this anatomical arrangement may result in a tendinitis, tenosynovitis, peritendinitis or bursitis.

Aetiology

The basic mechanism of the production of these lesions is similar although their anatomical site and clinical presentation may vary. In the upper limb, these injuries usually occur in any sport which involves hitting or propelling an object. In the lower limb they usually follow running. Inflammatory changes in tendons, tendinitis, are often associated with degenerative changes. These may result from ageing, vascular changes, attrition, impingement, calcification, and focal degeneration (see p. 182).

Degenerative changes in tendons are common and may relate to ageing changes or interference with the vascular supply. The blood supply to a tendon is derived from the musculotendinous junction, the periosteum and from the tenosynovium. Blood supply decreases with age, applied tension, vascular disease or from a relative vascular insufficiency following prolonged overuse. Focal degeneration, in which an area of approximately 10 mm of degenerated and damaged fibres is found within an area of normal tendon, was originally described in the Achilles tendon but a similar change may involve other tendons. The involved tendon fibres lose their normal structure and wavy outline, their nuclei become shrunken and pyknotic, and there is surrounding fibroblastic and inflammatory cell proliferation. This mesenchymoid reaction may also be a reaction to tissue hypoxia.

Complications

1   Tendon rupture may be partial or complete. As normal tendons can normally withstand large loads, ruptures usually involve an area of degeneration in the tendon. The tendons most commonly ruptured in sporting injuries are the Achilles tendon, the long head of the biceps may rupture in its bicipital groove, and the supraspinatus or infraspinatus tendon may rupture proximal to their insertion into the greater tuberosity.

2   Tendon avulsion usually follows an intense muscular contraction and occurs especially in children who are sprinting. The usual site of involvement is the lower leg around the superior or inferior iliac spine, the lesser trochanter of the femur, the ischial tuberosity or the tibial tuberosity. The diagnosis is clinical but should be confirmed from radiographs, showing the separated bone fragment.

3   Tendon calcification probably forms as part of the process of repair. It most commonly occurs in the rotator cuff tendons of the shoulder or in the gluteus medius tendon at its insertion into the greater trochanter.

4   Tendovaginitis occurs in two sites. De Quervain's disease involves the long abductor and short extensor tendons of the thumb over the radial styloid and occurs in sports that involve repetitive rolling action of the wrist, such as fencing. The other site is in the ankle, involving either the peroneus longus or the tibialis posterior tendon sheath, and occurs especially in ballet dancers or runners.

5   Dislocation of a tendon from its normal bony groove producing a painful clicking occurs especially in the biceps tendon in the shoulder and in the peroneal tendon around the ankle.

Tenoperiosteal lesions

The attachment of the tendon into the periosteum and underlying bone forms an enthesis, and is normally an area of relatively high metabolic activity. Degenerative changes, usually involving the anchoring collagen fibres, tend to occur in this site and may be associated with evidence of attempted repair. Inflammatory changes may then follow repeated muscle contractions, either concentric or eccentric, with consequent traction on the tenoperiosteal attachments. This lesion may predispose to acute tear. In the upper limbs, tenoperiosteal injuries occur mainly around the elbow, over the lateral epicondyle (tennis elbow), the medial epicondyle (golfer's elbow), the triceps insertion (javelin elbow), or over the medial joint compartment (baseballer's elbow). In the lower limb, tenoperiosteal lesions around the pelvis occur particularly in the origin of the hamstring both in sprinters and distance runners, particularly from running up hills. A common site of involvement is the origin of the tibialis posterior tendon from the medial border of the tibia.

Joints

Overuse conditions involving the joint include synovitis of the knee, which may occur in bicycle riders; lesions of the articular hyaline cartilage, e.g. in chondromalacia patellae; or a lesion of the bone around the joint margin as in talotibial exostoses.

Bone

Overuse injuries involving bone may result in a stress fracture. These injuries were originally encountered during the initial training of army recruits, most commonly as a fracture of the metatarsal shaft. 'March fracture' was altered to 'stress fracture' when it was realized that this relatively common injury occurred as a result of repeated overuse, and that a similar lesion may occur in almost any other bone. Bone responds to stress by constant remodelling with proliferation and resorption. Athletes are exposed to a complex combination of forces on the bone to which the normal response is bony thickening and so strengthening. Cortical bone is most resistant to compressive force, which is the normal force falling along a long bone. Compression stress fractures are not nearly so common and occur mainly in the under surface of the femoral neck.

Muscles normally absorb and store energy which helps to neutralize tensile forces but, during repeated activities, an additional force is applied to the bones as a result of repetitive strong contractions in the surrounding muscle groups. This movement can produce bending of the bone, which, if continued for sufficient time, will produce disruption of the bony trabeculae of the cortex exposed to the excess tensile force. Most stress fractures in the lower leg result from these excessive tensile forces and occur especially in metatarsals, fibula or tibia as an overuse condition.

Factors associated with excess loading include the running action, excessive or prolonged subtalar joint pronation with medial rotation of the tibia, muscle fatigue or imbalance, and altered patterns of gait. Alterations in the bone should also be considered

and in female athletes prolonged amenorrhoea may be a predisposing factor.

The usual history is one of regular strenuous activity but injury may also occur early in the athletic season when a sudden increased load is applied to the musculoskeletal system. Pain is the presenting problem. Often attempts are made to run through it but the pain eventually becomes so severe that the athlete is forced to rest. If activity is long continued, the repeated trauma may produce a complete fracture of the bone.

Diagnosis of stress fractures

The diagnosis of a stress fracture is essentially that of a clinically based history, including the type of activity, the degree of pain and local tenderness. This does require a high index of suspicion of its possible presence before changes become evident on radiographs. As stress fractures occur as a relatively gradual process, repair can take place simultaneously, so producing the typical radiological change with periosteal callus formation around the injured site. The diagnosis does, however, need to be confirmed by radiographs, CT scan or magnetic resonance imaging (MRI). Technetium bone scan is very sensitive but not very specific and is positive before radiographic changes.

Management of overuse injuries

Management depends on the grading of the overuse injury.

Grade 1

The balance between activity and recovery is starting to break down with some slight degree of resulting inflammation. There are no specific diagnostic aids; management consists of ice or local heat and non-steroidal anti-inflammatory drugs (NSAIDs). The athlete can continue the training but it will probably require some modification. This can be organized in consultation with the coach and is often an opportunity to look for and make some slight modification to training techniques.

Grade 2

Injuries can now be assessed clinically as soft tissue signs will be present (see Chapter 3). Management will require a continuation of the above methods with ice, heat or NSAIDs. Accurate clinical localization of the involved lesion to a small area allows the use of local corticosteroids and anaesthetic.

Activity will need to be modified to reduce the load on the involved part, usually by reducing the training volume by approximately 25%. Enquiries need to be made into training methods and techniques with the aim of increasing biomechanical efficiency.

Grade 3

Injuries occur when the balance between activity and recovery or adaptation is tilted, the load is excessive and activity will result in increasing inflammation. Rest to the involved part is therefore essential and needs to be continued until the pain settles. Other activities to maintain fitness may still be able to be carried out. Biomechanical aids or supports such as orthotic devices may be necessary.

Physiotherapy techniques include the use of pain-relieving techniques such as interferential or transcutaneous electrical nerve stimulation (TENS) machines.

Grade 4

Injuries, often with structural changes, e.g. stress fractures in bone, will require complete rest.

Prolonged conservative therapy will usually resolve these lesions but, if not, surgically correctable lesions should always be searched for, e.g. with Achilles tendinitis or impingement syndromes.

The training loads used today are quite likely to result in overuse injuries. Education about biomechanics and the effect of these loads remains the best prophylactic measure.

After-care is aimed at a carefully supervised, gradual return of the training loads after a period of time before a return to full activity. Alternative exercise programmes to correct muscle weakness and to improve flexibility and coordination may be added. Consultation with coaches and trainers may be necessary to improve training techniques and prevent recurrences by taking notice of any warning signs.

References

1 Eriksson, E. (1976) Sports injuries of the knee ligaments: diagnosis, rehabilitation and prevention. *Medical Science and Sports*, **8**, 133–144
2 Costill, D.L., Fink, W.S. and Habanski, A.J. (1977) Muscular rehabilitation following knee surgery. *Physician Sports Medicine*, **5**, 71
3 Dahners, L.E. and Muller, P. (1988) The effect of the application of tension on ligament growth. *Orthopaedic Research Society, Georgia*, **34**, 56
4 Dahners, L.E., Torka, M.D., Gilbert, J.A. *et al.* (1989) The effect of motion on collagen synthesis and fibre orientation during ligament healing. *Orthopaedic Research Society, Georgia*, **35**, 299
5 MacMillan, M., Sheppard, J.E. and Dell, P.C. (1987) An experimental flexor tendon repair in Zone 11 that allows immediate postoperative mobilization. *Journal of Hand Surgery*, **12**, 582–589
6 Shimizu, T., Videman, T., Shimazaki, K. *et al.* (1987) Experimental study on the repair of full thickness artic-ular cartilage defects: effects of varying periods of continuous passive motion, cage activity, and immobi-lization. *Journal of Orthopaedic Research*, **5**, 187–197
7 Zuran, B.H., Nelson, D.L., Sauer, J.A. *et al.* (1988) The effects of sheath repair and continuous passive motion on healing flexor tendons. *Orthopaedic Research Society*, **34**, 180
8 O'Driscoll, S.W., Kumar, A. and Salter, R.B. (1983) The effect of continuous passive motion on the clearance of a hemarthrosis from a synovial joint. *Clinical Orthopaedics and Related Research*, **176**, 305–311
9 Estwanik, J.J. and McAlister, J.A. (1990) Contusions and the formation of myositis ossificans. *Physician and Sports Medicine*, **18**, 53–64

3 Soft tissue lesions

History

History taking for musculoskeletal disorders is, as in the rest of medicine, of paramount importance and well repays the time spent in recording it accurately. This may allow an accurate assessment of the diagnosis, or at least narrow down the different diagnostic possibilities, before undertaking the clinical examination. It is worthwhile having a printed form with a body chart on which the site and distribution of the patient's symptoms can be charted. History taking requires a capacity to listen sympathetically to the patient and not to ask leading questions. However, some patients, because of either a natural reticence or circumlocution, need to be led to, and kept firmly on, the main points at issue. Nevertheless, even these patients should, as much as possible, tell the history in their own words. The actual events should be recorded and should not be confused with opinions of the patient or other interested parties.

The main consideration in this process is for the examiner to build up a pattern so that the behaviour of the patient's symptoms and his reactions to them can be identified. This includes an appreciation of the time relationship of the various symptoms, their onset and variability, some assessment of the patient as a person, his pain threshold, and the presence of any non-organic pattern or psychogenic overlay to his symptoms. This may be possible by observing the relationship between the patient's behaviour while speaking about his degree of pain. The patient is asked to describe his major complaint which is nearly always pain.

Pain

Worst problem

The patient should be asked about his worst current clinical problem in terms of pain and loss of function.

Site of pain

The patient should be asked to point to and map out the area of pain as accurately as possible. As a general rule, pain in the distal joints can be more accurately localized than pain in the proximal joints. It is also necessary to ensure whether pain is felt within the joint. The patient's original statement about his site of pain can be misleading. For example, pain in the shoulder may be to him any area from neck to upper arm, or pain in the hip may really be buttock pain, whereas hip pain may be referred to the knee.

Radiation

The area where the pain began, whether it is superficial or deep, where it is felt most, and where it radiates should also be mapped out. Pain and tenderness may be felt in one area of a limb but be referred from a more proximal site.

Quality of pain

The patient should be encouraged to describe the quality and character of his pain in his own words.

Musculoskeletal pain is usually described as deep, dull and aching or sharp, throbbing or stabbing. Bone pain is usually described as a severe, boring pain, often worse at night; otherwise it is usually difficult to differentiate between different qualities of musculoskeletal pain.

Severity

Severity may be difficult to assess as it depends mainly on the patient's description of and reaction to the pain. The degree of functional incapacity that results may be a good guide to severity; the patient may recognize that it is of nuisance value only or it may seriously interfere with and limit function.

Time relationships

The patient is asked how long pain has been present, whether it is constant, variable or intermittent. The duration of pain and the pain-free periods or the variation in pain throughout a 24-h period are of considerable relevance. Soft tissue pain typically has a diurnal variation. Pain from osteoarthritis is usually worse at the end of the day; in rheumatoid arthritis it is often worse early in the morning.

Night pain

Soft tissue pain may be worse at night and, if sufficiently severe, may disturb the patient's sleep. As a general rule, it reflects the intensity of the underlying inflammation and may occur in: (1) inflammatory arthritis, gout or septic arthritis; (2) polymyalgia rheumatica; (3) peripheral nerve entrapments, particularly of the median nerve in the carpal tunnel; (4) bone disorder, including avascular necrosis, Sudeck's atrophy, and malignancy; and (5) nocturnal pain, particularly common in capsulitis of the shoulder, osteoarthritis of the hip, and cysts of the meniscus in the knee, or in patients with depression.

Aggravating and relieving factors

The relationship of several factors in the patient's pain is of major significance. These include rest, movements of the affected part, exercise and posture. Musculoskeletal pain of mechanical origin is relieved by rest and aggravated by movement. Mechanical factors such as stretching or compress-ing the joint (e.g. by lying on it) may also cause pain. If the joint is painful at rest, it is usually because of the severity of the underlying inflammation.

Pain may also be related to posture and develop only after the patient has maintained a particular position over a considerable period. Pain may be related to different positions, or holding a joint comfortable in one position over a length of time and then moving from this position may produce sudden, sharp pain. Enquire if pain varies either in site or in intensity, and how long it takes for these symptoms to subside. If pain is aggravated or relieved by certain postures or movements it may be helpful to have these movements demonstrated.

Onset

The onset of pain may be spontaneous, either sudden or gradual, or follow trauma. In the latter, a detailed history is necessary in describing the position of the joint at the time of injury and the type of stress applied to the joint. In many patients with chronic degenerative or inflammatory conditions, the onset is gradual. However, symptoms often follow overuse and an assessment should be made of the total load applied by the patient to a joint, both at work and at play. A sudden onset of severe pain and swelling commonly occurs in patients with crystal synovitis or avascular necrosis of bone. Patients with psychogenically determined pain often lack this characteristic pattern of pain relief and aggravation.

Pattern of joint involvement

Whether one, several or multiple joints are involved is important. Enquire about the number of joints involved, the first joint and subsequent joints involved, the pattern of joint involvement, e.g. migratory, additive or simultaneous, and whether joint involvement is symmetrical or asymmetrical.

Effects of treatment

The patient is questioned about the results of any previous or current treatment and whether it relieved or aggravated the pain. He is asked about the name, dosage, duration of use, effects and side-effects of any medications or injections, and the results of any physiotherapy, including the type of therapy given, its duration, its effects, and whether it was beneficial or exacerbated symptoms.

Irritability

This is a most useful concept, especially beneficial for assessment of therapy. Irritability is the relationship of the degree of activity to the pain subsequently evoked. This pain is assessed both by its degree and by the length of time taken for this increased pain to subside to its usual level. A joint is 'irritable' if only a moderate degree of activity provokes an increase in pain lasting for approximately an hour. Examination should not then be prolonged and subsequent passive movement treatment must be gentle. Alternatively, a patient may suffer only a sharp momentary pain after a sudden jarring. This condition is not 'irritable' and subsequent examination and management by passive movements can be more forceful. Also, a previously 'irritable' joint that becomes non-irritable during treatment is patently improving.

Progress

The progress of the underlying condition may be: (1) intermittently present, (2) constantly present, (3) present in recurrent attacks, in which case the frequency, regularity and duration of attacks need to be known, and (4) progressively worse.

Related signs and symptoms

Related signs and symptoms include stiffness, swelling, crepitus, locking, instability, weakness and neurological symptoms. Stiffness is a symptom that implies an increased resistance to movement of a part throughout a given range. This range may not necessarily be restricted and so it is differentiated from limitation of movement, which is an objective sign. Hence it may be possible to demonstrate a restriction of movement in one direction, e.g. rotation of the neck to the right, but the patient may be more conscious of stiffness of movement in another direction, e.g. rotation of the neck to the left.

Points in the history include the distribution of the stiffness, how long it has been present and its relationship to pain. The duration of stiffness, especially the length of time that stiffness persists in the morning, is of prime importance. It is, moreover, an objective test of the degree of underlying inflammation in the joint because the duration of morning stiffness correlates well with this inflammatory change. Stiffness or 'articular gelling' may occur in patients with osteoarthritis or tendinitis; it lasts for only a few minutes and follows a period of prolonged immobilization, such as sitting in a chair. Neurological symptoms include sensory symptoms such as pins and needles or numbness. In patients who present with pain in the limb, the presence of such sensory symptoms is of major significance as it points to the diagnosis of neural compression.

Important points in the history include: (1) the distribution of sensory symptoms, (2) their relationship to the onset and distribution of pain, and (3) aggravating and relieving factors, especially spinal movements of posture.

General history

This includes the history related to:

1 Other systems: symptoms that may arise from the other bodily systems and any medications required should be checked.
2 Previous health: this includes details of previous trauma, operations, medical illnesses, and their investigations and treatments.
3 Precipitating factors: besides trauma, these may include infections, illnesses, surgery and stress.
4 Family history of any joint or systemic disorders.
5 Social history: the type of work that the patient does and any difficulty encountered in its performance; the type and intensity of any recreational or sporting activities.
6 Functional assessment: the loss of any function as the result of the current illness and its effect on the patient must be assessed.

Clinical assessment

Examination

Clinical signs in patients who complain of musculoskeletal pain are nearly always present and readily detectable. The main purpose of the clinical examination is to localize accurately the anatomical site that is involved. This depends on a knowledge of the anatomy and surface anatomy of the moving parts and an understanding of the usual traumatic, inflammatory and/or degenerative lesions commonly involved. The possible underlying pathological basis is determined to some extent from the patient's history and also from ancillary tests, such as radiography and blood tests. Radiographs of the affected area are usually of such importance that their use may also be considered as part of the normal joint examination.

Clinical examination to reveal the anatomical site of the lesion must be carried out using an orderly system comprising inspection, movement and palpation.

The limbs must be fully exposed and the unaffected limb is always examined before the affected one to gain the patient's confidence and assess the normal pain-free range of movement. Because the joints of a limb form part of a link system any alteration, weakness or tightness of one part of the link may be reflected in an alteration of another part. Also, pain may be referred from another, usually proximal, site. A common example is pain in the knee referred from a lesion in the hip joint, and pain in a limb may be referred from spinal joints. Hence the whole of the limb and the relevant part of the spine, referred to as the 'other joints in plan' [1] should also be examined. A general physical examination is also necessary and, in the limbs, special attention is given to the neurological and vascular systems. Clinical examination comprises:

1 Adequate exposure of the parts to be examined.
2 Examination of the normal side before the affected one.
3 Use of an orderly system comprising:
   (a) Inspection.
   (b) Movement.
   (c) Palpation.
4 Contraction, stretching or compression of the musculoskeletal parts by movements designed to be:
   (a) Active.
   (b) Passive.
   (c) Isometric.
   (d) Accessory.
5 Examination of other joints 'in plan'.
6 General physical examination.
7 Radiography.

Inspection

General examination

A great deal of information can be obtained from inspection which should commence as soon as the patient is first met; posture, gait, need to use supports or aids, deformities, ability or willingness to use certain joints, and how he sits down, undresses,

or gets on and off a couch may provide valuable information. His personality should also be assessed and an attempt made to gain a knowledge of his pain threshold and reaction to pain.

Inspection of posture may provide a clue to an underlying disorder. A patient with ankylosing spondylitis may have stiffness of spinal movements, kyphosis and forward flexion of the head. Patients with polymyalgia rheumatica, usually an elderly female, may have great difficulty in rising from a chair and may require someone to help them as movements are so painfully stiff. The hand is the arthritic's call-card and can reveal considerable information before the formal examination begins. A patient with gout in a metatarsophalangeal joint may have a classic sign: he may be well dressed except for wearing a sandshoe or a shoe with a hole cut in it.

Skin

The skin over the joint is examined for scars, sinuses, colour changes or rashes. An erythematous rash may occur over the joint in any of the connective tissue diseases and redness may also indicate an underlying inflammation. The skin over a joint involved with gout is red, hot and dry and may desquamate, indicating the intensity of the inflammation, whereas the skin over rheumatoid joints is often moist. Rashes may be due to psoriasis or other skin diseases and areas of pigmentation or depigmentation may be found.

Swelling

The presence of any swelling is often best appreciated by comparing the two limbs. A synovial effusion is usually better recognized by inspection than by palpation as it tends to bulge the synovium in a manner that is characteristic for each joint and is determined by the anatomical confines of the synovial membrane.

Deformities

Joint deformities are best seen on inspection and in the lower limb may be more apparent on weight bearing. The site of the deformity may be from alterations in the bones, joints or the soft tissues around them. A fixed deformity, a structural abnormality in which the joint cannot be voluntarily restored to its normal anatomical position, is usually a fixed-flexion deformity. Valgus and varus refer to angulation of the distal bone of the joint from and to the midline: valgus is a lateral inclination and varus a medial inclination.

Muscle wasting

With any severe degree of joint disease, especially in the hip, the surrounding muscles will become wasted and obvious on inspection. Wasting of the small muscles in the hand is very common in rheumatoid arthritis or in lower motor neurone lesions.

Movements

The neuromusculoskeletal system is made up of movable structures and it should be possible to reproduce symptoms by testing various movements. The fundamental rule in examination is to move parts so as to reproduce the patient's pain. This may not necessarily be experienced to the same degree and in exactly the same distribution as the patient's description, but the patient must recognize that it is the same type of pain of which he complains. Testing needs to be done in an orderly fashion: tension is applied to each of the structures around a joint so that it is moved by being contracted, stretched or compressed. The tension can be achieved by clinical testing using a sequence of active, passive, and isometric contractions. Accessory movements, described later, form an essential part of normal joint movements and should also be tested routinely.

The patient needs to undress so that the whole limb being examined can be observed. The unaffected limb is examined first before the affected one to provide a basis for comparison and allow the normal range of movement to be assessed. The patient is usually examined first while standing but also sitting or lying down. The examiner ensures that the patient is as relaxed as possible and enquires if any pain is felt while standing and, if so, to point to its site and distribution. The joint is then moved in each of its appropriate directions and the patient asked to report any alteration in his symptoms.

With this series of tests, a pattern of movement emerges. These consist of positive signs, the movements that are restricted and reproduce pain, and the negative signs, movements that are of full range and painless.

Active movements

As this name implies, the patient moves the parts himself. Active movements are performed within the patient's own limits of pain and should always be tested before passive movements as they indicate the degree of disability present and are a guide to the range of passive movement that can be reached without causing any undue discomfort. Active movements indicate that the musculotendinous structures which produce the movement are intact, for if they are completely ruptured active movement in the desired direction is usually impossible. They also indicate the patient's willingness to perform them.

The following observations are made:

1 The range of movement.
2 Whether they reproduce or provoke pain in a related site.
3 The behaviour of pain.
4 The rhythm of the movement.
5 The effect of rapid movements.
6 The effects of compression.

The range of movement is best measured with a goniometer and may be normal, decreased, increased or abnormal. The normal range depends mainly on anatomical features and varies according to age, sex and individual variation.

The patient is asked whether the movements are painless or whether pain is reproduced on certain movements, and to relate the pain to the point in the joint range in which it is felt. The relationship of pain to any loss of joint movement should always be assessed. The site, type, degree of pain, and any alteration in pain throughout the joint range is recorded and one of three patterns may emerge: (1) pain may be felt before the limit of the range, (2) pain may be felt at the limit of the range, or (3) the range may be limited but not painful unless over-pressure to the joint is applied. These patterns add little to the clinical diagnosis but they are of importance when considering the type of manual therapy to be used.

An arc of pain may sometimes be present. In the shoulder an arc of pain may be felt on abduction of the shoulder through the range of approximately 60–120 degrees but no pain is felt on abduction before or after this middle range.

The rhythm of the movement should be assessed. This involves the changes in relationships between the moving parts and the movements usually need to be repeated several times while observing the normal joint rhythm. It may not be possible to perform repeated movements if movement is very painful.

If pain is not provoked by a full range of movement performed at the usual speed, the movements should be retested using a series of rapid movements as these may then reproduce the pain.

The effect of compression on the joint may be tested. As an example, knee movements may be tested by having the patient squat.

Passive movements

Passive movements, as their name implies, are performed by the examiner. As the patient plays no active role in producing these movements, they can also be performed in the presence of a ruptured musculotendinous structure and the effect of any compression of the joint surfaces by the contraction of surrounding muscle is also eliminated. The starting position in which the joint is positioned is similar to that used for active movements and the patient should be as relaxed as possible, preferably while lying supine. Extreme gentleness is necessary when handling the joints to ensure that undue pain is not provoked and to allow a proper 'feel' of the parts being moved.

The following observations are made:

1   The range of movement.
2   Whether any movement provokes or reproduces pain.
3   The position in the range where pain and muscle spasm are first felt and the subsequent behaviour on passively increasing the range. The more rapidly and the earlier in the range that the pain increases, the more severe is the underlying lesion and the greater the need for more care and gentleness in the examination.
4   The end-feel of the movement: the range of passive movements is usually somewhat greater than the range of active movements and is associated with a normal amount of 'give' in the musculoskeletal structures. This elasticity may be felt as a sense of end-feel and practice is necessary to develop an appreciation for the normal characteristic type of end-feel in each joint. The normal types of end-feel may be caused by approximation of soft tissues around the joint which gives a soft, springy type of feel; or by a bony block owing to approximation of the bones around the joint; or to ligament tightening.

Abnormal end-feel may be produced by: (a) muscular spasm, (b) joint stiffness owing to capsular thickening, ligamentous adhesions or muscular shortening, and (c) a cartilaginous loose body.
5   Over-pressure may be applied at the end of the passive range by using small oscillatory movements to test the small extra range normally available. This may be the only movement to reproduce pain and so no joint can be assessed as being normal unless over-pressure at the end of the range can be applied painlessly.
6   Ligaments: the strength and stability of the ligaments are tested by applying a passive stretching force to the joint.

Isometric tests

The musculotendinous structures and their insertions around a joint are tested by the use of isometric contractions in which the muscle is contracted strongly but the joint itself does not move. The joint being examined first needs to be positioned accurately and it is necessary to demonstrate to the patient what is required.

One of three positions of the joint may be used as the starting position. (1) The joint is placed in the neutral position and the examiner resists the patient's attempt to move it in the desired direction. (2) The examiner initially passively stretches the musculotendinous structure and then actively resists the patient's attempt to return the joint to the neutral position. (3) The examiner places the joint in a position midway through its active range and the patient holds it steady in this position while the examiner attempts to return it to the neutral position.

The examiner palpates the muscle and its tendon with his other hand to assess its bulk and continuity. The observations to be made are: (1) the strength of the movement, and (2) whether it reproduces pain.

One of three patterns should emerge. (1) The resisted movements may be strong and painless; if so, the musculotendinous structure involved can be considered normal. (2) The movement may be weak and painless; this may result from a complete rupture of the musculotendinous apparatus or an interruption in its motor nerve supply. (3) The movement may reproduce pain; this indicates that the musculotendinous structure being tested is at fault. An assessment of the degree of the underlying lesion may be obtained from the strength of the contraction, for if the movement is weak and painful it usually indicates a more severe degree of damage than if the movement is strong and painful.

Patterns of movement

By testing active, passive and isometric contractions a pattern of movement emerges that should allow the anatomical site and type of lesion to be identified. The usual or typical findings are summarized as follows.

In arthritis and capsulitis the usual patterns are: (1) The active and passive ranges of movement are decreased and usually painful, especially at the limits of the range. However, there are exceptions to this finding, especially in early cases of arthritis when movement may be lost mainly in one or two directions only. Ultimately movements are lost in a proportionate degree that varies depending on the severity of the underlying inflammation. (2) Resisted movements should be painless.

In tendinitis: (1) Pain is best reproduced by fully resisted movements. (2) Pain may also be reproduced by stretching the tendon. (3) The range of active movement is often normal but pain may also be produced during or at the end of the range.

With complete rupture of musculotendinous structure: (1) Active range of movement is lost. (2) Passive range is normal. (3) Resisted movements are weak and painless.

With ligament sprains: (1) Pain is reproduced on passively stretching the ligament, especially with over-pressure. (2) The range of active and passive movements is usually decreased and painful. (3) Resisted movements are normal.

With complete ligament rupture, abnormal joint movement is present on passive movement.

With muscle lesions, pain may be present on resisted movement or appropriate isometric tests and stretching the muscle produces a painful loss of movement.

In patients with hypermobility, the active and passive range is increased but resisted movements are normal.

With an intra-articular loose body, pain is of sudden onset; active and passive movements in one direction, usually extension, are blocked but other movements are full.

Accessory movements

These joint movements, which cannot be performed voluntarily or in isolation, are a necessary component of normal joint function. Although their range of movement is small, a full range of accessory movements is essential for normal active and passive joint movements. Accordingly, a loss of an accessory movement produces a restriction in the normal range of joint motion. For example, when the hand grasps an object such as a ball, as the grip is tightened rotation occurs at the metacarpophalangeal joints. The normal physiological movements in this joint are flexion, extension, adduction and abduction, and rotation is an accessory movement produced during the active movement. Rotation can also be tested passively and the range produced is then greater if the left index finger is held relaxed in a position midway between the limits of flexion, extension, abduction and adduction. The proximal phalanx is supported by the thumb and forefinger of the right hand which are then used to move the proximal phalanx through quite an appreciable range of either medial or lateral rotation.

Another example of accessory movement is in the glenohumeral joint. With the arm hanging loosely by the side, the head of the humerus occupies the upper portion of the pear-shaped glenoid cavity, from which it is separated by a small gap. To move the arm into flexion, the surrounding muscles contract and the first accessory movement in the joint is a compression of the joint surfaces. When the shoulder is flexed, the humeral head is involved in a second accessory movement as it glides downwards and slightly backwards in the glenoid fossa. Some accessory movements can never be produced actively, e.g. a distraction of one joint surface away from another.

The articular surfaces of many joints are normally incongruent in most positions of the joint. They become congruent only at one extreme of the joint ranges as tension in the capsule and ligaments is increased, so that joint surfaces are brought into maximal contact and are tightly compressed. No movement is then possible in this close-packed position. In all other positions of the joint the articular surfaces are not congruent, the capsule is more lax and the joint is in a loose-packed position so that movement at the joint surfaces can more readily take place. The range of accessory joint movements is greatest when the muscles acting over the joint are relaxed and the joint is positioned midway between the limits of its different directions of active movements.

Clinical testing

The patient is placed in a relaxed position with the joint to be tested adequately supported. The starting position ensures relaxation of the surrounding muscles and joint, in the position in which the joint capsule has its greatest laxity. Usually the proximal bone forming the joint is fixed and the more distal bone is moved. The different accessory movements present in each joint and their method of clinical testing will be described later.

When testing accessory movements, different areas of adjacent surfaces of hyaline cartilage will be opposed when the joint is positioned in different ranges. For example, if the arm is kept by the side and a posteroanterior accessory movement of the head of the humerus in the glenoid cavity is tested, particular areas of the articular surface of the humerus will be opposed to particular areas of the articular surface of the glenoid cavity. However, if the arm is then abducted by 30 degrees and the same posteroanterior accessory movement is produced, a different area on the articular surface of the head of the humerus will now contact the same area of the articular surface of the glenoid.

When accessory movements are performed in different positions of the joint, different joint structures are placed on stretch. Accordingly, when testing accessory movements it may be necessary to perform each accessory movement with the joint placed in different positions if restrictions of movement, pain with movement and smoothness of movement between the opposing joint surfaces are to be determined accurately.

Clinical importance

The importance of accessory movements is: (1) They play an essential role in the production of normal joint movement. (2) Loss of accessory movements is associated with loss of normal joint movement. (3) Normal or restricted accessory movements can be detected by appropriate clinical testing. (4) At times, a restriction in their range (hypomobility) may be the only detectable relevant clinical finding. (5) They are used to treat painful or stiff joints by a passive movement technique using gentle rhythmical oscillations (mobilization). The range of joint movement is increased by this method, rather than by directly trying to force an increase in the passive joint range.

The clinical importance of accessory movements may be considered in three different types of joint:

1   In joints such as the shoulder or knee, with a large range of movement, a lesion is usually associated with loss of the normal range of active and passive movements. If so, the accessory movements will also be lost and testing should also reveal a painful restriction in their range.

2   In small single joints, active and passive joint movements may not be painful but testing accessory movements may reveal that they are restricted and reproduce pain.

3   In the integrated movements of several small joints, such as the carpus, active and passive wrist movements may reproduce pain but do not accurately localize the affected joint. This may be localized by testing the accessory movements of all the intercarpal joints.

An example of the importance of accessory movements may be given by considering movements between the capitate and hamate bones, which can easily be grasped by the examiner. These two bones can then easily be made to glide backwards and forwards against each other and the normally pain-free joint movement can be readily felt. In some patients wrist pain may be produced with movement either of the capitate or the hamate.

Assessment

During the testing of accessory movements three factors need to be assessed: stiffness, smoothness and pain.

1   Stiffness: the available range of accessory movement is assessed and any restriction in the range noted. This is tested with the joint placed in two positions: first, midway between the limits of all active ranges, and second, with the joint placed at the limit of any one or all directions of active movement.

2   Smoothness: this implies the friction-free feel of the accessory movements through the full amplitude of joint range from the limit of the range in one direction to the limit of the range in its opposite direction. The test for normal smoothness of movement is performed with the joint positioned midway between the limits of all its active ranges and the joint surfaces in a relaxed relationship to each other. The smoothness of movement should be compared with that felt when the joint surfaces are compressed and then moved through the same range.

3   Pain: an assessment should be made of any pain or discomfort experienced as the accessory movement is taken from one limit of its range to the other. It should be first made when the joint surfaces are relaxed and then compared with pain or discomfort experienced with the joint surfaces compressed.

Palpation

Palpation forms an essential part of the examination and requires a knowledge of the surface anatomy of each of the joint structures. These are palpated in an orderly sequence and the examiner confirms the presence of any alterations, deformity or muscle wasting that have been noted on inspection and detects the presence of any warmth, swellings, crepitus and tenderness.

Warmth

The presence of warmth over the joint surface should be sought for underlying inflammation or haemarthrosis. The customary teaching is to elicit warmth with the dorsal surface of the fingers but it is better appreciated by palpating the area with the palmar surface of the whole hand.

Swellings

Swellings may be either intra- or extra-articular. Intra-articular swellings may be either soft or hard. Soft tissue swellings may be due to either fluid or synovial thickening. A synovial effusion is usually better recognized on inspection but palpation is necessary to confirm its presence and that the swelling is fluid. Synovial thickening from a chronically inflamed synovium produces a characteristically firm and 'doughy' feel, best felt by rolling the fingers across the area of attachment of synovium to underlying bone.

Hard intra-articular swellings are due to bone and may be caused by osteophytic outgrowths around the edge of the joint, joint subluxations, intra-articular bony foreign bodies, bone tumours or bone deformities. In Freiberg's disease, an osteochondrosis involving the head of the second metatarsal, the irregular and deformed bone ends may be easily palpable.

Extra-articular swellings may be caused by oedema, haematoma formation, fat deposits, synovial swellings in bursae or tendon sheaths, calcific deposits, nodules or tophi. Swellings should be palpated to record their size, shape, consistency, surface, edges and attachments to superficial or deeper structures.

The tendons and their muscle bellies should also be palpated for the presence of any localized swelling. Tears in muscles or tendons may be felt as a localized gap, often with a nearby swelling from the rolled-up portion of the torn muscle or tendon tissue. Localized areas of thickenings in the muscle belly may be found with healing of recent tears. The bones around the joint are palpated for any swellings, irregularities or thickening.

Crepitus

Crepitus is a noise that may be heard or felt on a movement. A coarse, grating crepitus palpable with the hand over the joint surface indicates articular cartilage degeneration, often best felt in the knee. A fine crepitus is felt with synovial thickening and is often best felt in patients with tenosynovitis. Clicks such as the normal vacuum click felt in the joint are usually of no significance and are particularly common in hypermobile joints. A painful click may indicate the presence of a torn meniscus. Snapping may be heard or felt around joints as tendons or ligaments slip over bony prominences. This is often loud and disturbing to the patient but is usually of no clinical significance. A coarse 'clunking' type of noise may accompany joint subluxation or instability. This may be produced by degenerative changes in the joint or can be found particularly in rotary instability of the knee.

Tenderness

The structure being examined should be carefully palpated for tenderness while simultaneously observing the patient's face to gauge the degree of any painful reaction. Palpation is usually carried out by the examiner using his thumb or forefinger and it is essential that a firm even pressure be used. This can usually be judged to be sufficient if a blanching of the distal aspect of the examiner's thumb becomes apparent during the palpation.

Considerable difficulties arise in the correct assessment of tenderness. The point at issue is not that locally inflamed or damaged tissues may be tender but that correct interpretation of this sign requires considerable experience and expertise. Tenderness can often be a misleading sign because it is in part subjective. Many normal structures can often be made to feel tender, especially if the patient is not sufficiently relaxed. Moreover, tenderness may at times be referred and is associated with referred pain, so that the site of the causative lesion may be more proximal.

The mistake most commonly made is to seek for tenderness as the first sign in the clinical examination. Tenderness should be used only as a confirmatory test after the site of the underlying lesion has been identified by appropriate movement tests. If examination using active, passive and isometric test movements has demonstrated the presence of tendinitis then tenderness over the involved tendon is most useful as a confirmatory sign. However, to commence the examination of a patient with joint pain by first palpating for tenderness will most often lead to an incorrect diagnosis.

References

1   Maitland, G.D. (1990) *Peripheral Manipulation*, 3rd edn, Butterworth-Heinemann, Oxford

4 Management of soft tissue injuries

Management may be classified under the following headings:

1 Rest.
2 Orthotics and supports.
3 Medications.
4 Injections.
5 Physical therapy:
  (a) Heat.
  (b) Ice.
  (c) Massage.
6 Pain-relieving modalities:
  (a) Transcutaneous electrical nerve stimulation (TENS).
  (b) Interferential therapy.
7 Exercise and hydrotherapy.
8 Stretching.
9 Manual therapy.
10 Surgery.
11 Aftercare and prophylaxis.

Rest

Direct or indirect sporting injuries treated with prolonged rest lead to a longer period of rehabilitation and disability. The realization that athletes can be treated with quite vigorous early treatment programmes, including active exercises and passive stretching, has enabled the athlete to return to sport more rapidly without having lost any general level of fitness (see Chapter 2).

The management of overuse injuries is more complex. A generalized medical prescription for rest is usually ignored by an athlete to whom rest is anathema. They may prefer to change their doctor than to change their training schedule. None the less, in overuse injuries, treatment regimens rarely succeed unless some modification to the total load placed on neuromusculoskeletal structures is achieved and the athlete is convinced he cannot continue to exercise through the pain. Many patients with other degenerative or inflammatory soft tissue or joint disorders are encouraged to exercise too early in the belief that 'exercise is good for you'.

If pain and inflammation are sufficiently severe, restriction of the particular activity causing overuse is necessary. The degree of rest needed will vary according to the degree of inflammatory reaction present and the cooperation of the patient. The art is to arrange rest to the overused musculoskeletal structure without inhibiting more generalized activities.

Orthotics and supports

Orthotic devices are used to obtain a functional control of any biomechanical dysfunction present during the different phases of stance by providing normal muscular action about a stable lever system. In the treatment of foot disorders their advantage over conventional types of arch supports is in controlling the function of both the rear foot and the fore foot simultaneously so that the normal angular relationship between the bones of the rear foot to the fore foot is retained. The orthotic forms a system with the foot that moves with it and not against it and also permits the rear foot to act as a shock absorber. Orthotic devices are available in different forms of increasing rigidity that vary in effectiveness and patient acceptability. (1) Soft devices are usually made of felt or rubber and are used particularly in running-shoes. (2) Semi-flexible devices are usually made of leather or firmer rubber. (3) Rigid devices are made of thermally pliable plastic constructed from a neutral balanced cast of the patient's foot.

They extend from the heel to behind the metatarsal head and provide stability during the heel strike and midstance phases of gait. They may need to be balanced by posts or wedges at either the rear foot or fore foot, or both. For example, patients with either rear foot varus or valgus deformities will require pronatory or supinatory wedging of the heel. Care must be taken during the making of the cast to ensure that the foot is in a neutral position relative to the lower leg, i.e. neither supinated nor pronated (see p. 207).

Other aids may be used to support a painful joint or to help transfer the body-weight from one leg to the pain-free one. The large variety of supports will not be considered here but some general examples are given. In the lower limb, these include: (1) Crutches, sticks, and walking frames. (2) Knee braces that may help to support a painful, weakened or unstable knee. (3) Callipers that may be 'long leg' with weight-bearing under the ischial tuberosity or 'short leg' used to support the ankle or subtalar joint with a T-strap. (4) Ankles may need to be strapped.

In the upper limb slings, triangular bandages or a collar and cuff bandage may be used to rest the shoulder or elbow.

Medications

Medication may be used to produce either an analgesic or an anti-inflammatory effect. As pain is such a common problem in musculoskeletal disorders, it is not unreasonable to prescribe simple non-narcotic drugs for pain relief. Paracetamol, salicylates or dextropropoxyphene are commonly used, often in combination tablets.

Non-steroidal anti-inflammatory drugs (NSAIDs) are often of benefit in the management of soft tissue injuries. These medications have analgesic, anti-pyretic properties and the ability to reduce inflammation in animal models. Inflammation is characterized by a complex series of events produced by chemical mediators, such as prostaglandins and kinins, resulting in vasodilation, tissue oedema and pain. All NSAIDs inhibit these chemical mediators.

NSAIDs are absorbed from the gastrointestinal tract so are very effective when taken orally. They vary in their duration of action with some medications such as ibuprofen having a short half-life while piroxicam and tenoxicam have half-lives of over 24 h. Naproxen, diclofenac and ketoprofen have intermittent half-lives. The frequency of dosing will depend on the half-life of the medication involved. Providing the dosage is appropriate and the interval between doses is selected according to the half-life, there is no reason why a similar degree of anti-inflammatory effect cannot be obtained with any of these medications.

Prostaglandins are also involved in the auto-regulation of other organ systems, in particular the kidney and gastrointestinal tract, and so prolonged use of NSAIDs is likely to affect these areas. Common side-effects may include indigestion, nausea or vomiting and the development of gastric ulceration. Fluid retention may occur and is particularly a problem in those people who have pre-existing renal, hepatic or cardiac disease.

Injection therapy

Shortly after corticosteroids were first introduced in 1949, it was realized that a low dose of this preparation, deposited at a site of inflammation, could obviate some of the problems caused by a large oral dose. The original corticosteroid used, cortisone, was ineffective for local use as it needs to be converted in the liver to hydrocortisone. Several synthetic analogues of hydrocortisone have since been manufactured. Taken by mouth, these drugs have different degrees of potency and side-effects that are not necessarily reflected in their usefulness as local preparations either topically or as local injections. For example, triamcinolone given by mouth has considerable side-effects but is a most useful form of local injection. Acetate, tertiary butyl acetate or phosphate salts are used in local injections: their different properties are related to their solubility and chemical preparation. Crystalline forms, which may themselves produce an intense crystal synovitis, and long-acting preparations are now available.

Injections must be given using thorough aseptic techniques, including scrubbing of the hands and sterilization of the skin. Similarly, local injections must never be given in the presence of any skin infections. It is good practice to swab the skin at least twice with an antiseptic skin solution and an alcohol swab may be left on the skin with the finger placed over it to palpate the site of the injection. The use of disposable syringes and needles and small phials of local anaesthetic and corticosteroid preparations have undoubtedly been major advances. The injections may be given either into joints or into surrounding soft tissues. They are especially useful in traumatic or inflammatory synovitis and are of great value in treating crystal synovitis, particularly if it involves the larger joints. The joint surfaces are palpated and the patient suitably postured so that the synovium bulges at the site of injection. The optimum site for injection varies with each joint but is usually found on the extensor surface and will be described in subsequent chapters. The size of the needle used varies with the size of the joint but in small joints a 25-gauge needle may be used and in large joints, such as the knee, a 20-gauge needle is usually sufficient for aspiration and injection.

If the bony outlines of the joint have been carefully palpated it is usually possible to insert the needle directly into the synovial cavity without having to guide it along the bony surfaces so that entering a distended synovial space can be as easy as puncturing an inflated balloon. Any synovial fluid present should be aspirated and submitted for routine analysis of its cell count, protein content and the presence of any crystals.

Occasionally, folds of synovium or fibrinous intrasynovial deposits block the tip of the needle and prevent easy withdrawal of fluid. Should this happen, the needle is withdrawn slightly and gently moved about within the joint. Any fluid that has already been aspirated may be reinjected through the needle to clear it or a few ml of local anaesthetic solution may be injected.

Dosage is determined by the volume of the joint to be injected. Small joints such as the finger joints usually take approximately 0.5 ml of solution, the wrist and elbow about 1 ml, larger joints such as the elbow or ankle about 2 ml and a large synovial joint such as the knee 2–3 ml.

If the needle has been correctly placed inside the cavity the injection of corticosteroid can be made easily without any sense of resistance. If not, the needle has probably been placed outside the synovial cavity. Inside the synovial cavity the corticosteroid solution spreads evenly, mixes with the synovial fluid and bathes the cells of the synovial membrane. It acts by blocking the inflammatory reaction which may be related to its effect in stabilizing lysosomal enzymes. Hence, it is important in treating joint

diseases that the corticosteroid preparation is deposited within the synovial cavity. Once the injection has been given, the needle is rapidly withdrawn, the skin area again swabbed and a small protective dressing applied.

In the soft tissues, local corticosteroid injections are of most value in the overuse type of inflammatory lesions involving the bursae, ligaments or musculotendinous structures, and in the nerve entrapment syndromes. In injuries from direct or indirect trauma, their use is much more limited as they are never given in the early stages as they may induce further bleeding. At a later stage in the healing, a small area of fibrous tissue thickening may form that limits movement and promotes an inflammatory reaction with use of the part. These areas in muscles, tendons or ligaments can usually be readily felt with careful palpation and often respond well to local corticosteroid injection.

In soft tissue lesions the injection must be deposited accurately at or around the involved site and this presupposes an accurate clinical diagnosis and knowledge of the anatomy and surface landmarks. For soft tissue injections the optimum position for injection depends on suitable posturing of the patient so that the area to be injected can be accurately palpated. As a general rule, they should be given with the structure to be injected put on stretch. Soft tissue landmarks and the site of injection vary for each joint and will be considered in greater detail in other chapters. Local anaesthetic, usually 1% Xylocaine (lignocaine), is also added to the corticosteroid solution as it eases any pain. If this injection has been accurately sited the patient's pain should be relieved and retesting the active, passive or resisted movements should no longer reproduce the pain.

Patients should be warned that as the effect of the local anaesthetic wears off, some pain or discomfort may be experienced for 1 or possibly 2 days but that subsequently there should be considerable improvement in their symptoms. Also, to prevent further damage they should not overuse the part while the analgesic effect of the local anaesthetic is still present.

Injection therapy forms only a part of the overall management and the injected area should be rested after the injection is given. The practice of giving a local corticosteroid injection and allowing the athlete to exercise immediately afterwards should be condemned.

There is no absolute rule as to how often an injection should be repeated but as a general rule injections are best given with as long an interval as possible between the injections. In the weight-bearing joints injections should be limited to two or three times a year.

Injections should never be given:

1 In the presence of any infections.
2 At a late stage of articular diseases when irreparable joint damage is present.
3 If a haemarthrosis is present.
4 If a fracture involves the joint surfaces.
5 Before a definitive diagnosis has been reached.
6 If a psychogenic cause of the patient's symptoms is suspected.
7 If previous injections have failed to produce any prolonged benefit.

Advantages

In most of the soft tissue lesions for which local corticosteroid injections are indicated, a considerable degree of relief of symptoms can usually be expected. In the chronic joint diseases these injections obviously do not represent a cure but as they help to suppress the inflammatory reaction they can provide at least a temporary relief of pain and swelling. This may permit the use of other pharmacological and physical methods to improve the functional status of the patient.

Inflammatory arthritis injections are of considerable value in the total management of the patient. They should be used only if: (1) a few joints are affected, (2) a few joints are actively inflamed, (3) a few involved joints prevent active rehabilitation of the patient, e.g. a patient may have severe joint disease but only synovitis in the knee prevents him from becoming ambulant, and (4) the use of NSAIDs is contraindicated.

In degenerative joint disease, injections are most unlikely to produce any lasting effect or alter the underlying pathological process. They may occasionally be of value when there is a superadded inflammatory element, such as in Heberden's nodes.

Complications

The complications of intra-articular injections should always be remembered, particularly as these injections are so easy to perform.

Infection

Infection introduced with the injection is a major tragedy, although fortunately quite rare. As *Staphylococcus aureus* is the most common infecting organism, the need for constant attention to maintaining asepsis is of paramount importance.

Acute crystal synovitis

If the corticosteroid solution is microcrystalline an intense crystal synovitis may be produced, which lasts for a few days.

Systemic absorption

The synovial cavity is a highly vascular structure and so the local injection is never retained wholly within the joint cavity but is partly absorbed.

Articular cartilage damage

Corticosteroids, whether given by mouth or injection, can inhibit the metabolism of cartilage by their effect on chondrocytes and glycosaminoglycan metabolism. Damage to joint hyaline cartilage after the use of local steroid injections may result in overuse of the joint due to alleviation of the pain. Gibson *et al* [1] injected a large dose of methylprednisolone into *Macaca* monkeys over 12 weeks and failed to demonstrate any significant degree of cartilage damage. In humans infrequent injections would probably not accelerate cartilage damage and the benefits in reducing synovial inflammation could far outweigh any problems caused by cartilage damage.

Repeated injections may result in cartilage and bone destruction, producing an aseptic necrosis of the bone, or a destructive Charcot-type of arthropathy. This appears to be more common in the hip but may follow repeated injections in any joint.

Tendon rupture

An injection must never be given directly into the tendon substance as there is at least a theoretical consideration that it may weaken the collagen fibres. Any swelling may compress the relatively tenuous vascular supply. The area of tenderness, usually near the tendon origin or on its surface, should be found by careful palpation and the needle is then directed obliquely along the side of this area.

To summarize: the use of local corticosteroid injections is still controversial but:

1 They are of immense value in soft tissue injuries after trauma or overuse if properly administered into the locally affected area.
2 In degenerative joint disease their use is short lasting and adds little to the total management of the patient.
3 In chronic inflammatory arthritis they are of considerable value as an adjunct to the total management of the patient, especially when combined with joint aspiration.
4 In acute crystal synovitis involving large joints, e.g. the knee, their use combined with aspiration of the joint is usually the treatment of choice.
5 The advantages of their use outweigh their complications, which must none the less never be ignored.
6 They must be used only as one part of a total programme of management.

Physical therapy

Physical methods of therapy have a time honoured role in the management of these musculoskeletal disorders.

Heat

Heat may be used to relieve the symptoms of musculoskeletal disorders but will obviously play little part in their cure. It may be used for its analgesic properties, and is especially useful when given before exercise therapy as a form of warm-up procedure. The physical intricacies of the various forms of therapeutic heat will not be considered here but factors in its application include depth of penetration beneath the skin and the convenience and availability of application.

Simple methods of producing heat for home treatment include infrared lamps, hot packs, paraffin wax baths, showers or contrast baths in which heat is alternated with the use of cold. More complex methods include the following.

Microwaves

These are electromagnetic radiations with a wide frequency range produced by a microwave machine with applicators placed a few centimetres from the skin surface to direct a beam of radiation. It is an easy method to use but the depth of heating is largely superficial.

Ultrasound

This employs an acoustic vibration that is produced when a high-frequency oscillatory voltage is passed through a quartz crystal to produce an electrical effect. The crystal is contained in a metal head that produces a cylindrical beam and so allows optimal ultrasound transmission. Its main effect is probably as a form of heat produced particularly at the intersurface between tissues such as muscle layers.

Ultrasonic therapy is believed to increase the permeability of semipermeable membranes and so disperse any accumulation of fluid and improve the rate of healing independent of any heating effect. Ultrasound given to tissue culture stimulated an increased protein synthesis in fibroblasts [2]. It also may produce a local micromassaging effect that may help to disperse fibrous tissue and so is useful in the chronic stage of many soft tissue injuries.

Its concentrated use can produce tissue damage from a localized mechanical destructive force but this potential danger is overcome by moving the point of application gradually over a field of several square centimetres at any one time. It may, however, produce a rapid rise in the temperature of the deep tissues without producing any skin heating or sensation of warmth, so that a correct knowledge of its use and method of application is essential.

Short-wave diathermy

This undoubtedly produces the deepest penetration of heat but requires expensive equipment and supervision by a physiotherapist. It uses high-frequency currents and the patient is placed within the electrical circuit to produce an impedance. Two methods are available which use either an induction coil or a condenser field. The machine needs to be tuned to adjust the total impedance so that the frequency of oscillation in the machine resonates with the patient's circuit.

All clothing, jewellery and metallic objects must be removed from the patient before treatment and this form of therapy cannot be used if the patient has had a metal implant inserted surgically. The accumulation of any sweat on the skin can also result in local burning.

Ice therapy

Ice has been used as a therapeutic agent for many years but only recently has it been used in treating musculoskeletal disorders. Its main indication appears to be in the immediate treatment of sporting injuries where the proposed rationale for its use is cooling of the deeper tissues with vasoconstriction and reduction of the localized bleeding. The depth of cooling probably depends on the length of time that the ice is applied. Ice may also be used in the treatment of chronic musculoskeletal conditions, including the healing phase of musculotendinous injuries, and can replace the traditional role played by heat.

Method of application

The ice is finely crushed and placed in a wet towel which is then placed over the area to be treated and kept in place with a crêpe bandage for approximately 20 min. Some patients cannot tolerate this because of an intense burning sensation but most report only minor, tolerable discomfort or numbness. The ice is taken off after 20 min but may be reapplied every 2 h.

Ice is easy, safe, simple to apply, cheap, convenient and may be used as a home treatment.

Indications

1 The immediate treatment of most sports injuries.
2 Long continued treatment of sports injuries, including overuse injuries.
3 To relieve muscular spasm.
4 Preparatory to exercise therapy or stretching.
5 Acute bursitis, e.g. acute subacromial bursitis where heat often produces an exacerbation of the pain.
6 To reduce oedematous swelling, e.g. in the hand.

Precautions

Prolonged or often repeated ice therapy should not be used and it must never be placed over or near a branch of a nerve. Complications of its use cannot be predicted. It may damage the skin, the so-called 'ice burn', which produces painful, red skin blotches that usually disappear within a few days if ice is not reapplied. More extensive damage may occur in the subcutaneous tissues owing to fat necrosis and persists for some weeks. In one series of 1000 cases [3] 15 patients had a skin reaction but only one developed subcutaneous fat damage.

Contraindications

Ice should never be used if there is any impairment of the local blood supply, such as peripheral vascular disease or Raynaud's phenomenon, or if the patient is known to be unduly sensitive to the effects of cold.

Massage

Massage by rubbing a painful area has the longest history among the physical methods of treatment. It is used in different forms but these are variants of a single theme and have been glorified by the use of French names. They include stroking (effleurage), kneading (pétrissage) and percussion (tapotement). They will not be described here as they are of little practical value but one form of massage that may be useful is deep pressure (friction) massage.

Deep pressure massage uses intermittent pressures over the soft tissues in which the therapist's finger and the patient's skin and subcutaneous tissues are moved simultaneously over the deeper structures in varying directions. The pad of the operator's index finger is usually used and force is applied by the flexor tendon and not by pressure from the terminal interphalangeal joint. This action may be strengthened by laying the pad of the middle finger over the dorsum of the index finger.

The action of deep pressure massage appears to be mainly as a form of counter-irritation but it may improve the local blood supply and provide some degree of reaction in chronic ligamentous sprains or in chronic tendinitis. It should never be used in the early stages of healing of an injury or in the presence of acute inflammation.

Pain-relieving modalities

Transcutaneous nerve stimulation

Transcutaneous nerve stimulation is a simple and safe method used to control pain. An electric current is applied to the skin through electrodes connected to a small battery-operated pulse generator. This apparatus was originally developed as a screening device to test a patient's response to electrical stimulation before surgical implantation of a nerve stimulator but it was found to relieve pain itself in many cases. It has since been used in the control of chronic pain arising from many different disorders. Its mode of action is controversial with both gate control and endorphin theories postulated to explain its pain modulation.

The electric current is produced by a small pulse generator which can be carried by the patient and has controls for adjusting the electrical output, frequency and duration. This is connected to two cables attached to flexible electrodes that are strapped to the patient's skin over a painful area or over a peripheral nerve proximal to it. An electrode gel is first applied to the skin and the electrodes are then taped in place. The stimulator is switched on and the output control slowly adjusted until stimulation is felt. This is then adjusted so that the most comfortable sensation with the maximum pain relief is obtained. Pain relief may be obtained on the first application or only after several weeks. It may last only while the current is turned on or it may last for hours or days after the current is turned off. The machine can be used while carrying out daily activities.

Interferential therapy

This form of electrotherapy was introduced in 1959. The machine used is electrically operated and is small, light and easily portable. It uses a wide variety of low-frequency currents delivered into the deeper structures but without any sensory stimulation of the skin. The intensity of the combined current increases and decreases rhythmically so that in the area of the body where the currents mix a medium-frequency current is produced that changes in intensity to a low-frequency rhythmical beat. By adjusting these low-frequency rhythms, different structures are stimulated and varying therapeutic effects produced. Thus these rhythms may be used to produce analgesia whereas at another frequency swelling and oedema may be assessed. This form of therapy may be useful in treating pain and swelling arising as a result of various musculoskeletal conditions or as a precursor to more active therapy.

Exercise therapy

The cornerstone of active rehabilitation is exercise therapy as the evidence is overwhelming for activity rather than inactivity to restore muscle function. Modern exercise therapy is predicated on a knowledge of muscle fibre types. Broadly they are white or red fibres which develop different tensions because of their properties. White fibres are larger, fast

twitch, have a low myoglobin content and an anaerobic energy system with explosive power. Red fibres are smaller, slow twitch, have a high myoglobin content, dense capillary network and an aerobic energy system which may sustain effort over a long period of time.

Aims

1 To restore strength in weakened muscles, e.g. after injury or around an inflamed joint.
2 To restore mobility or increase the range of movement. This occurs especially after a muscle injury with a loss of flexibility.
3 To correct postural faults.
4 To prevent joint deformity.
5 To improve joint stability, e.g. with a cruciate ligament rupture, increased knee stability may be obtained with thigh muscle exercises. This is even more important if the quadriceps have become rapidly wasted, as usually happens.
6 After passive movement techniques have relieved joint pain in order to restore a full range of physiological movement.
7 An active exercise programme may have little role to play while joint pain is the major problem but passive exercises can then still be of help.

Exercises may be (1) static or isometric, and (2) dynamic: isotonic, isotonic variable resistance, and isokinetic. These are described in Chapter 2.

A hydrotherapy pool can be of great assistance in allowing exercise without the effect of gravity in a warm and relatively friction-free environment.

Requirements of an exercise regimen

The practice of handing a patient a sheet of printed exercises and giving the general advice that exercises should be performed is to be deplored. To be effective, an exercise regimen requires:

1 A medical prescription. The first requirement is a proper medical prescription because, as with drug medication, too little exercise therapy can be of no value and too much is harmful.
2 Assessment. This prescription can only be made after a proper assessment of the patient's disabilities, deformities and muscle strength. The assessment then needs to be related to the patient's future needs, work requirements and capacity to undertake such work.

3 Individualization. An exercise regimen needs to be prepared and tailored to these individual deficits and requirements.
4 Specificity. Specificity of exercises is necessary to obtain a training effect.
5 Motivation. The patient must be properly motivated. This can be difficult at times as a long period of therapy is necessary before any great degree of improvement is observed. A detailed explanation of the aims of therapy is required and often great enthusiasm on the part of the physiotherapist.
6 Supervision. The programme needs to be supervised by a physiotherapist to ensure that the exercises are properly taught and carried out.
7 Progression. The exercise programme needs to be gradually progressed and increased in its intensity.
8 Effectiveness. The regimen should produce its desired result without producing any prolonged period of pain or undue fatigue; should it do so, the treatment programme needs to be revised.

Stretching

Stretching is a passive technique used to increase the flexibility of musculoskeletal tissues and hence aid movement and activity, improve performance and decrease the incidence of sporting injuries. Stretching exercises are also necessary in the treatment of musculoskeletal sporting injuries to relieve pain and to restore or increase the range of movement. Stretching should be performed both before activity, as a warm-up procedure and after activity as a warm-down procedure.

Prolonged static stretching is the preferred technique. The musculotendinous structure is moved slowly and gently to a position of stretch and held there for up to 60 s. The muscle can then usually be stretched out a little further without pain and with little chance of injury. Sudden, forced movements are contraindicated. The stretching programme should be preceded by a warm-up as this allows a greater degree of flexibility to be gained.

Usually most muscle groups around a joint are stretched but at times the regimen may be concentrated on improving range in one direction only, e.g. in ballet dancers to increase external rotation at the hip, i.e. turn-out.

Passive stretching also needs to be used with active exercises to increase and retain the joint range that has been attained.

In people with soft tissue injuries, the restoration of full muscle power may be inhibited by pain, the presence of an effusion or by loss of the normal passive over-pressure. Normally the passive range of a joint is greater than the active range and a further small range can be attained with passive over-pressure. This extra range is often lost in muscle injuries and can be restored by passive stretching with over-pressure (see p. 7).

The strength of passive stretching is dependent on the diagnosis and assessment of the degree of the injured tissue and the pain response.

Stretching movements should be commenced early in the management of soft tissue lesions within the limit of pain. In grade 1 or 2 ligament sprains early gentle passive stretching should be used, governed by the pain response. Grade 1 injuries can be stretched much more strongly than grade 2 injuries.

If joint restriction remains a problem, stretching is first taken just to the point of pain, then further into the painful range and is then released. This is repeated four to six times. The patient can then repeat these movements taking the joint to its maximal stretch and then actively contracting the agonist muscle. This cycle is then repeated a few more times.

However, if the range is painfully restricted, the irritability (see p. 17) of the disorder must first be assessed. Stretching is then taken with some discomfort or pain into the restricted range. This position is sustained and small, slowly performed oscillations are carried out and allow some increase in range. Slow larger amplitude movements are then performed. This combination is repeated several times in a session which itself may be repeated three or more times a day.

The behaviour of the pain response during and after this technique must be carefully assessed. Ideally, treatment should continue until passive stretching can be performed very strongly and without pain with the same strength of stretch as that on the normal side.

Other stretching techniques have been described but are not generally as effective or as safe. These include proprioceptive neuromuscular facilitation (PNF) and ballistic or bouncing stretching movements.

Passive movements such as continuous passive motion (CPM) play an important role in the early management of musculoskeletal injuries [4] to improve healing in injuries to joints, ligaments and tendons [5]. In particular, it can promote repair to articular cartilage whereas joints that are immobilized show no repair [6].

Manual therapy

Manual therapy is a passive movement technique that can be classified into either joint manipulation or mobilization.

Manipulation is a sudden movement or thrust of small amplitude; it is performed at the end of the joint range at such a speed that the patient is unable to prevent it. In disorders of the peripheral joints, a joint may be manipulated with or without an anaesthetic. Without anaesthesia, the procedure may be modified using a steady, controlled movement to stretch a stiff joint in an attempt to increase the joint range.

Mobilization is defined as a passive movement technique performed so that the movements are at all times within the control of the patient who can prevent them if he wishes. They are performed mainly as slow oscillatory movements in the physiological and accessory range of a joint and the joint surfaces may be held either distracted, compressed or midway between these two positions. Distraction is applied by pulling the bone ends apart at right angles to their joint surfaces. Compression is applied in the opposite direction to push the joint surfaces together. The oscillatory movements are usually used in one of two methods: (1) as large or small amplitude movements, at a rate of two or three per second, and applied anywhere within the joint range; or (2) combined with sustained stretching as small amplitude oscillations applied at the limit of the joint range.

Method

The patient should be as relaxed and comfortable as possible. The joint to be moved is held and stabilized in a firm grasp so that the joint movement can be appreciated. This requires the therapist to be comfortably positioned so as to control the movements with a minimum of effort and ensure that no undue pain is produced. The joint to be mobilized is placed in a starting position that ensures relaxation of the joint and its surrounding muscles, usually in the midposition of the joint. The proximal bone forming the joint surface is usually fixed and the distal bone is moved. The movements produced must be very gentle, the amount of treatment given in the first few sessions must be limited and continual assessment is essential.

Grades of movement

Any part of a range of movement may be used in treatment and widely varying amplitudes may be chosen. It is time consuming to refer to a treatment movement as a 'large amplitude movement performed in the early part of the range' or as a 'small amplitude movement performed firmly at the limit of the range'. To overcome this and make the recording of treatment quicker and simpler, a system of grading the movement is used. Grades I and IV are used to describe the treatment movements but, like all similar gradings (e.g. rating of muscle power), the values overlap and so there is also a place for plus and minus values. The grades of movement described below can be depicted by a straight line representing a full range of movement (Figure 4.1).

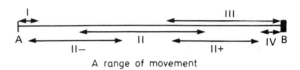

Figure 4.1 Grades of movement. A, neutral position at the beginning of movement; B, end of normal, average range of movement

Grade I is a small amplitude movement performed at the beginning of the range.

Grade II is a large amplitude movement performed within the free range but not moving into any resistance or stiffness. If the movement is performed near the beginning of the range it is expressed as II–; if it is taken deeply into the range but is still free of resistance it is expressed as II+.

Grade III is a large amplitude movement performed up to the limit of the range. This movement can also be expressed with plus and minus values. If the movement knocks vigorously at the limit of the range it is expressed III+ but if it nudges gently at the limit of the range it is expressed as III–.

Grade IV is a small amplitude movement performed at the limit of the range. This too can be expressed as IV+ or IV– depending on the vigour with which it is used.

If a joint disorder limits the normal range of joint movement, grades III and IV are restricted to smaller amplitudes (Figure 4.2).

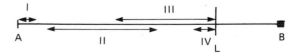

Figure 4.2 Restricted grades of movement. A, neutral position; B, average anatomical limit; L, pathological limit of range

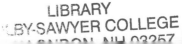

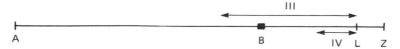

Figure 4.3 Grades of movement in a hypermobile joint. A, neutral position; B, average anatomical limit; L, pathological limit of range; Z, limit of normal hypermobile range

Similarly, pain may arise from a hypermobile joint that has become slightly stiff. This alters the positions of grade III and IV movements, as shown in Figure 4.3.

The oscillatory treatment movements may be smooth and regular or performed with an irregular rhythm. When the treatment movement is carried into the painful range and the patient finds it difficult to relax, the treatment movement must be regularly performed a little slower than usual with an even rhythm. The patient will then realize exactly how his joint is to be moved and will find it easier to relax. Some patients have difficulty in relaxing completely even when pain is minimal and may periodically tense their muscles without realizing they are doing so. If large amplitude treatment movements are then hindered movements of broken rhythm and changing amplitude are used to attempt to trick the muscles. Sometimes the movements need to be performed almost as a flick. At first the joint is moved in an exploratory manner to determine the response of the joint. Treatment movements are continually modified to meet the changing circumstances and will vary in depth, gradually moving deeper or receding, according to what is felt at different depths.

Many techniques are performed in positions similar to those used for the joint examination. Many directions of movement are tested during examination, each movement being performed only once or twice. This usually indicates the best position for treatment. In treatment the movement is repeated many times in only one direction, although the position may then be altered after such a sequence.

Assessment of mobilization

A balance needs to be maintained between the firmness of the treatment, the amount of improvement produced in symptoms and any reaction suffered by the patient. This requires constant reassessment of symptoms and signs, which are checked after each treatment and again before the next treatment session. Symptoms should never be checked by asking the patient direct questions. The active and passive ranges of movements are retested to determine any increase in their range and whether pain is reproduced. Provided that joint range is improving, treatment may be continued but constant reassessment is still necessary. If there is no improvement, or if pain is aggravated, a different treatment technique should be selected.

Indications for manipulative therapy

1   Replacement of a joint dislocation, e.g. a dislocated shoulder, or a joint subluxation, e.g. in a child with a pulled elbow.
2   Reduction of an internal derangement of a joint, e.g. in the knee, where a torn meniscus or loose body produces blocking of joint movements, and manipulation can re-position the torn meniscus to allow normal movements.
3   Stretching or breaking down adhesions. Joint stiffness may follow a sprained ligament with pain and tenderness over the ligament. In capsulitis of the shoulder, mobilization and manipulation may be used to break down periarticular adhesions to increase joint mobility.
4   Restoring normal joint range in patients with painful and/or stiff joints with associated loss of the normal accessory movements and some degree of spasm in the surrounding muscles.

Choice of techniques

The choice of techniques depends on whether the patient suffers from joint stiffness, pain, spasm or combinations of these.

Treatment of joint stiffness

A patient with joint stiffness alone may be treated by mobilization using either the physiological or accessory joint movements; in practice both of these movements are usually used. The physiological movements are used first with any of the normal movements for the particular joint. All normal joint movements are used if the degree of stiffness is marked. Alternatively, only one of the reduced physiological movements may be used in treatment and if so it is often found that as the range of this movement increases the range of all other joint movements also increases.

Treatment is first performed using physiological movements at the limit of the available joint range with small amplitude oscillatory movements for approximately 2 min. Then, while still holding the joint at the limit of the range, the accessory joint movements are also mobilized with small amplitude movements. This cycle of treatment with physiological and then accessory movements may be repeated three or four times in a treatment session. Any subsequent soreness in the joint can be relieved by repeating the physiological movement and using a large amplitude movement within the pain-free joint range.

Treatment of joint pain

A patient with joint pain alone, or joint pain and stiffness in which pain is predominant, is treated mainly by mobilization using accessory movements. When the pain is the dominant factor the joint being treated needs to be supported in a neutral position at first and accessory movements should be performed in the pain-free range. If pain or discomfort is provoked during the first treatment session treatment must continue in the pain-free range and smaller amplitude movements must be used. As the condition improves, movements may be increased, taken into the painful range and increased in amplitude. Provided improvement is maintained, physiological movements can be introduced and performed slowly through a large amplitude.

Treatment of painful and stiff joints

Most patients requiring treatment will have both painful and stiff joints. The painful component is best treated first, using the accessory joint movements with small amplitude movements and with the joint positioned in a neutral pain-free position. These movements are initially used in a range that does not provoke pain but may be increased as the pain improves and ultimately may be performed in the painful range also. The direction of the treatment movement is selected according to the type of lost accessory movement as found on clinical examination.

Stiffness in the painful joint may also be treated with gentle grade IV movements applied at the limit of range, so stretching the joint. If these are not successful manipulation of the joint under an anaesthetic should be considered.

Treatment of muscular spasm

Patients with joint pain may be found to have a marked muscle spasm at the limit of the available range. This is best treated by moving the joint at the limit of the physiological range until spasm commences and using small amplitude grade IV movements; this may also be combined with active relaxation techniques.

References

1 Gibson, T., Burry H.C., Poswillo, D. *et al* (1977) Effect of intra-articular corticosteroid injections on primate cartilage. *Annals of Rheumatic Disease*, **36,** 74–79
2 Harvey, W., Dyson, M., Pond, J.B. *et al* (1975) The stimulation of protein synthesis in human fibroblast by therapeutic ultrasound. *Rheumatology and Rehabilitation*, **14,** 237
3 Laing, D.R., Dalley, D.R. and Kirk, J.A. (1973) Ice therapy in soft tissue injuries. *New Zealand Medical Journal*, **78,** 155–157
4 O'Driscoll, S.W., Kumar, A. and Salter, R.B. (1983) The effect of continuous passive motion on the clearance of a hemarthrosis from a synovial joint. *Clinical Orthopaedics and Related Research*, **176,** 305–311
5 Zuran, B.H., Nelson, D.L., Sauer, J.A. *et al* (1988) The effects of sheath repair and continuous passive motion on healing flexor tendons. *Orthopaedic Research Society*, **34,** 180
6 Richardson, W.J. and Garrett, W.E. (1985) Clinical use of continuous passive motion. *Contemporary Orthopaedics*, **10,** 75–79

5 Shoulder

The glenohumeral joint is a ball and socket joint surrounded by a loose capsule which inferiorly forms a wide pouch-like axillary recess. This arrangement allows the shoulder greater mobility than any other joint. The shoulder is unique in that it has an accessory joint, the subacromial joint, formed between the humerus and a superior arch made up of the acromion process and the coracoid process of the scapula joined by the stout coracoacromial ligament (Figure 5.1). This arch is lined by the synovial membrane of the subacromial bursa. In this space runs the rotator cuff, comprising the tendinous insertions of the subscapularis, supraspinatus, infraspinatus and teres minor muscles (Figure 5.2). These tendons blend intimately with the subacromial bursa and the shoulder capsule and help to provide shoulder stability (see p. 60). The muscles function in the relatively confined subacromial space where they are subject to impingement and trauma [1].

Shoulder movements occur as a combination of angular and rotational movements in all three degrees of freedom. Most functional shoulder movements take place in diagonal planes providing a complex series of movements in the glenohumeral, clavicular and the gliding scapulothoracic joints. All these joints are involved, for example, in abduction in which the arm is raised to the side of the head through a range of 180 degrees with the palm of the hand facing medially and the thumb facing posteriorly. This position of the hand is also the same as that reached on forward flexion of the arm.

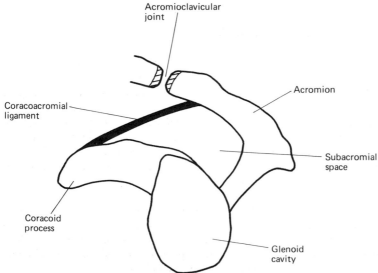

Figure 5.1 Components of the subacromial joint

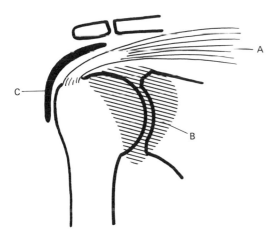

Figure 5.2 The supraspinatus muscle (A) runs through the subacromial space and its tendon is inserted into the greater tuberosity. The tendon blends with the capsule of the joint (B) and the subacromial bursa (C)

The position of the palm of the hand during abduction shows that the shoulder rotates laterally after approximately 90 degrees of abduction. This rotation is necessary to prevent impingement between the bony surfaces of the acromion and the greater tuberosity, allowing the tuberosity to slide under the more spacious posterior part of the subacromial arch. The joint capsule is voluminous and lax to accommodate lateral rotation of the head of the humerus, which amounts to almost 180 degrees.

Concomitant movements in the scapulothoracic and clavicular joints are necessary to achieve full elevation of the arm. This requires a smooth integration of all these joints which function simultaneously once movement is initiated. The scapula glides smoothly over the thoracic wall, ribs and intercostal muscles and this scapulothoracic area may be looked on as a joint. The plane of the scapula runs obliquely in an anteroposterior and mediolateral direction to form an angle of 30 degrees with the frontal plane. This is important as the position of function in abduction is also at an angle of 30 degrees, usually with the elbow flexed, e.g. when writing at a desk [2]. The proportion of glenohumeral to scapulothoracic joint movement in attaining full elevation is of the order of two to one. After 30 degrees, rotation of the scapula becomes more marked, and the scapulothoracic movement contributes approximately 60 degrees to full elevation of the arm in abduction. As the arm is abducted the scapula rotates so that its inferior angle moves laterally and the glenoid fossa now faces upwards.

Simultaneous movements take place in the clavicle which acts as a strut to prevent the scapula moving medially. The clavicle is attached to the scapula through the acromioclavicular joint and two strong ligaments, the conoid and trapezoid, which bind the outer third of the clavicle to the coracoid process of the scapula. Thirty degrees of rotation about the long axis of the clavicle can occur in each of these two clavicular joints. As the arm is abducted, the clavicle rolls upwards and backwards and the clavicular joints are elevated mainly after shoulder abduction has reached 90 degrees.

The rotator cuff acts as a functional unit, initially depressing the humeral head, stabilizing it against the glenoid fossa. Abduction of the arm is initiated by supraspinatus contraction [3] which then works in synchrony with the deltoid; external rotation with the arm abducted above 60 degrees is achieved by the infraspinatus.

The muscles of the rotator cuff provide rotation of the humerus and are also involved in stability of the glenohumeral joint. The scapular rotators, e.g. serratus anterior, coordinate scapular movement so that the rotator cuff is not impinged against the acromial arch during abduction.

For ease of description, the component movements are usually taken separately but in a normal shoulder with a full and painless range at each joint and normal musculotendinous coordination, a smooth integrated movement termed scapulohumeral rhythm is observed. A disturbance of this normal rhythm may readily be observed in patients with lesions of these structures, with an altered or 'jerky' type scapulohumeral rhythm.

Shoulder pain

Shoulder pain is a very common symptom [4]. The glenohumeral joint normally has considerable mobility and degenerative changes commonly develop in surrounding soft tissue structures. Pain may arise from intrinsic shoulder disorders or be referred from extrinsic causes such as the cervical spine or visceral structures. Shoulder pain may be referred from the neck and then may occur in one of the three clinical settings:

1 The patient may present with pain in the neck radiating to the shoulder. This usually causes no clinical confusion as neck movements reproduce the patient's pain whereas shoulder movements are normal and painless.

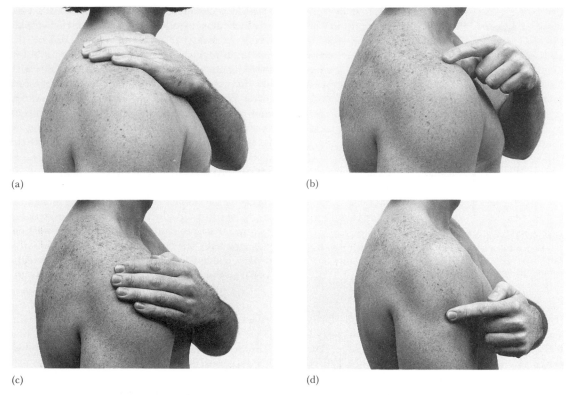

Figure 5.3 (a) Usual site of shoulder pain referred from the neck; (b) acromioclavicular pain is usually localized; (c) usual site for intrinsic shoulder disorders such as capsulitis; (d) site of referred shoulder pain in area of deltoid insertion

2   The patient may have shoulder pain alone in the absence of any neck pain. However, neck movements will reproduce pain whereas shoulder movements do not. This is often associated with a hypomobility lesion at the C4–5 or C5–6 level and on testing, these joints are restricted, feel thickened and painful. Treatment to the neck, especially mobilization techniques, should alleviate shoulder pain.

3   An uncommon, unexplained variation is shoulder pain alone, and testing shoulder movements do cause pain at the limits of range. Neck movements are either normal or produce only slight pain or restriction. Testing of the passive accessory intervertebral movements of C4–5 or C5–6 produces deep neck pain and a local restriction of movement on the same side as the painful shoulder. In this group, treatment to the neck for up to 3 days should relieve the patient's shoulder symptoms. If not, and especially if neck signs have improved, it should be abandoned and treatment confined to the shoulder.

Shoulder pain may also be the presenting symptom in visceral diseases, an important, although uncommon, cause of confusion. Visceral causes arise from intrathoracic or intra-abdominal diseases as the phrenic nerve, arising from the C3, C4, and C5 segments, also shares in the innervation of the shoulder structures. Associated symptoms such as cough, chest pain or abdominal symptoms should be sought and a full clinical examination and radiographs undertaken.

The majority of shoulder lesions involve the soft tissues, musculotendinous structures and capsule surrounding the shoulder. Although arthritis may involve the shoulder as part of a generalized disease or may even commence in the shoulder, this is relatively uncommon.

The site of pain may provide a clue to the source of the underlying lesion (Figure 5.3). The patient with shoulder pain referred from the neck often clasps his opposite hand over the trapezius area. When referred from visceral structures pain may be felt diffusely in the scapular region. In acromioclavicular joint disorders the patient usually places one finger over the upper part of this joint. Pain from intrinsic disorders of the glenohumeral joint may be felt deeply inside the joint and the patient clasps his hand over the lateral aspect or tip of the joint. Many patients indicate that the site of pain is felt around the area of the deltoid insertion and may be difficult to persuade that this is not really the source of pain. Pain felt here is referred from the shoulder and when severe may radiate down the outer side of the arm.

Other symptoms include stiffness and loss of range of movement. Instability, 'coming out', is common in athletes (see p. 60). The 'dead arm' refers to a sensation of weakness and/or paraesthesiae with sudden severe pain for seconds to minutes during sporting actions. It is diagnostic of instability. Complaints of weakness or swelling are rare.

Examination

Relevant information may be obtained from the way the shoulder moves while undressing to bare the neck, arms and scapular regions. The neck should first be examined to assess its range and whether movement is painful or reproduces shoulder pain. The whole arm is examined for evidence of any neurological or vascular abnormality, arthritis, swelling or vasomotor disturbances.

Examination of the shoulder joint

1 Inspection – observe especially:
   (a) Shape and contour of the shoulder.
   (b) Muscle wasting.
   (c) Swelling.
2 Movements.
   (a) Active.
   (b) Passive.
   (c) Locking and quadrant tests.
   (d) Accessory.
   (e) Isometric.
3 Palpation.

Inspection

The examiner should at first stand behind and then in front of the patient to compare the soft tissue contours of the shoulder, to observe any muscular

wasting over either the deltoid, or the supraspinous or infraspinous fossae of the scapula. Synovial effusion, if present in small amounts, is difficult to detect but a moderate effusion is seen to bulge anteriorly. A synovial swelling localized over the lateral aspect of the joint as a result of an effusion in the subacromial bursa is rare but there may be a combined swelling if the glenohumeral joint communicates with the subacromial bursa.

Movements

Active

The patient stands with the arms by the side in neutral rotation with the thumbs placed anteriorly. The examiner stands behind the patient and asks whether any pain is experienced in this position and, if so, to indicate its site.

Forward flexion

The arm is moved forwards to a position of 180 degrees with the palm facing inwards. Observe:

1 The range of this movement.
2 Whether the pain is reproduced.
3 Scapulohumeral rhythm.
4 Whether the affected arm can be moved as quickly as the unaffected one or is now moved more slowly because of pain.
5 Whether the patient needs to carry the arm into some degree of abduction to perform the movement.
6 If this abnormal movement is produced it should be repeated with pressure over the lateral aspect of the elbow so that the arm is now flexed forwards directly in the sagittal plane. The movement may now be restricted and reproduce pain.

Abduction

This is best tested in its position of function with the arm in the plane of the scapula with 30 degrees of horizontal flexion. The examiner stands behind the patient who is asked to raise the arm sideways to above the head. This combined glenohumeral and scapulothoracic movement should approach 180 degrees. During this movement observe:

1 The extent of this range.
2 Whether pain is provoked or reproduced.

3   The presence of an arc of pain.
4   The scapulohumeral rhythm.

Extension

The patient stands with the arm by the side and the elbow extended. The arm is carried backwards into extension and the range observed.

Medial rotation

This is tested with the arm by the side and the elbow flexed to 90 degrees. The hand is then carried inwards towards the abdomen.

Lateral rotation

This is tested with the arm by the side and the elbow flexed to 90 degrees. The hand is then carried outwards.

Horizontal flexion

This is tested by the patient stretching the arm horizontally across the body with the hand reaching posteriorly behind the opposite acromion. The elbow should easily be able to pass the chin.

Combined movements

These are useful as a screening test and to measure the progress of treatment. The hand is placed behind the back to reach upwards as far as possible. This involves mainly medial rotation but also extension and adduction. Next, abduct the shoulder, place the hand behind the neck and reach downwards as far as possible.

Passive movements

The five basic movements are again tested passively with the patient lying supine and the arm moved in the same direction as for active movements. Horizontal flexion is also tested by the examiner placing his hand over the posterior aspect of the patient's elbow joint and passively flexing the glenohumeral joint to 90 degrees. The patient's arm is then passively abducted across the chest so that his hand reaches towards the opposite shoulder (Figure 5.4).

Five findings are noted:

1   The range of each movement.
2   Whether pain is provoked or reproduced.

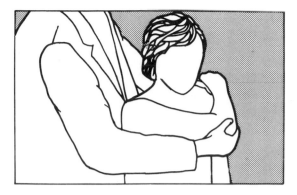

Figure 5.4 Passive horizontal flexion

3   The presence of an arc of pain.
4   Over-pressure is applied at the limit of the normal range to assess whether pain is produced and the end-feel of movement, normally felt as a springing-type sensation.
5   Compression. While compressing the head of the humerus into the glenoid cavity these movements are retested and pain response compared.

Locking and quadrant tests

Both these tests [5] refer to the position of the greater tuberosity of the humerus in relation to the acromial arch and the posterior and superior margin of the glenoid. In the locking position the greater tuberosity is caught within the subacromial space so that any further movement into lateral rotation, abduction or flexion is impossible. In this position the shoulder joint is locked. The term quadrant position is derived from the fact that the arm can normally move through an arc of 360 degrees of circumduction which requires the greater tuberosity of the humerus to move so that it does not impinge in the subacromial space. The area being tested forms one quadrant of this total 360 degrees.

These movements are usually the first lost during the early stages of many shoulder conditions. A normal painless range must be present if the glenohumeral joint is to be considered normal. Their clinical significance is in an intermittent or minor degree of shoulder pain when routine testing of shoulder movements does not reproduce pain. Examination of these two positions may then provoke or reproduce pain and demonstrate a small but significant loss of movement which may at times be the only clinical abnormality found. They are also used as the starting position for several passive movement techniques.

Starting position

The patient lies supine and the examiner stands by the side with his forearm placed medial to the patient's scapula and the fingers extended over the trapezius to prevent shoulder shrugging. With his other hand he first flexes the elbow and places the shoulder in a slight degree of medial rotation and extension.

METHOD

The arm is moved from alongside the patient's side into abduction and towards a position of full flexion. It is moved until the humerus reaches a position where it becomes locked and further movement is impossible (Figure 5.5).

SIGNIFICANCE

The normal shoulder can easily be placed in this locking position without pain. In some shoulder abnormalities this position may not be attainable because of pain or stiffness.

Quadrant position

This small arc of movement may be felt by the examiner as the arm is released from the locking position and is taken towards full flexion [5].

METHOD

The shoulder is placed in the locking position. The arm is then carried towards full flexion by first relaxing the pressure on the abducted and extended arm so that it can be moved slightly anteriorly from the coronal plane. Lateral rotation of the shoulder can then take place as the movement into abduction continues. The small arc of movement that can be felt during this anterior and rotational movement is known as the quadrant position, felt at approximately 30 degrees lateral to the fully flexed position when the arm moves anteriorly from the locked position. The humeral head is now unlocked and the arm can continue its normal movement into full flexion (Figure 5.6).

The following observations are made in the quadrant position: the site and degree of pain and then with over-pressure; the range of this movement in the sagittal plane between the humerus and the plane of the scapula; and the degree of prominence of the head of the humerus in the axilla.

Accessory movements

There are five accessory movements in the shoulder:

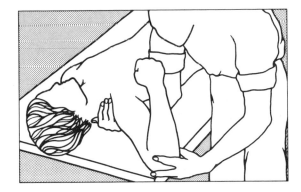

Figure 5.5 Locking position

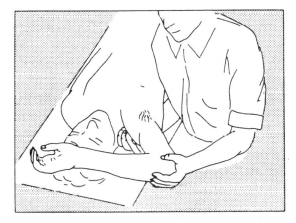

Figure 5.6 Quadrant position

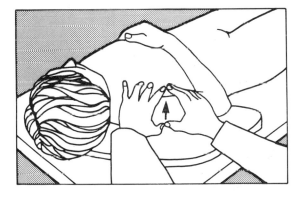

Figure 5.7 Posteroanterior accessory movement

1 Posteroanterior movement produced by pressure on the posterior surface of the humeral head (Figure 5.7).
2 Anteroposterior movement produced by the palm of the hand over the anterior surface of the humeral head (Figure 5.8).

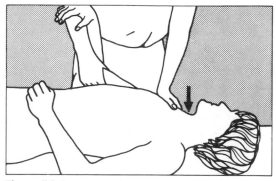

Figure 5.8 Anteroposterior accessory movement

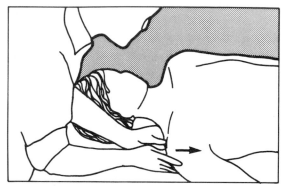

Figure 5.9 Longitudinal caudad accessory movement

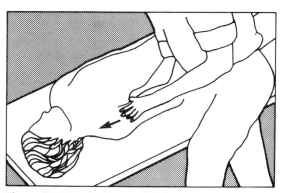

Figure 5.10 Longitudinal cephalad accessory movement

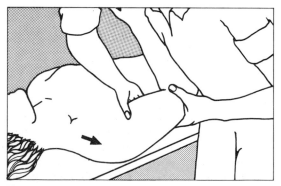

Figure 5.11 Lateral accessory movement

3 Longitudinal caudad movement produced by pressure over the head of the humerus (Figure 5.9) or by a longitudinal pull on the arm.
4 Longitudinal cephalad movement produced by compression upwards of the humerus (Figure 5.10).
5 Lateral movement produced by movement of the humeral head away from the glenoid cavity (Figure 5.11).

It is also necessary to test these accessory movements in other positions of the glenohumeral joint, e.g. at 90 degrees of abduction or at the limit of any range.

Isometric tests

Four isometric tests are assessed routinely: abduction, medial rotation, lateral rotation and flexion. The examiner notes the strength of these movements and whether they reproduce pain, while carefully palpating the tendon being tested with his other hand.

Resisted abduction

This tests primarily the supraspinatus tendon.

STARTING POSITION
The patient sits with the glenohumeral joint abducted to 30 degrees, the elbow flexed to 90 degrees and one hand is placed on the lateral side of the elbow. The tendon should be tested in varying positions and degrees of abduction. The best of these is with the shoulder abducted to 90 degrees then placed in 30 degrees of forward flexion with the palm facing the floor (the empty beer can sign) (Figure 5.12).

METHOD
The tendon should be tested in varying positions and degrees of abduction. The best of these is with the shoulder abducted to 90 degrees then placed in 30 degrees of forward flexion with the palm facing the floor (the empty beer can sign). The patient's attempt to move the arm outwards into abduction is fully resisted while the tendon is palpated over its insertion into the greater tuberosity.

Resisted medial rotation

This tests primarily the subscapularis tendon.

STARTING POSITION
The patient stands with the upper arm by the side, the elbow flexed to 90 degrees and held firmly by the

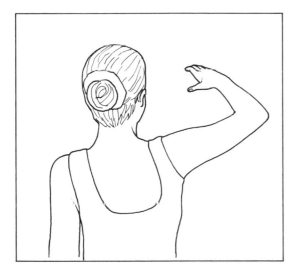
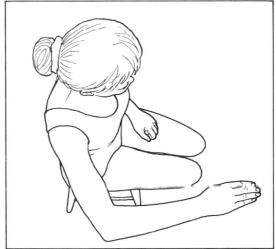
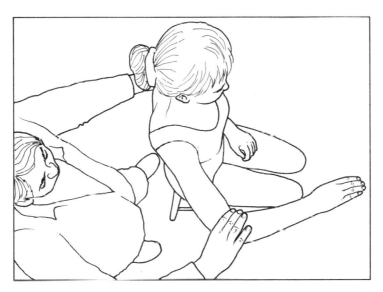

Figure 5.12 Testing for supraspinatus tendinitis: the 'empty beer can sign'

side with the palm of the hand facing inwards. The examiner stands in front with his palm over the palmar surface of the patient's wrist.

METHOD

The patient's attempt to move the forearm medially is fully resisted while the subscapularis tendon is palpated over its insertion into the lesser tuberosity.

Resisted lateral rotation

This tests primarily the infraspinatus tendon.

STARTING POSITION

The patient stands with the shoulder abducted to 90 degrees and the elbow flexed to 90 degrees.

METHOD

The shoulder is then fully medially rotated so that the palm of the hand faces backwards. The examiner places the palm of his hand over the dorsum of the wrist (Figure 5.13) and fully resists the attempt to bring the hand forward, this laterally rotating the shoulder.

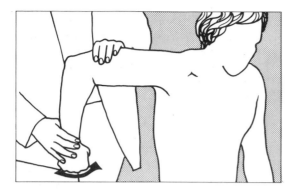

Figure 5.13 Resisted lateral rotation

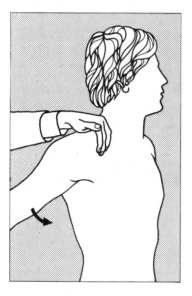

Figure 5.14 Palpation of the biceps tendon. The shoulder is extended and the examiner simultaneously resists forward flexion of the shoulder

Forward flexion

This tests primarily the biceps tendon (Figure 5.14).

STARTING POSITION
The patient stands with the shoulder fully extended to stretch the tendon; the elbow is fully extended with the forearm pronated so that the hand faces backwards. Place the hand over the dorsum of the patient's wrist.

METHOD
The attempt to move the arm forwards is fully resisted by the examiner, who palpates the biceps tendon in its groove.

Additional tests of the biceps may be carried out by making use of its action of flexing the elbow and supinating the forearm (see p. 54).

Palpation

Many of the bony landmarks and the soft tissue structures around the shoulder can be readily palpated. The scapula is subcutaneous and ends laterally in the broad rectangular-shaped acromion process. This process articulates with the clavicle, also subcutaneous, at the acromioclavicular joint that is easily palpated just lateral to the enlarged outer end of the clavicle. By palpating two finger-breadths medially and two finger-breadths caudally from this joint the bony outline of the coracoid process may be felt. The anterior part of the glenohumeral capsule lies just lateral to this process and overlies the joint line.

A finger-breadth distal to the lateral border of the acromion lies the greater tuberosity of the humerus with the tendinous insertions of the rotator cuff. Two finger-breadths medial to the anterior aspect of the greater tuberosity lies the tendon of the long head of the biceps in the bicipital groove, easily felt to move as the shoulder is abducted to 90 degrees and then rotated medially and laterally. Just medial to the biceps tendon lies the lesser tuberosity of the humerus and its attached subscapularis tendon.

Palpation is used to confirm the presence of any crepitus, heat, swelling or tenderness. Soft tissue crepitus may be palpable in patients with rotator cuff degeneration and a bony crepitus with osteoarthritis. Both shoulders should be palpated for heat and synovial swelling. The supraspinatus tendon insertion is palpated easily by standing behind the patient and placing two fingers of one hand over the greater tuberosity (Figure 5.15) and passively rotating the arm medially and laterally with the other hand, while also applying distraction. The normal tendon insertion can be felt to move as a firm cord. This area should be palpated carefully for an area of tenderness and at times a gap may be felt if the tendon has been ruptured.

The infraspinatus tendon is best palpated while the patient's arms is held with the glenohumeral joint at 90 degrees of forward flexion and the elbow also flexed to 90 degrees. Two fingers are then placed over the posterior aspect of the joint just below the acromion and behind the posterior border

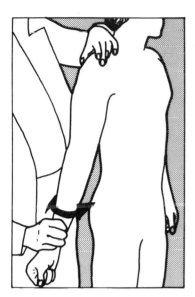

Figure 5.15 Palpation of the supraspinatus tendon

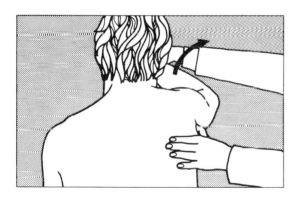

Figure 5.16 Palpating the infraspinatus tendon. The shoulder is in medial rotation

of the deltoid. The arm is then passively rotated medially and laterally while palpating deeply over the humeral head for tenderness (Figure 5.16).

The tendinous insertion of the subscapularis is palpated over the lesser tuberosity just medial to the tendon of the long head of biceps with the arm held in about 20 degrees of extension. The long head of the biceps is easily palpated in its groove. The gleno-humeral joint is firstly abducted to 90 degrees with

the elbow held flexed also at 90 degrees. The examiner places two fingers over the bicipital groove while the patient's arm is medially and laterally rotated and palpated for the presence of any tenderness (Figure 5.14).

Patterns of movement

Clinical examination of the shoulder usually allows the anatomical site of the underlying lesion to be localized. By the use of active, passive and isometric tests, certain patterns of shoulder movements can be built up. Three distinct patterns are usually differentiated:

1. Pain on active and passive movement, usually with restriction of shoulder movement in each plane, which may be of sudden or gradual onset. A sudden onset of severe shoulder pain and restriction of movement in each plane is usually caused by an acute calcific bursitis. A more gradual onset of pain and restriction of movement in each plane may be due to either a capsulitis or arthritis of the shoulder. Radiographs help to differentiate between these two conditions.
2. Pain may be present on movement in only one of the planes tested, usually both on active and on passive movements. It may also be associated with a painful weakness or restriction on isometric testing of the movement. This pattern is produced by a tendon lesion.
3. A painless weakness of movement in one plane only may result from either a rupture of the musculotendinous insertion or a neurological lesion, e.g. a painless weakness of shoulder abduction usually indicates a complete rupture of the supraspinatus tendon. Less commonly, a C5 nerve root palsy with paralysis of shoulder muscles may be present.

By the systematic use of clinical methods an accurate clinical diagnosis should be possible in most patients [6]. There does remain, however, a small percentage of patients in whom a definitive diagnosis cannot be readily made. This includes patients in whom signs are equivocal and difficult to detect or a prolonged period of observation with repeated testing is necessary and in some patients there may be shoulder pain without obvious clinical signs. Additional information is then obtained with ancillary methods [7], such as radiography and special views, arthrography, radionuclide scans, CT scans, especially combined with arthrography, ultrasound, MRI and arthroscopy.

Classification of shoulder lesions

1 Impingement syndromes.
2 Tendon lesions.
   (a) Rotator cuff tendons
      (i) Tendinitis.
      (ii) Incomplete rupture.
      (iii) Complete rupture.
      (iv) Calcification.
   (b) Biceps tendon.
      (i) Tendinitis.
      (ii) Tenosynovitis.
      (iii) Subluxation.
      (iv) Rupture.
3 Bursitis.
   (a) Subacromial bursitis.
      (i) Chronic bursitis.
      (ii) Acute calcific bursitis.
   (b) Subcoracoid bursitis.
4 Capsulitis.
5 Instability of the shoulder joint.
6 The shoulder–hand syndrome.
7 Entrapment neuropathies.

Impingement syndromes

Impingement of the soft tissues in the subacromial space with loss of their normal gliding mechanism is a common, important cause of shoulder pain [8–10]. Because the functional range of shoulder movement is in the anterior plane, anterior structures such as the supraspinatus, subacromial bursa and the biceps tendon may be entrapped between the humeral head below and by the anterior acromion, coracoacromial ligament or the acromioclavicular joint above. The most common causes are a prominent anterior acromion [6] or bony spurs from under the acromion [11], or arising from the acromioclavicular joint [12]. The tuberosity impinges mainly anteriorly under the acromion during forward flexion. In no other part of the body are tendons so entrapped between two bones.

Impingement may occur at any age, in young athletes or weekend sportspeople whose activity involves repeated overhead actions such as

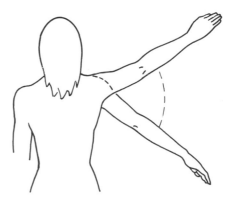

Figure 5.17 Painful arc on abduction

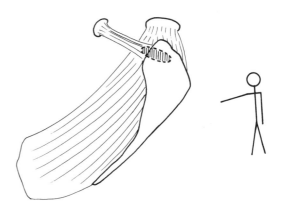

Figure 5.18 Critical zone impinging in the subacromial space on abduction

swimming, throwing or tennis [12–14], or in more elderly people working with their arm repeatedly in a horizontal position during abduction and elevation.

Impingement first results in oedema and inflammatory changes in the supraspinatus tendon [2,15], followed later by cuff degeneration, weakness and ultimately rupture [16]. The biceps tendon may also be involved [17]. Pain on shoulder movements and at times stiffness or weakness are the major symptoms.

The painful arc refers to impingement of the supraspinatus felt in the middle range of abduction (Figure 5.17). As the greater tuberosity approaches the acromion, structures between these two bony prominences are impinged on, producing pain (Figure 5.18). As the arm is raised further the painful tissues are accommodated and pain ceases. A painless range of movement occurs up to approximately 70–80 degrees of abduction, followed by an arc of pain to approximately 120 degrees, after which movement becomes painless. Pain may be felt on active or passive abduction, or as the arm is raised or lowered. This is often best observed while lowering the arm and a sudden hitch in the movement is produced.

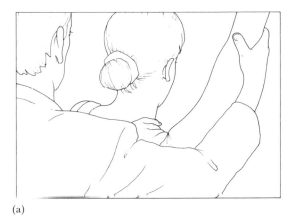

(a)

Examination

The patient may have evidence of wasting of the supraspinatus or infraspinatus fossae. A full range of active shoulder movement is usually present but a sharp arc of pain is experienced in forward elevation or abduction and at times during rotation.

Impingement signs

1 The patient is seated and the examiner holds the patient's scapula down with one hand. The patient's arm is fully passively flexed which brings the greater tuberosity around to impinge under the acromion and so reproduce pain (Figure 5.19).
2 The arm is put into forward elevation of 90 degrees and the elbow is then flexed to 90 degrees. The shoulder is then put into a maximal internal rotation until pain is reproduced (Figure 5.20).

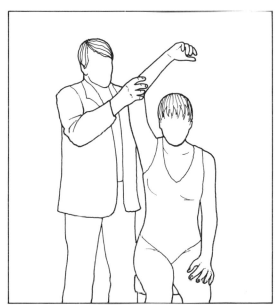

(b)

Figure 5.19 Testing for impingement. The arm is fully flexed while the scapula is held down

Management

Prophylaxis requires a proper knowledge of biomechanics [2]. Some people, especially those using their arms above shoulder level [12,18], as in throwing sports, are at greater risk because of the repetitive, strenuous nature of their sporting activity. Attention must be paid to flexibility, stretching and strengthening exercises and warm-up procedures.

Early or mild cases may respond to conservative therapy [19–21] including:

1 Rest from activities known to aggravate pain, especially swimming or serving at tennis, with the arm in abduction and external rotation.

2 Non-steroidal anti-inflammatory agents are used to control inflammation and pain.
3 Infiltration of 2–3 ml of local anaesthetic and 1 ml of corticosteroid into the subacromial space may be expected to control the inflammatory component even though they do not alter anatomical changes. A lateral approach is used with a 23-gauge needle inserted under the lateral surface of the acromion into the bursa. It may be repeated at monthly intervals for three to four injections.

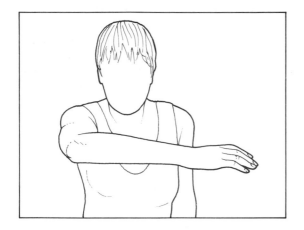

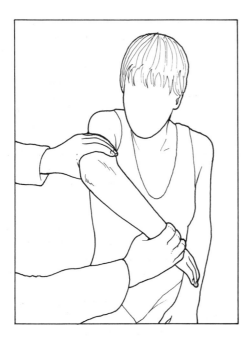

Figure 5.20 Testing for impingement. Pain is also reproduced on resisting external rotation

4   Physical therapy including ice, heat and ultrasound is used to ease pain.
5   Mobilization techniques are used to restore the passive range of motion and restore normal scapulohumeral rhythm. This must be followed by stretching, especially of the posterior capsule, and strengthening exercises done in a pain-free range.

Surgery

Considerations for surgery include age, severity and duration of pain, type of activity and future aspirations and response to conservative therapy. The main goal of surgical decompression is pain relief and improved function may be secondary [2]. Surgery is indicated in patients with chronic or recurrent pain, cuff tears or biceps tendon involvement [22]. An anterior acromioplasty with removal of osteophytes, the coracoacromial ligament and acromioclavicular joint osteophytes may be performed either by open or preferably arthroscopic surgery [14,23–26].

The return to sport needs to be gradual and carefully supervised with special attention to technique and training methods.

Lesions of the supraspinatus tendon

Symptoms may arise from: (1) supraspinatus tendinitis, (2) subacromial bursitis, (3) incomplete rupture of the tendon, (4) complete rupture of the tendon, and (5) calcification.

Supraspinatus tendinitis

This common cause of shoulder pain usually follows impingement or overuse involving a degenerated supraspinatus tendon. Degeneration may follow wear and tear with friction and attrition of the tendon in the subacromial space with hyaline degeneration of the tendon collagen fibres [27].

Peculiarities in the microvascular supply, an area of relative avascularity in the tendon just proximal to its insertion, also play a role even in young people. This 'critical zone' (Figure 5.21) is the site at which degenerative changes, tendinitis, calcification and spontaneous rupture tend to occur. Vascular compression occurs with the arm by the side, so stretching the tendon over the head of the humerus. Pain is usually felt over the outer aspect of the shoulder but may radiate to the region of the deltoid insertion or may be felt in this site only. It may disturb sleep.

Major signs

Pain is reproduced on active and/or passive abduction of the shoulder, usually felt as an arc of pain in the midrange of movement. When the patient brings the arm down from full abduction to the side, pain is again usually felt in this range of the arc owing to

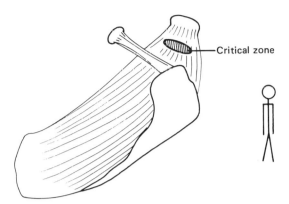

Figure 5.21 The supraspinatus tendon viewed from above, with arm by the side

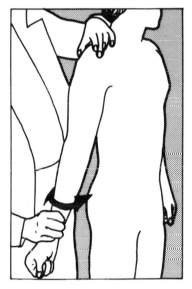

Figure 5.22 Palpation of the supraspinatus tendon

the same mechanism. At this point a characteristic sign may be present in which the patient suddenly allows his shoulder to drop past this painful spot. Pain may also be reproduced on isometric contraction of the supraspinatus muscle.

Confirmatory signs

A disturbance of the scapulohumeral rhythm may be evident during abduction. The supraspinatus tendon may be palpated easily as a tender cord between the examiner's finger and the greater tuberosity while the shoulder is depressed by applying traction to the arm and then laterally and medially rotating the shoulder (Figure 5.22).

Radiographs of the shoulder are usually normal but degenerative changes may lead to an area of sclerosis or pitting on the greater tuberosity. Other investigations [28,29] include ultrasound [30–38], arthrography [30,39], CT arthrography [40–42] or CT arthrotomography [43], MRI [10,16,30,44–49] and arthroscopy [25,41,50–55].

Management

1 The natural history of this condition is one of exacerbations and remissions over the years. Rest from movements known to aggravate pain is usually required.
2 Non-steroidal anti-inflammatory drugs are used to control inflammation and relieve pain [56].
3 Local infiltration of corticosteroids around the tendon may be expected to control the inflammatory component, even though they have no effect on any underlying degenerative changes. The tendon can be palpated by passively rotating the arm medially and laterally. A 23-gauge needle is inserted under the lateral surface of the acromion along the line of the tendon to lie under the acromion; 1 ml of corticosteroid with 2–3 ml of local anaesthetic are injected. The injection may be repeated several times at intervals up to 4 weeks, depending on the degree of improvement.
4 Physical therapy [21], ice or ultrasound applied directly over the site of local tenderness can produce an improvement in symptoms. Exercise into the painful range of movements is contraindicated.
5 Three passive movement techniques may be used.
   (a) Uses accessory movements of the head of the humerus, especially posteroanterior movement (Figure 5.7).
   (b) Is a movement of the head of the humerus away from and then towards the undersurface of the acromion process (Figure 5.11).
   (c) The quadrant position may be used; the technique is performed as very small range movements carried into some degree of discomfort for 1 min.
6 With conservative therapy, symptoms gradually improve but may recur when the patient returns to activity. With chronic disability or frequent recurrences, various surgical procedures have been advocated whose main aim is to increase the subacromial space and prevent impingement. This may include removal of the anterior

acromion, division of the coracoacromial ligament and excision arthroplasty of the acromioclavicular joint.

Chronic subacromial bursitis

Chronic subacromial bursitis is usually associated with an underlying supraspinatus tendinitis. The supraspinatus tendon forms the major part of the floor of the bursa, and the tendon and bursa work together as a functional unit in the subacromial space.

Incomplete rupture of the supraspinatus tendon

The degenerated tendon is easily torn [57,58], causing a partial rupture either on its superior or inferior aspect [50,58]. It is much more common in the elderly but may also occur as an acute injury in younger people, such as labourers or sportspeople, and may go on to become a full thickness tear [59]. The clinical findings are usually indistinguishable from those of supraspinatus tendinitis, as the same symptoms, signs and investigations are common to both. Further investigations are described above (p. 49).

Management

This is also similar to that of supraspinatus tendinitis. Local corticosteroid injections help in relieving pain. Surgery is not indicated in the elderly. In younger athletes it should be considered, for the tear is liable to produce chronic disability. The impingement is decompressed and direct closure with excision of any degenerative areas of tendon is usually possible [3,31,60,61]. Early post-operative movement is essential.

Complete rupture

A complete rupture may be acute or chronic [60,62,63] and may occur in elderly patients with a history of previous supraspinatus tendinitis [60]. In athletes the onset may be spontaneous but usually follows injury. The site of rupture is usually through the 'critical zone' of the tendon [88] (Figure 5.21), although occasionally the tendon may be avulsed from its insertion. The patient may be conscious of having heard or felt a sudden painful 'snap' in the shoulder. Pain remains for some time afterwards

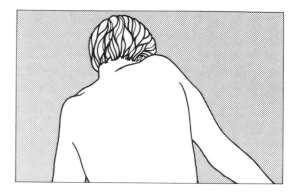

Figure 5.23 Complete rupture of the supraspinatus tendon – active movement

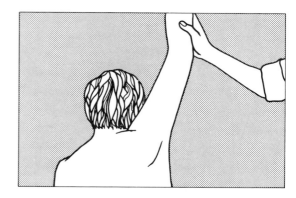

Figure 5.24 Complete rupture of the supraspinatus tendon – passive movement

then usually eases gradually with loss of strength and mobility in the shoulder. It may be associated with a haemarthrosis [65].

Major signs

There is a marked disparity between the active, passive and isometric tests. Active range of shoulder abduction is lost so that the shoulder can be abducted to only approximately 20 degrees. This movement is accompanied by a considerable degree of scapular movement and an upwards shrugging of the shoulder (Figure 5.23). This movement may be produced by the action of the deltoid, acting without the stabilizing effect of the supraspinatus, which results in elevation of the shoulder. It may also be due to the serratus anterior muscle, which rotates the scapula and produces an abduction movement of 20 degrees at the glenohumeral joint. The shoulder can be fully passively abducted by the examiner

(Figure 5.24). On isometric tests a marked painless weakness of abduction is found.

Confirmatory signs

The humeral head appears prominent as it can ride upwards. A gap in the tendon may be felt by palpation between the acromion and the greater tuberosity. After some time, atrophy of the muscle can be observed in the supraspinous fossa.

Investigations

Plain radiographs of the shoulder are usually normal unless the tendon has been avulsed with a small fragment of bone. Double contrast arthrography or ultrasound demonstrates the rupture, which allows a communication between the glenohumeral joint and the subacromial bursa [28,32,66] (Figure 5.25).

Management

Surgery is considered if pain is a problem [67,68] but should be undertaken within 6–12 weeks of the injury. However, in most cases, diagnosis is delayed [69]. In younger athletes a decompression operation is performed and direct repair is attempted [3,17]. If this is not possible, part of the biceps tendon may be used as a graft [70]. In the elderly, pain usually settles with conservative treatment and, although the physical signs do not alter, the resultant functional disability may not be sufficient to warrant surgery.

Late complications: cuff arthropathy

The supraspinatus is responsible for the superior stabilization of the glenohumeral joint and when its integrity is lost the humeral head can sublux upwards [71]. The greater tuberosity of the humerus becomes attenuated as it loses the traction from the supraspinatus tendon. In time, degenerative changes may be found in the glenohumeral joint itself and there is erosion and a thinning out of the lower surface of the acromion with osteophyte formation (Figure 5.26). Degenerative changes may also develop in the acromioclavicular joint.

Calcification

Calcification develops in the area of degenerated tendon just proximal to the tendon insertion in approximately 8% of routine shoulder radiographs

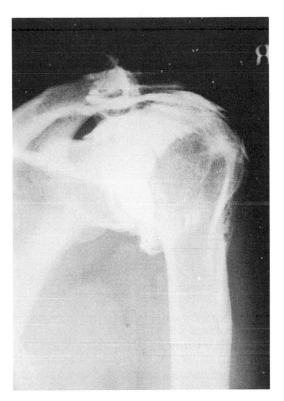

Figure 5.25 Arthrogram to show a ruptured cuff with contrast present outside the glenohumeral joint. Dye is also present in the acromial joint ('Geyser sign')

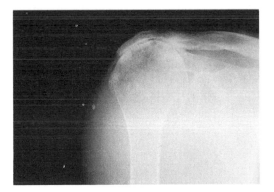

Figure 5.26 Cuff arthropathy follows loss of the supraspinatus tendon

(Figure 5.27). The calcific deposits are usually firm and granular, single or multiple, about 10 mm in size, but may at times have a linear appearance spreading along the tendon and may be bilateral. Similar calcific deposits may also be found in the trochanteric bursa.

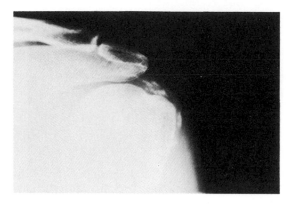

Figure 5.27 Calcification in the supraspinatus tendon and subacromial bursa

Calcification may:

1 Be asymptomatic and a chance radiographic finding only.
2 Be associated with supraspinatus tendinitis. The signs are identical with those of uncomplicated tendinitis, as described above.
3 Be of a sufficient size to produce a mechanical block to full shoulder abduction, as the calcified mass impinges beneath the acromion.
4 Produce an acute calcific bursitis, one of the most painful and dramatic events in clinical practice. It is relatively common and may occur in the younger more active age group. It follows a calcific tendinitis with rupture of microcrystals of calcium hydroxyapatite into the subacromial bursa, producing an acute inflammatory crystal synovitis. There is no adequate explanation for this sudden rupture, as the calcific deposits may have been present in the tendon for some years.

Patients present with intense, sudden onset of shoulder pain, often radiating down the upper arm and rapidly becoming worse. Pain is made worse by any shoulder movement and disturbs sleep. Patients are unable to use their arm owing to a painful limitation of shoulder movements in all directions, and the arm usually needs to be supported in a sling. Indeed, it is virtually impossible to attempt to examine these movements but some swelling may be obvious over the lateral aspect of the joint, which is exquisitely tender and warm on palpation.

Radiographs confirm the presence of the calcific deposits, which may still be present as a granular deposit but are more commonly seen as a hazy,

poorly defined appearance within the bursa. The size of the calcific deposits does not usually bear any direct relationship to the acuteness or severity of the attack and at times only small deposits are visible. Enlargement of the soft tissue shadow of the subacromial bursa and displacement downwards of the humeral head may also be evident. A radiograph taken after the condition has resolved often shows that the calcific deposit has disappeared. If so, it may reaccumulate over several years so that another acute attack may occur.

Management of calcific bursitis

Rest to the shoulder is essential and a sling needs to be worn for several days. Anti-inflammatory drugs must be given in a relatively high dosage to control the intense crystal synovitis. Indomethacin, up to 200 mg per day for 2 or 3 days, is used until the intense pain begins to settle and the dose gradually reduced. Analgesics are also needed to control pain and ensure sleep. Heat, exercises or massage are contraindicated, but ice applied locally to the shoulder region may provide some pain relief. Local anaesthetic and corticosteroid may be injected directly into the subacromial bursa. Although this may be painful at the time, the patient is usually most grateful for the relief obtained. Alternatively, two 19-gauge needles may be inserted into the calcific mass using a lateral approach after first anaesthetizing the skin. An injection of 10 ml of local anaesthetic is given rapidly into one needle and the calcific deposit, which resembles gritty tooth-paste, may be extruded through the other needle.

With conservative treatment most cases resolve over 4 or 5 days. Subsequent radiographs usually show that the calcific deposit has disappeared. Surgery to curette the calcific mass may be indicated if the acute bursitis does not resolve rapidly. At operation, an inflamed bursa is found with a granular deposit of calcific material bulging into it.

Infraspinatus tendinitis

This is not as common as supraspinatus tendinitis and pain is associated with underlying degenerative changes, usually after overuse of the shoulder. It occurs most commonly in labourers and in sports such as swimming or tennis. The site of the lesion may be over its insertion or at its musculotendinous junction. The patient usually presents with pain over the posterior aspect of the shoulder, made worse by most shoulder movements, and, when severe, the

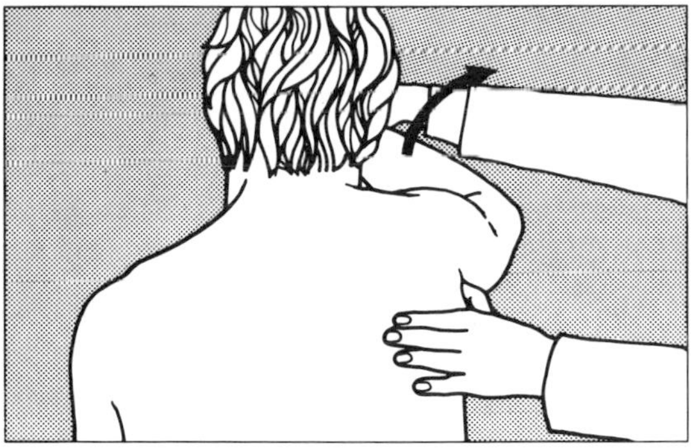

Figure 5.28 Palpating the infraspinatus tendon. The shoulder is in medial rotation

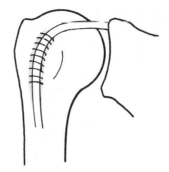

Figure 5.29 Long head of the biceps running in the bicipital groove

pain may radiate down the posterior aspect of the upper arm.

Major signs

The patient's pain may be reproduced by either contracting or stretching the infraspinatus tendon. Isometric contractions of the tendon are tested by the examiner fully resisting lateral rotation of the shoulder (Figure 5.13) and a painful weakness of this movement may be demonstrated.

Confirmatory signs

The arc of pain in the middle range of abduction may be felt as the tendon impinges under the acromion. The tendon may be palpated by placing the shoulder at 90 degrees of forward flexion with the elbow at 90 degrees of flexion and rotating the arm medially and laterally (Figure 5.28). Tenderness may be felt either at the tendon insertion or at the musculotendinous junction. In patients with a lesion at the musculotendinous junction, a tender area of thickening may be palpable at this site.

Management

This is similar to that outlined for supraspinatus tendinitis.

Injection of the infraspinatus tendon

The patient sits with the arm held across the lower chest to bring the posterior portion of the greater tuberosity into prominence and stretch the tendon. The insertion is palpated deep to the deltoid a finger-breadth lateral to the posterolateral border of

the acromion. A 23-gauge needle is used, directed under the lateral surface of the acromion, and the area around the tendon is injected with 1 ml of corticosteroid solution and 2–3 ml of local anaesthetic.

Complete rupture of this tendon usually occurs suddenly and the patient complains of pain over the posterior aspect of the shoulder. Clinical findings reveal a marked disparity between active, passive and resisted movements. The normal range of active lateral rotation of the shoulder is lost but the passive range remains full. Testing the resisted movement by isometric contraction reveals a painless weakness of lateral rotation. After a time, wasting of this muscle in the infraspinous fossa of the scapula becomes evident.

Bicipital tendinitis

The biceps tendon in the bicipital groove is the second most common cause of shoulder tendinitis (Figure 5.29). The tendon takes part in all shoulder movements and is subjected to degenerative processes of wear and tear and attrition [70,72]. The tendon may be impinged against the acromial arch during many of the functional patterns of shoulder movements [17] and tendinitis usually occurs after overuse. It may also be associated with tenosynovitis of its investing synovial sheath which will produce the same symptoms and signs as tendinitis, and is usually chronic and recurrent. An avulsion of its attachment to the labrum of the superior glenoid may occur in association with labral damage – the SLAP lesion.

Symptoms

Pain in the shoulder is usually well localized anteriorly over the joint but may radiate down the arm.

Pain may be produced on shoulder movement especially when the arm is abducted with the shoulder laterally rotated as in the action of throwing a ball or in overarm swimming. Other signs of impingement should be looked for.

Major signs

Pain is produced by stretching or contracting the biceps tendon. Stretching the tendon is usually best achieved by having the patient stand with the elbow extended and the forearm pronated so that the hand faces backwards and the examiner fully passively extends the shoulder. Pain may be produced by this manoeuvre or by actively resisting the patient's attempt to move the arm into forward flexion. The bicipital groove is palpated with the other hand (Figure 5.14).

Confirmatory signs

Two isometric tests rely on the action of the biceps which flexes the elbow and supinates the forearm. In the first, the examiner resists active flexion of the elbow while the patient stands with the elbow at 90 degrees and the forearm supinated. In the second, the patient stands with the elbow flexed to 90 degrees and the forearm in the midposition while the examiner resists active supination of the forearm (Yergason's sign).

The tendon may also be stretched by abducting the arm to 60 degrees with the elbow flexed at a right angle and then passively rotating the shoulder laterally. Pain may be reproduced at the extreme of this movement.

The biceps tendon can be palpated in most patients with the patient's arm abducted to approximately 90 degrees and the elbow flexed to 90 degrees (Figure 5.30a). The shoulder is then medially and laterally rotated while palpating the tendon with the other hand (Figure 5.30b). The tendon may be felt to roll under the fingers as a tender cord-like structure in the bicipital groove. Radiographs of the shoulder are usually normal [73], but ultrasound gives good definition [37].

Management

The general management is basically similar to that of supraspinatus tendinitis and includes the use of rest, anti-inflammatories, ice and passive movements.

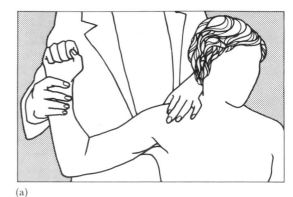

(a)

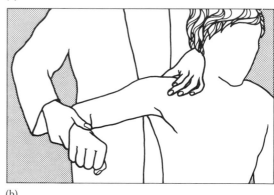

(b)

Figure 5.30 Palpation of the biceps tendon while rotating the shoulder

Injections

The site of maximal tenderness should be found (Figure 5.30) as the patient sits with the arm hanging loosely by the side. A 23-gauge needle is inserted at the proximal end of the bicipital groove above the tender area and is then slid down the groove until the tender area is reached. Then 1 ml of corticosteroid solution and 2 ml of local anaesthetic are injected around and not into the tendon.

Surgery

If symptoms persist or are recurrent, tenodesis and decompression may be performed [70,74].

Rupture of the biceps tendon

Rupture of the long head of the biceps tendon in its groove, usually in male patients, middle-aged or older with a history of bicipital tendinitis, is not uncommon. The rupture may occur spontaneously or follow lifting or a fall on the outstretched hand. The patient is usually conscious of a sudden tearing or snapping in the shoulder. The shoulder may be painful or difficult to move and bruising may appear over the upper arm after some days. Pain usually settles over a short period of time. There is little weakness or functional disability as the short head of the biceps remains intact. The distal belly of the biceps muscle rolls up to appear as a lump in the anterior part of the upper arm which may be seen to bulge when the muscle is made to contract, as by bringing the hand up to the mouth or by resisting flexion of the elbow (Figure 5.31). The gap in the tendon is easily seen and felt over the bicipital groove. In young sportsmen surgery may be warranted but in older patients with little functional incapacity surgery is not indicated [75].

Subluxation of the biceps tendon

The long head of the biceps may sublux out of its groove. This usually follows trauma and the patient feels a sudden painful click especially on rotation. It needs to be differentiated from the much more common subluxation of the shoulder joint itself. Treatment is surgical [70,73,76,77].

Subscapularis tendinitis

This condition is uncommon. The patient presents with pain in the front of the shoulder, usually after an overuse injury that involves excessive internal rotation of the shoulder.

Pain should be reproduced on isometric contraction of the subscapularis muscle by fully resisting medial rotation of the patient's arm. Tenderness is found in a localized area medial to the lesser tuberosity of the humerus. Radiographs are usually normal but calcification, if present, may only be evident on an axial view. Patients usually respond readily to local corticosteroid injection.

Bursitis

Subacromial bursitis

A diagnosis of subacromial bursitis is commonly made but it is rarely a primary disorder and is secondary to impingement and lesions in the rotator cuff. The patient experiences a painful arc in the

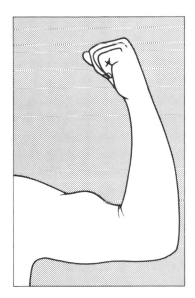

Figure 5.31 Ruptured long head of biceps

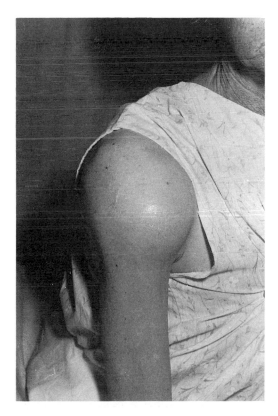

Figure 5.32 Combined shoulder joint and subacromial bursa effusion

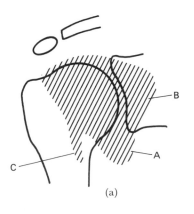

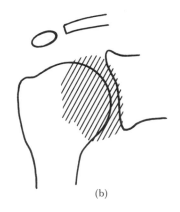

(a)

(b)

Figure 5.33 Outlines of arthrograms. (a) Shows (A) the axillary recess, normally the joint can be injected with 20–30 ml of contrast medium, (B) the subcapsularis recess, and (C) extension around the biceps tendon; (b) capsulitis of the shoulder, only 5–10 ml can be injected with greater force, and the normal capsular recesses, especially the axillary recess, is lost

mid-range of active and passive shoulder abduction. Resisted abduction should not reproduce pain, which should distinguish it from supraspinatus tendinitis (Figure 5.32).

Chronic subacromial bursitis is usually associated with supraspinatus tendinitis and its management is similar. The bursa is injected with the patient sitting with the arm hanging loosely by his side. The posterolateral angle of the acromion is identified and a 23-gauge needle is slid under it in an anterior direction to lie free in the subacromial space. Then 1 ml of local corticosteroid and 3 ml of 1% local anaesthetic are injected easily.

Subcoracoid bursitis

This rare condition may follow impingement [78,79] and overuse with repeated shoulder medial rotation as in table-tennis players or truck drivers. Pain is usually well localized over the anterior aspect of the shoulder, just distal to the coracoid process of the scapula. Pain may be reproduced on lateral rotation of the shoulder at the extreme of range or on passive horizontal flexion of the arm across the chest. Resisted movements are usually painless. Tenderness is well localized to just below the tip of the coracoid process. Injection of corticosteroid into this area usually produces marked relief of symptoms.

Capsulitis

Capsulitis is an inflammatory lesion of the glenohumeral joint capsule that leads to thickening and contraction with consequent loss of joint volume [80]. Clinically it results in a painful stiffness of the active and passive range of all shoulder movements. The unfortunate term 'frozen shoulder' is a glib medical malapropism, an anachronism that has led to considerable confusion about the nature and management of this condition.

It may involve one shoulder, then, after a variable time, involve the other shoulder in approximately 10% of cases, or rarely may commence in both shoulders simultaneously. Once an attack has resolved, second attacks in the same shoulder are quite rare.

The pathology is an inflammatory synovitis that progresses to thickening and retraction of the capsule [81]. Radiographs are essentially normal but may show osteoporosis or small cystic inclusions and are necessary to differentiate it from osteoarthritis which may have similar clinical findings. Arthrography (Figure 5.33) or arthroscopy are definitive ancillary investigations.

It occurs most commonly in middle-aged females and its aetiology is unknown [82]. No theory has been proposed for its relative frequency in the shoulder joint, whereas it is most rare in other joints. It is not associated with an increased incidence after middle age so that degenerative changes in the capsule seem most unlikely. Capsulitis rarely complicates existing shoulder lesions such as supraspinatus tendinitis and is quite a different condition to them [75]. Other theories have ascribed capsulitis to adhesion in the subacromial bursa, the biceps tendon or joint surfaces but these are not present on arthroscopy [84]. It is considered a primary condition affecting the capsule so that the pain and stiffness in conditions that result in prolonged immobilization such as trauma, neurological lesions, myocardial infarction or other intrathoracic disease or diabetes [85,86] may be a separate condition [84].

The onset of capsulitis is usually gradual although it may, at times, be sudden. It usually goes through

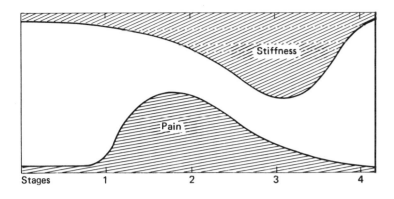

Figure 5.34 Stages of capsulitis of the shoulder

four stages and the typical findings of pain and restriction of movement in all planes vary according to the particular stage that has been reached (Figure 5.34).

Stage one

There is a mild erythematous fibrinous synovitis over the entire joint [81,84]. Pain is experienced usually in or around the glenohumeral joint, made worse by shoulder movements, especially rotation, but stiffness is not usually noticed by the patient.

Major signs

Active and passive movements are of almost full range but pain is reproduced at the extremes of all movements and over-pressure applied at the limits of the passive range produces increased pain. Isometric tests are strong and do not produce pain. Accessory shoulder movements at the limit of range are restricted and painful.

Stage two

In stage two inflamed, thickened, adhesive synovitis grows over the axillary recess onto the humerus. Pain becomes more intense, is present at night and disturbs the patient's sleep, especially if he rolls onto the affected shoulder. Most shoulder movements produce pain and sudden movements or jarring are intensely painful. Pain is commonly felt deep in the shoulder and may radiate further down the arm, although usually not below the elbow, and the shoulder becomes increasingly stiffer. This painful restriction of shoulder movement results in a severe functional disability; the patient experiences great difficulty in dressing, working, driving a car, or hanging clothes on the line.

Major signs

Active movements become more limited and painful in every plane of movement. Passive movements are similarly restricted and over-pressure produces considerably more pain. The accessory shoulder movements become more restricted, particularly lateral and inferior glide. Fully resisted movements should remain painless.

Stage three

This shows adhesive capsulitis, especially involving the axillary recess and little synovitis [81]. There is now little spontaneous pain at rest, although pain still may be experienced on suddenly stretching the joint. However, the degree of shoulder stiffness has now become much more pronounced owing to contracture of the thickened shoulder capsule. Surrounding muscles, supraspinatus and infraspinatus, become wasted. If ever the term 'frozen shoulder' is to be used, it should be reserved to describe this stage in which pain is not a feature but there is marked restriction of shoulder movements.

Major signs

The range of the active and passive glenohumeral movements is greatly restricted in all planes but, even in its most severe degree, some degree of scapular movement remains so that some movement at the shoulder is possible.

Stage four

In this stage there is a gradual resolution of the shoulder stiffness with a gradual return of shoulder mobility in most patients.

Course

Capsulitis runs a protracted course [83], which varies in length from approximately 9–24 months, and the length of any of the above four stages is also variable. As an approximation, each of the first three stages lasts from a few weeks up to about 2 months, and the fourth stage starts about the fourth or fifth month of the disease and lasts approximately 6–12 months, although there are variations to this general theme. Although the natural tendency is towards complete resolution, up to 20% of patients may be left with some degree of residual shoulder stiffness.

Management

Management remains controversial. Many different regimens have been advocated and no single method will cure this condition. Management should be considered in relation to its natural history, with four distinct stages. Much of the controversy results from the failure to relate available treatments to each of these stages. In the first two stages inflammation and pain is the dominant problem and in the next two stages stiffness is the major problem. The therapeutic approach to these two different clinical problems must be varied accordingly [87].

Stages one and two

Rest

Rest to the shoulder is essential [88] as forced movements will increase pain, especially at night. In stage one, when pain and restriction of movement are not yet marked, rest from excessive use of the shoulder, especially at the limit of the range, may be sufficient. In stage two, pain is usually severe. Rest is obtained with a sling, which needs to be worn continuously, with the arm held next to the skin so that it is not disturbed while dressing and undressing. The arm may be supported in any position that provides maximal relief and the hand may be used by placing it through a blouse or shirt. The sling needs to be worn for approximately 3 weeks until nocturnal pain has abated. This treatment will undoubtedly tend to increase the shoulder stiffness, but if active exercises are given with the aim of relieving stiffness at this stage they will inevitably increase the degree of the patient's pain.

Medications

Analgesics are needed to control pain. Non-steroidal anti-inflammatory drugs are also usually prescribed but are not often very successful in controlling pain. Oral corticosteroids may then be used and prednisolone, 20 mg daily, is given for approximately 2 weeks, and the dose is then gradually reduced until pain settles.

Injections

Intra-articular corticosteroids may be given once a week for several weeks to help control the inflammatory symptoms [56].

Physical methods

Ice may also be used to control pain but heat to the shoulder is usually of no benefit; exercises, massage and forcible movements are contraindicated. Pain-relieving modalities, such as TENS, should be considered with painless accessory movements.

Mobilization techniques

Treatment with mobilization techniques designed to ease the degree of pain in the first two stages must be extremely gentle. They should be discontinued if they produce any exacerbation of pain. No treatment is given on the day the patient is first seen lest the initial clinical examination causes exacerbation of pain. Subsequently, treatment is given on a daily basis dependent on any provoked joint reaction. Selection of technique is determined by the range of pain-free forward flexion of the arm. If this range is limited to less than 90 degrees, the accessory glenohumeral movements are used as a large-amplitude slow oscillatory movement.

Stages three and four

In the third and fourth stages pain is not the major problem but the shoulder is now stiff. Routine physical methods used to increase the joint range include mobilizations using physiological and accessory movements at the end of range, stretching and exercises. Heat or ice may be applied to the shoulder before their use. Rarely, a manipulation under an anaesthetic may be indicated.

Mobilization techniques

These are the main method of treatment in stages three and four. Forward flexion is usually chosen first as the treatment position.

In the starting position, the patient lies supine without a pillow under the head and the therapist supports the patient's fully flexed arm. Longitudinal, posteroanterior and anteroposterior accessory movements are used as small-amplitude movements at the limit of the available range. Treatments should not provoke any excessive pain and are carried out for approximately 3 min. The patient then stands and symptoms and range of movements are reassessed. This technique may be repeated once or twice provided there has been some improvement in range. This whole cycle is repeated daily if no painful reaction is provoked.

Stretching

The patient lies supine and the therapist first stabilizes the scapula with one hand and then fully flexes the shoulder by the elbow with the other hand.

For this technique, small-amplitude oscillatory movements are used at the end of the range and then by gradually increasing the pressure the shoulder is stretched to a limit tolerated by the patient for approximately 1 min. This technique is then changed to accessory movements applied at the end of the range, as described above. These two treatments, used alternately, may be repeated two or three times in a treatment session.

Exercises

These increase or maintain any increase in range obtained by the passive techniques and also increase the strength of the shoulder muscles. Exercise programmes should be carried out in a set routine, supervised by a physiotherapist. Several different methods are available:

1 Isometric exercises.
2 PNF techniques, using rotary movements in normal patterns of motion for the upper limb in which the patient contracts and then relaxes the agonist and then the antagonist muscles.
3 Pendular exercises are antigravity exercises with the patient flexed forward at the hips so that the arm hangs freely down. A weight is carried in the hand to produce traction on the glenohumeral joint, so stretching the capsule. By moving the trunk, the shoulder can be moved so that there

is no muscular activity around the glenohumeral joint. The arm can then be moved like a pendulum in a forwards and backwards, lateral or circumduction plane.
4 Active assisted exercises may be given, using either an apparatus such as a pulley or a rotation disc.
5 The patient may also force flexion and abduction by supporting the affected arm against a wall and 'climbing up' the wall with the fingers. This should not be accomplished by any 'trick' movements, such as shoulder shrugging. This point is marked, and the patient lifts his hand off the wall, retaining the same range. He then places his hand on the wall and attempts to stretch higher. The process of lifting off then stretching higher is repeated.

Manipulation

In most patients, a slow steady increase in the range of shoulder movements may be expected. Occasionally, treatment produces an early improvement but after some weeks it fails to effect any further improvement in the range. Should this occur, a manipulation under an anaesthetic may be used in an attempt to stretch the shoulder capsule [84]. The advantage of anaesthesia is that the shoulder muscles are relaxed and no great force is needed as it may dislocate or fracture the humerus.

Movements are controlled by the therapist, who holds the patient's shoulder in one hand with his palm under the posterior aspect of the patient's shoulder and his thumb over the anterior aspect of the joint. The manipulation consists of a passive stretching of the capsule in which adhesions can and should be felt to tear. These may be brief and sound like a piece of wood snapping or a sound like the tearing of wet blotting paper. The following movements are used in an orderly routine with great care and gentleness:

1 Traction on the arm while held at approximately 10 degrees of abduction.
2 Forward flexion of the shoulder.
3 Full adduction across the chest.
4 Abduction of the shoulder.
5 Lateral rotation of the shoulder with the patient's arm at 90 degrees of abduction and the elbow held at a right angle.
6 Medial rotation of the shoulder with the arm in the same position as in (5).

An intra-articular injection of corticosteroid is given after the manipulation to dampen down any subsequent inflammatory reaction. A single manipulation only rarely results in a full range of shoulder movements being restored. More commonly, the manipulation will allow the range of movements to start to improve once again and this improvement can then be maintained with the continued use of mobilization techniques and active exercises.

Prophylaxis

Prevention should be paramount as any prolonged immobilization of the shoulder may result in capsular contraction with shoulder stiffness. This is especially apt to occur in cardiac, thoracic or neurological disorders. Shoulder stiffness may occur as a complication of these disorders and prophylactic measures, such as encouraging the patient to move the shoulder and passive shoulder movements, should be undertaken.

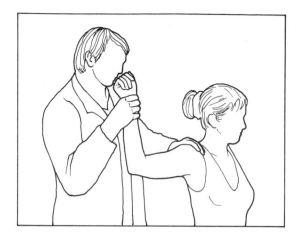

Figure 5.35 Testing recurrent subluxation of the shoulder

Instability of the shoulder

Instability is a common cause of shoulder pain in athletes [18]. Previously diagnosed only with recurrent shoulder dislocation, it is now recognized that recurrent subluxation of the joint is more common [89]. Subluxation may be recurrent, transient, follow one traumatic event or repetitive microtrauma, in contact or non-contact sports [90], in hypermobile patients or be voluntary or involuntary. It is usually anterior, less often posterior or multidirectional [91–94].

The shoulder joint is inherently unstable as the surface area of the glenoid fossa is only 20% of the humeral head. Stability depends on the surrounding soft tissues. The capsule, thin and lax, is supported by the muscles and tendons of the rotator cuff that intimately blends with it. Three glenohumeral ligaments, superior, middle and inferior, form as thickenings in the capsule. The inferior ligament forms as a sling to provide the major stabilizer of the humeral head. Instability results from soft tissue and osteochondral lesions. The labrum may be torn, detached or attenuated [50,95]; the anterior capsular–ligamentous complex may be torn; or there may be capsular laxity, which may result from repetitive microtrauma [42].

Recurrent anterior dislocation [47] usually occurs as a complication in patients who have had an acute anterior dislocation, usually following detachment of the glenohumeral ligament–labrum complex or of the capsule. A fracture of the posterosuperior head

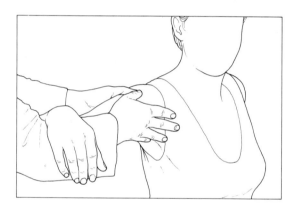

Figure 5.36 Testing for recurrent inferior subluxation of the shoulder

of humerus, the Hills–Sachs lesion, or the glenoid lip may be evident on radiographs.

With recurrent anterior subluxation the patient presents with a history of recurrent, sudden attacks of shoulder pain and clicking on shoulder movement. The attack may be momentary, the patient is conscious of 'the shoulder slipping out' and it then reduces spontaneously. In some cases the history is not so definite, and the patient says the shoulder catches, locks, feels weak, or has symptoms consistent with impingement. 'Dead arm' refers to a sudden severe pain, lasting for seconds or minutes, associated with a sensation of weakness and/or paraesthesiae coming on during a sporting activity. It is diagnostic of instability. Multidirectional instability may occur in active sports people, especially swimmers.

Major signs

With instability there may be some loss of range of external rotation. The abnormal shoulder movement should be demonstrated by the examiner positioning the patient's arm in abduction and lateral rotation and applying pressure in an anterior direction to the back of the head of the humerus (Figure 5.35). This manoeuvre may reproduce pain and the shoulder joint may be felt to begin to 'give' or sublux and there is inhibition of the movement with apprehension. This test should also be performed by placing the shoulder in many different positions including the quadrant position and stressing the shoulder also in posterior and inferior directions (Figure 5.36). Downward traction on the arm may produce a gap below the acromion with anteroinferior laxity – the sulcus sign.

Investigations

Routine radiographs of the shoulder are usually normal and special views may be needed [96–98].

Double contrast computed arthrotomography [42,43,89,96,99–101], MRI [47], cineradiography [94,102], examination under anaesthesia [18,96,103] and arthroscopy [18,41,57,101,104] are more definitive.

Management

After acute symptoms settle, conservative treatment consisting of intensive muscle strengthening and flexibility exercises must be commenced. Weakness is assessed using Cybex or Kin Corn machines. Major emphasis is then placed on stabilizing medial and lateral rotators by exercises [105]. Any stiffness is treated by mobilization techniques. Surgery is indicated if these methods are unsuccessful. Numerous procedures have been described [106] but it is no longer a technique of personal choice but an anatomical reconstruction of the observed defect [33,81,89,104, 108–110]. Arthroscopic repair may be performed with suturing or a replaceable rivet [105,112].

Shoulder–hand syndrome

The essential clinical features of this syndrome are shoulder pain, usually associated with stiffness of the shoulder, and pain and vasomotor disturbances in the corresponding hand. This combination allows this condition to be differentiated from other conditions causing pain radiating down the arm from the shoulder. It is the result of disturbance of the sympathetic nerve control of the vascular supply to the hand and has three distinct phases. In the first, pain and stiffness in the shoulder may precede, accompany or follow pain in the hand. The hand is painful, stiff, extremely tender, sweaty, oedematous and warm. The palm is usually pink, red or cyanotic. This stage, owing to a state of increased vasodilatation, lasts approximately 3–6 months. Although it may resolve spontaneously it usually proceeds to the second stage when the hand becomes less swollen and painful but stiffness becomes more marked. The palm appears pale and dry with atrophy of muscles, skin and its appendages. The shoulder becomes increasingly more painful and stiff and clinically behaves like a capsulitis. This stage lasts approximately 3–6 months. In the third stage the hand becomes stiff and atrophic without any vasomotor changes and a flexion deformity of the fingers develops. The shoulder remains stiff with wasting of surrounding muscles. This stage may last for some years.

Radiographic changes in the shoulder and hand are the result of patchy osteoporosis. Blood studies are normal but the erythrocyte sedimentation rate may be elevated. A nuclide bone scan in the early stages shows an increased uptake in the involved hand.

Entrapment neuropathy

An entrapment neuropathy causing shoulder pain may arise from the thoracic outlet syndrome or entrapment of the suprascapular nerve [113].

Suprascapular nerve entrapment

The suprascapular nerve, derived from C5 and C6, supplies motor innervation to the supraspinatus and infraspinatus muscles and sensory innervation to the posterior shoulder capsule and the acromioclavicular joints. At the upper border of the scapula it runs through the suprascapular notch before entering the supraspinous fossa. The site of compression of this nerve is in the suprascapular notch, which is enclosed by a transverse ligament [114]. Entrapment may follow trauma, especially traction or overuse of the shoulder, e.g. by painting a house, and may complicate rotator cuff injuries [115]. Pain is felt mainly in the posterolateral aspect of the shoulder but may also radiate down the arm. It is often severe but only vaguely localized. Wasting of the supraspinatus and infraspinatus muscles may follow.

Major signs

Pain should be reproduced by compressing the nerve, by passively adducting the arm fully across the chest and applying over-pressure at the end of range. Alternatively, it may be produced by elevating the arm above the head and then depressing the shoulder girdle.

Confirmatory signs

Prolonged pressure over the nerve in its suprascapular notch at the junction of the outer quarter of the spine of the scapula with the inner three-quarters reproduces the patient's pain. The diagnosis should be confirmed by electromyography to show an increased latency or a decreased amplitude [116].

Management

Rest to the shoulder is essential. An injection of 5 ml of local anaesthetic and 1 ml of corticosteroid solution may be given around the nerve as it runs through the suprascapular fossa [114]. The site of injection is located just above the spine of the scapula at the junction of the outer quarter with the inner three-quarters of the spine.

A 23-gauge needle is used and inserted distally in the supraspinous fossa until it hits the scapular spine. The needle is then withdrawn slightly and the injection given over a wide area. Pain should be relieved within a few minutes. The injection usually needs to be repeated several times at fortnightly intervals.

If conservative measures fail division of the transverse ligament is necessary [116].

References

1   Bland, J.H., Merrit, A. and Boushey, D.R. (1977) The painful shoulder. *Seminars in Arthritis and Rheumatism*, **7**, 21–47

2   Hawkins, R.J. and Abrams, J.S. (1987) Impingement syndrome in the absence of rotator cuff tear (Stages 1 and 2). *Orthopedic Clinics of North America*, **18**, 373–382

3   Post, M., Silver, R. and Singh, M. (1983) Rotator cuff tear. *Clinical Orthopaedics and Related Research*, **173**, 78–91

4   Withrington, R.H., Girgis, F.L. and Seifert, M.H. (1985) A comparative study of the aetiological factors in shoulder pain. *British Journal of Rheumatology*, **24**, 24–26

5   Maitland, G.D. (1990) *Peripheral Manipulation*, 3rd edn, Butterworth-Heinemann, Oxford

6   Butters, K.P. and Rockwood, C.A. Jr (1988) Office evaluation and management of the shoulder impingement syndrome. *Orthopedic Clinics of North America*, **19**, 755–765

7   Heron, C.W. (1990) Imaging the painful shoulder. *Clinics in Radiology*, **41**, 376–379

8   Neer, C.S. II. (1983) Impingement lesions. *Clinical Orthopaedics*, 70

9   Cone, R.O. III, Resnick, D., Danzig, L. (1984) Shoulder impingement syndrome: radiographic evaluation. *Radiology*, **150**, 29–33

10 Seeger, L.L., Gold, R.H., Bassett, L.W. *et al.* (1988) Shoulder impingement syndrome: MR findings in 53 shoulders. *American Journal of Radiology*, **150**, 343–347

11 Newhouse, K.E., El-Khoury, G.Y., Nepola, J.V. *et al.* (1988) The shoulder impingement view: a fluoroscopic technique for the detection of subacromial spurs. *American Journal of Roentgenology*, **151**, 539–541

12 Cahill, R. (1985) Understanding shoulder pain. *American Academy of Orthopedic Surgeons*, **34**, 332–336

13 Brunet, M.E., Haddad, R.J. and Porche, E.B. (1982) Rotator cuff impingement syndrome in sports. *The Physician and Sportsmedicine*, **10**, 86–94

14 Tibone, J.E., Jobe, F.W., Kerlan, R.K. *et al.* (1985) Shoulder impingement syndrome in athletes treated by an anterior acromioplasty. *Clinical Orthopedics*, **198**, 134–140

15 Watson, M. (1989) Rotator cuff function in the impingement syndrome. *Journal of Bone and Joint Surgery*, **71**, 361–366

16 Reeder, J.D. and Andelman, S. (1987) The rotator cuff tear: MR evaluation. *Magnetic Resonance Imaging*, **5**, 331–338

17 Neviaser, T.J. (1987) The role of biceps tendon in the impingement syndrome. *Orthopedic Clinics of North America*, **18**, 383–386

18 Jobe, F.W. and Kvitne, R.S. (1989) Shoulder pain in the overhand or throwing athlete. The relationship of anterior instability and rotator cuff impingement. *Orthopaedic Reviews*, **18**, 963–975

19 Hardy, J.R., Vogler, J.B. III and White, R.H. (1986) The shoulder impingement syndrome: Prevalence of radiographic findings and correlation with response to therapy. *American Journal of Radiology*,, **147**, 557–561

20 Carson, W.G. Jr (1989) Rehabilitation of the throwing shoulder. *Clinical Sports Medicine*, **8**, 657–689

21 Nicholson, G.G. (1989) Rehabilitation of common shoulder injuries. *Clinical Sports Medicine*, **8**, 633–655

22 Neviaser, T.J. (1987) Arthroscopy of the shoulder. *Orthopedic Clinics of North America*, **18**, 361–372

23 Johansson, J.E. and Barrington, T.W. (1984) Coracoacromial ligament division. *American Journal of Sports Medicine*, **12,** 138–141

24 Gartsman, G.M., Blair, M.E. Jr., Noble, P.C. *et al.* (1988) Arthroscopic subacromial decompression. An anatomical study. *American Journal of Sports Medicine*, **16**, 48–50

25 Ellman, H. (1988) Shoulder arthroscopy: current indications and techniques. *Orthopedics*, **11**, 4551

26 Bjorkenheim, J.M., Paavolainen, P., Ahovuo, J. *et al.* (1990) Subacromial impingement decompressed with anterior acromioplasty. *Clinics in Orthopaedics*, **252**, 150–155

27 Brewer, B.J. (1979) Ageing of the rotator cuff. *American Journal of Sports Medicine*, **7**, 102–110

28 Crass, J.R. (1988) Current concepts in the radiographic evaluation of the rotator cuff. *CRC Critical Reviews and Diagnostic Imaging*, **28**, 23–73

29 Bernageau, J. (1990) Roentgenographic assessment of the rotator cuff. *Clinics in Orthopaedics*, **254**, 87–91

30 Crass, J.R., Craig, E.V. and Feinberg, S.B. (1988) Ultrasonography of rotator cuff tears: a review of 500 diagnostic studies. *Journal of Clinical Ultrasound*, **16**, 313–327

31 Lanzer, William L. (1988) Clinical aspects of shoulder injuries. *Radiologic Clinics of North America*, **26**, 157–160

32 Hodler, J., Fretz, C.J., Terrier, F. *et al.* (1988) Rotator cuff tears: correlation of sonographic and surgical findings. *Radiology*, **169**, 791–794

33 Collins, R.A., Gristina, A.G., Carter, R.E. *et al.* (1987) Ultrasonography of the shoulder: Static and dynamic imaging. *Orthopedic Clinics of North America*, **18**, 351–360

34 Mack, L.A., Nyberg, D.A. (1988) Sonographic evaluation of the rotator cuff. *Radiologic Clinics of North America*, **26**, 161–177

35 Bretzke, C.A., Crass, J.R., Craig, E.V. *et al.* (1985) Ultrasonography of the rotator cuff. Normal and pathologic anatomy. *Investigative Radiology*, **20**, 311–315

36 Furtschegger, A. and Resch, H. (1988) Value of ultrasonography in preoperative diagnosis of rotator cuff tears and postoperative follow-up. *European Journal of Radiology*, **8**, 86–95

37 Middleton, W.D., Reinus, W.R., Totty, W.G. *et al.* (1986) Ultrasonographic evaluation of the rotator cuff and biceps tendon. *Journal of Bone and Joint Surgery*, **68A**, 440–450

38 Farin, P.U., Jaroma, H., Harju, A. *et al.* (1990) Shoulder impingement syndrome: Sonographic evaluation. *Radiology*, **176**, 845–849

39 Neviaser, T.J. (1987) Adhesive capsulitis. *Orthopedic Clinics of North America*, **18**, 439–443

40 Beltran, J., Gray, L.A., Bools, J.C. *et al.* (1986) Rotator cuff lesions of the shoulder: Evaluation by direct sagittal CT arthrography. *Radiology*, **160**, 161–165

41 Callaghan, J.J., McNiesh, L.M., Dehaven, J.P. *et al.* (1988) A prospective comparison study of double contrast computed tomography (CT), arthrography and arthroscopy of the shoulder. *American Journal of Sports Medicine*, **16**, 13–20

42 Rafll, M., Firooznia, H., Bonamo, J. *et al.* (1987) Athlete shoulder injuries: CT arthrographic findings. *Radiology*, **162**, 559–564

43 Faithfull, G.R. and Sonnabend, D.H. (1988) Computerised arthrotomography of the glenohumeral joint. *Australasian Radiology*, **32**, 111–116

44 Kursunoglu-Brahme, S. and Resnick, D. (1990) Magnetic resonance imaging of the shoulder. *Radiology Clinics of North America*, **28**, 941–954

45 Holt, R.G., Helms, C.A., Steinbach, L. *et al.* (1990) Magnetic resonance imaging of the shoulder: Rationale and current applications. *Skeletal Radiology*, **19**, 5–14

46 Buirski, G. (1990) Magnetic resonance imaging in acute and chronic rotator cuff tears. *Skeletal Radiology*, **19**, 109–111

47 Kieft, G.J., Sartoris, D.J., Bloem, J.L. *et al.* (1988) Magnetic resonance imaging of the glenohumeral joint diseases. *Skeletal Radiology*, **16**, 285–290

48 Meyer, S.J. and Dalink, M.K. (1990) Magnetic resonance imaging of the shoulder. *Orthopedic Clinics of North America*, **21**, 497–513

49 Tsai, J.C. and Zlatkin, M.B. (1990) Magnetic resonance imaging of the shoulder. *Radiology Clinics of North America*, **28**, 279–291

50 Andrews, J.R., Broussard, T.S. and Carson, W.G. (1985) Arthroscopy of the shoulder in the management of partial tears of the rotator cuff: A preliminary report. *Arthroscopy*, **1**, 17–22

51 Kneisl, J.S., Sweeney, H.J. and Paige, M.L. (1988) Correlation of pathology observed in double contrast arthrotomography and arthroscopy of the shoulder. *Arthroscopy*, **4**, 21–24

52 Pattee, G.A. and Snyder, S.J. (1988) Sonographic evaluation of the rotator cuff: Correlation with arthroscopy. *Arthroscopy*, **4**, 15–20

53 Ogilvie-Harris, D.J., Wiley, A.M. (1986) Arthroscopic surgery of the shoulder. A general appraisal. *Journal of Bone and Joint Surgery*, **68**, 201–207

54 Paulos, L.E. and Franklin, J.L. (1990) Arthroscopic shoulder decompression development and application. A five year experience. *American Journal of Sports Medicine*, **18**, 235–244

55 Gartsman, G.M. (1990) Arthroscopic acromioplasty for lesions of the rotator cuff. *Journal of Bone and Joint Surgery*, **72A**, 169–180

56 Petri, M., Dobrow, K., Neiman, R. *et al.* (1987) Randomized, double-blind, placebo-controlled study of the treatment of the painful shoulder. *Arthritis and Rheumatism*, **30**, 1040–1045

57 Goss, T.P. (1988) Anterior glenohumeral instability. *Orthopaedics*, **11**, 87–95

58 Fukuda, H., Hamada, K. and Yamanaka, K. (1990) Pathology and pathogenesis of bursal-side rotator cuff tears viewed from en bloc histologic sections. *Clinics in Orthopaedics*, **254**, 75–80

59 Hawkins, R.J., Misamore, G.W. and Hobeika, P.E. (1985) Surgery for full-thickness rotator-cuff tears. *Journal of Bone and Joint Surgery (Am)*, **67**, 1349–1355

60 Neviaser, R.J. (1987) Ruptures of the rotator cuff. *Orthopedic Clinics of North America*, **18**, 387–394

61 Levy, H.J., Uribe, J.W. and Delaney, L.G. (1990) Arthroscopic assisted rotator cuff repair: Preliminary results. *Arthroscopy*, **6**, 55–60

62 Rosenberg, P.S. and Clarke, R.P. (1986) Chronic rotator cuff tears. *Orthopaedic Review*, **15**, 280–289

63 Petersson, C.J. (1984) Ruptures of the supraspinatus tendon. *Acta Orthopaedica Scandinavica*, **55**, 52–56

64 Stiles, R.G., Resnick, D., Sartoris, D.J. *et al.* (1988) Rotator cuff disruption: Diagnosis with digital arthrography. *Radiology*, **168**, 705–707

65 Ishikawa, K., Ohira, T. and Morisawa, K. (1988) Persistent hemarthrosis of the shoulder joint with a rotator cuff tear in the elderly. *Archives of Orthopedic and Trauma Surgery*, **107**, 210–216

66 Hamada, K., Fukuda, H., Mikasa, M. *et al.* (1990) Roentgenographic findings in massive rotator cuff tears. A long term observation. *Clinics in Orthopaedics*, **254**, 92–96

67 Watson, M. (1985) Major ruptures of the rotator cuff. The results of surgical repair in 89 patients. *Journal of Bone and Joint Surgery*, **67**, 618–624

68 Tibone, J.E., Elrod, B., Jobe, F.W. *et al.* (1986) Surgical treatment of tears of the rotator cuff in athletes. *Journal of Bone and Joint Surgery* (Am), **68**, 887–891

69 Lanzer, W.L. (1988) Clinical aspects of shoulder injuries. *Radiologic Clinics of North America*, **26**, 157–160

70 Warren, R.F. (1985) Lesions of the long head of the biceps tendon. *Instructional Course Lectures*, **34**, 204–209

71   Neer, C.S., Craig, E.V. and Fakuda, H. (1983) Cuff-tear arthropathy. *Journal of Bone and Joint Surgery*, **65A**, 1232–1244

72   Ahovuo, J., Paavolainen, P. and Slatis, P. (1985) Radiographic diagnosis of biceps tendinitis. *Acta Orthopaedica. Scandinavica*, **56**, 75–78

73   Ahovuo, J., Paavolainen, P. and Slatis, P. (1985) Radiographic diagnosis of biceps tendinitis. *Acta Orthopaedica Scandinavica*, **56**, 75–78

74   Dines, D., Warren, R.F. and Inglis, A.E. (1982) Surgical treatment of the lesions of the long head of the biceps. *Clinical Orthopedics*, **164**, 165–171

75   Sturzenegger, M., Beguin, D., Grunig, B. *et al.* Muscular strength after rupture of the long head of the biceps. *Archives of Orthopedics and Trauma Surgery*, **105**, 18–23

76   Slatis, P. and Aalto, K. (1979) Medial dislocation of the tendon of the long head of the biceps brachii. *Acta Orthopaedica Scandinavica*, **50**, 73–77

77   O'Donoghue, D.H. (1982) Subluxing biceps tendon in the athlete. *Clininical Orthopaedics and Related Research*, **164**, 26

78   Gerber, C., Terrier, F., Zehnder, R. *et al.* (1987) The subcoracoid space. An anatomic study. *Clinical Orthopedics*, **215**, 132–138

79   Dines, D.M., Warren, R.F., Inglis, A.E. *et al.* (1990) The coracoid impingement syndrome. *Journal of Bone and Joint Surgery*, **72B**, 314–316

80   Neviaser, R.J. and Neviaser, T.J. (1987) The frozen shoulder. Diagnosis and management. *Clinical Orthopedics*, **223**, 59–64

81   Johnson, L.L. (1987) The shoulder joint. *Clinical Orthopaedics and Related Research*, **223**, 113–125

82   Murnaghan, J.P. (1988) Adhesive capsulitis of the shoulder: current concepts and treatment. *Orthopedics*, **11**, 153–158

83   Reeves, B. (1975) The natural history of the frozen shoulder syndrome. *Scandinavian Journal of Rheumatology*, **4**, 193–196

84   Neviaser, R.J. (1987) Radiologic assessment of the shoulder. Plain and arthrographic. *Orthopaedic Clinics of North America*, **18**, 343–349

85   Morien-Hybbinette, I., Moritz, U. and Scherstien, B. (1986) The painful diabetic shoulder. *Actaica Medica Scandinavica*, **219**, 507–514

86   Pal, B., Anderson, J., Dick, W.C. *et al.* (1986) Limitation of joint mobility and shoulder capsulitis in insulin- and non-insulin-dependent diabetes mellitus. *British Journal of Rheumatology*, **25**, 147–151

87   Schneider, G. (1991). Personal communication.

88   Nitz, Arthur J. (1986) Physical therapy management of the shoulder. *Physical Therapy*, **66**, 1912–1919

89   Goss, T.P. (1988) Anterior glenohumeral instability. *Orthopaedics*, **11**, 87–95

90   Garth, W.P. Jr., Allman, F.L. Jr. and Armstrong, W.S. (1987) Subluxations of the shoulder in non-contact sports. *American Journal of Sports Medicine*, **15**, 579–585

91   Schwartz, E., Warren, R.F., O'Brien, S.J. *et al.* (1987) Posterior shoulder instability. *Orthopedic Clinics of North America*, **18**, 409–419

92   Norwood, L.A. and Terry, G.C. (1984) Shoulder posterior subluxation. *American Journal of Sports Medicine*, **12**, 25–30

93   Hawkins, R.J., Koppert, G. and Johnston, G. (1984) Recurrent posterior instability (subluxation) of the shoulder. *Journal of Bone and Joint Surgery (Am)*, **66**, 169–174

94   Ozaki, J. (1988) Glenohumeral movement of the involuntary inferior and multi-directional instability. *Clinical Orthopaedics and Related Research*, **233**, 107–111

95a McMaster, W.C. (1986) Anterior glenoid labrum damage: A painful lesion in swimmers. *American Journal of Sports Medicine*, **14**, 383–387

95b Rafii, M., Minkoff, J., Bonamo, J. *et al.* (1988) Computed tomography (CT). Arthrography of shoulder instabilities in athletes. *American Journal of Sports Medicine*, **16**, 352–361

96   Cofield, R.H. and Irving, J.F. (1987) Evaluation and classification of shoulder instability. *Clinical Orthopaedics and Related Research*, **223**, 32–33

97   Horsfield, D. and Stutley, J. (1988) The unstable shoulder – a problem solved. *Radiography*, **54**, 74–76

98   Pring, D.J., Constant, O., Bayley, J.I.L. *et al.* (1989) Radiography of the humeral head in recurrent anterior shoulder dislocations: brief report. *Journal of Bone and Joint Surgery*, **71B**, 141–142

99   Resch, H., Helweg, G., zer Nedden D. *et al.* (1988) Double-contrast computed tomographic examination techniques in habitual and recurrent shoulder dislocation. *European Journal of Radiology*, **8**, 6–12

100 Singson, R.D., Feldman, F. and Bigliani, L. (1987) CT arthrographic patterns in recurrent glenohumeral instability. *American Journal of Roentgenology*, **149**, 749–753

101 Nottage, W.M., Duge, W.D. and Fields, W.A. (1987) Computed arthrotomography of the glenohumeral joint to evaluate anterior instability: correlation with arthroscopic findings. *Arthroscopy*, **3**, 273–276

102 Maki, N.J. (1988) Cineradiographic studies with shoulder instabilities. *American Journal of Sports Medicine*, **16**, 362–364

103 Adolfsson, L. and Lysholm, J. (1989) Arthroscopy and stability testing for anterior shoulder instability. *Arthroscopy*, **5**, 315–320

104 Wiley, A.M. (1988) Arthroscopy for shoulder instability and a technique for arthroscopic repair. *Arthroscopy*, **4**, 25–30

105 Dalton, S.E. and Snyder, S.J. (1989) Glenohumeral instability. *Baillières Clinics in Rheumatology*, **3**, 511–534

106 Rao, J.P., Francis, A.M., Hurley, J. *et al.* (1986) Treatment of recurrent anterior dislocation of the shoulder by DuToit Staple capsulorrhaphy. Results of long-term follow-up study. *Clinical Orthopedics and Related Research*, **204**, 169–176

107 Rowe, C.R. (1987) Recurrent transient anterior subluxation of the shoulder. The dead arm syndrome. *Clinical Orthopaedics*, **223**, 11–19

108 Collins, K.A., Capito, C. and Cross, M. (1986) The use of the Putti-Platt procedure in the treatment of recurrent anterior dislocation. With special reference to the young athlete. *American Journal of Sports Medicine*, **14**, 380–382

109 Hodgkinson, J.P. and Case, D.B. (1987) The modified staple capsulorrhaphy for the correction of recurrent anterior dislocation of the shoulder. *Injury*, **18**, 51–54

110 Matthews, L.S., Vetter, W.L., Oweida, S.J. *et al.* (1988) Arthroscopic staple capsulorrhaphy for recurrent anterior shoulder instability. *Arthroscopy*, **4**, 106–111

111 Morgan, C.D. and Bodenstab, A.B. (1987) Arthroscopic Bankart suture repair: Technique and early results. *Arthroscopy*, **3**, 111–122

112 Yahiro, M.A. and Matthews, L.S. (1989) Arthroscopic stabilization procedures for recurrent anterior shoulder instability. *Orthopaedic Reviews*, **18**, 1161–1168

113 Herring, S.A. (1989) Secondary causes of shoulder pain. *Sports Training, Medicine and Rehabilitation*, **1**, 141–143

114 Emery, P., Bowman, S., Wedderburn, L. *et al.* (1989) Supracapsular nerve block for chronic shoulder pain in rheumatoid arthritis. *British Medical Journal*, **299**, 1079–1080

115 Kaplan, P.E. and Kernahan, W.T. Jr. (1984) Rotator cuff rupture: management with suprascapular neuropathy. *Archives of Physical Medicine and Rehabilitation*, **65**, 273–275

116 Post, M. and Mayer, M.D. (1986) Suprascapular nerve entrapment. *Clinical Orthopaedics and Related Research*, **223**, 126

6 Clavicular joints

Acromioclavicular joint

The acromioclavicular joint moves during all movements of the glenohumeral joint and the scapula.

During glenohumeral movement, rotary movement takes place in the acromioclavicular joint [1]. With shoulder flexion, the clavicle rotates by approximately 40 degress [2]. With abduction, the clavicle elevates by some 20 degrees.

During movement of the scapula on the thorax, shrugging or depressing the shoulder or protraction or retraction of the scapula, a gliding movement takes place in the acromioclavicular joint and the clavicle elevates with minimal rotation [2].

Joint pain is usually well localized over the joint and is only rarely referred distally into the upper arm or proximally into the neck. The patient, if asked to put one finger over the site of pain, usually places it accurately over the upper surface of the joint. Pain is usually made worse by movements of the shoulder [1], especially horizontal flexion or by wearing shoulder straps.

Glenohumeral, scapular and neck movements are first tested routinely. The clinical examination involves: (1) inspection; (2) movements: active, passive and accessory; and (3) palpation.

Inspection

The subcutaneous acromioclavicular joint is easy to inspect. The examiner stands in front of the seated patient to observe the presence of any joint swelling or subluxation upwards of the outer end of the clavicle.

Movements

Active movement

Active movement is best tested by horizontal flexion of the patient's arm across the chest. The examiner stands behind the patient and passively flexes the shoulder to 90 degrees by holding under the flexed elbow (Figure 6.1). The arm is horizontally flexed across the chest so that the hand reaches past the opposite shoulder. The range of this movement is assessed by comparing both arms and noting the position reached by the point of the elbow in relation to the opposite shoulder.

Passive movement

Passive movements are tested by the same movements, with over-pressure produced by oscillatory movements at the end of the range to reproduce pain. Pain may also be reproduced by movement of the glenohumeral joint, especially flexion from full extension or abduction, or on scapulothoracic movements, elevation, depression, protraction, retraction and rotation of the scapula on the chest wall.

Accessory movement

There are six accessory movements in the acromioclavicular joint:

1 Anteroposterior movement, produced by pressure over the anterior surface of the outer third of the clavicle (Figure 6.2).

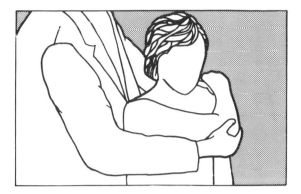

Figure 6.1 Horizontal flexion

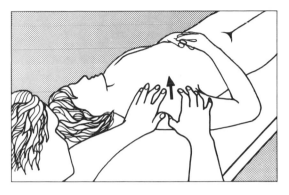

Figure 6.3 Posteroanterior accessory movement

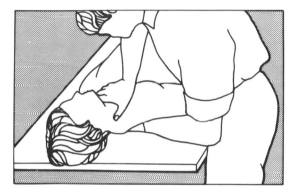

Figure 6.2 Anteroposterior accessory movement

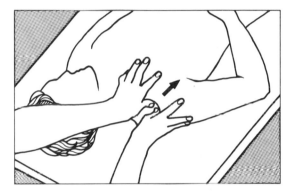

Figure 6.4 Longitudinal caudad accessory movement

2 Posteroanterior movement is produced by pressure over the posterior surface of the clavicle (Figure 6.3).
3 Rotation is produced when the arm is flexed above the head.
4 Transverse lateral movement is produced by distraction of the joint.
5 Transverse medial movement is produced by compressing the joint.
6 Longitudinal movement is produced by pressure over the superior surface of the joint (Figure 6.4).

Palpation

The acromioclavicular joint is subcutaneous and its joint margins, osteophytes and any malalignments can easily be felt and palpated for tenderness. Old injuries may be felt as slightly tender chronic thickenings over the anterior joint capsule and in the space below. Crepitus or clicking may indicate degenerative changes.

Lesions of the joint

1 Injuries.
   (a) Ligaments.
   (b) Intra-articular meniscus.
2 Bone osteolysis of the outer clavicle.
3 Arthritis.
   (a) Inflammatory.
   (b) Osteoarthritis.

Injuries

Ligaments

The acromioclavicular joint is commonly injured either by a direct lateral blow to the shoulder or indirect injuries. The latter occur in all body-contact sports or after a fall from a speeding object such as a horse or motor cycle. An indirect injury to the joint may follow a fall onto the outstretched hand or a fall onto the outer side of the shoulder, which may follow

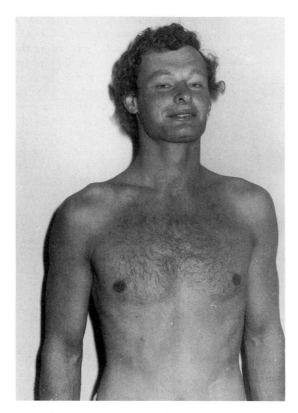

Figure 6.5 Grade 2 subluxation of the acromioclavicular joint

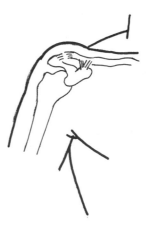

Figure 6.6 Second degree rupture of acromioclavicular ligament

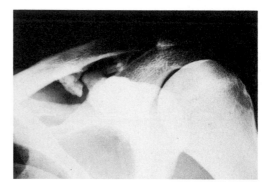

Figure 6.7 Calcification in the ruptured conoid and trapezoid ligaments

twisting sideways to avoid a head-on collision. The force is usually transmitted through the glenoid cavity, to the acromioclavicular ligaments and finally to the coracoclavicular ligaments. Injuries are divided into three grades or degrees.

Minor or first degree

This is produced by a tear of some fibres of the acromioclavicular ligaments without any joint displacement. Pain, swelling and tenderness are localized over the joint and no obvious deformity or instability is present. Passive shoulder movements, especially horizontal flexion of the arm across the body, usually reproduce the patient's pain.

MANAGEMENT

Treatment consists of initial rest from active shoulder exercises, the use of analgesics and ice. Pain usually settles within a few days after which active exercises can be commenced.

Moderate or second degree

This damage is associated with disruption of the capsule and acromioclavicular ligament fibres which allows the joint to sublux, so that the clavicle moves slightly upwards. A slight step deformity in the joint is present and abduction of the arm beyond 80 degrees is usually painful. Pain is also reproduced on horizontal flexion of the shoulder.

MANAGEMENT

Treatment consists of rest from shoulder movements and supporting the arm in a sling, such as the Kenny–Howard splint [2–4], until pain settles. This usually takes 7–10 days and analgesics are usually required.

Injections are most helpful for pain relief. The patient sits with the arm hanging loosely by the side and laterally rotated. A 25-gauge needle is inserted into the joint space, palpable distally to the bony enlargement of the clavicle. The needle needs to be angulated according to the different shapes of the joint surfaces. Then 1 ml of local anaesthetic and 1 ml of corticosteroid are injected.

Mobilization techniques involving slow, pain-free accessory movements should be introduced as pain settles over the next few weeks. Active arm exercises are commenced and the injection may be repeated if necessary.

Severe or third degree

In this the ligaments that stabilize the acromioclavicular joint are disrupted so that the clavicle becomes dislocated upwards on the acromion (Figure 6.7). The acromioclavicular ligaments and usually the coracoclavicular ligaments and attachments of deltoid and trapezius muscles are ruptured, allowing further elevation of the clavicle. The patient complains of severe pain at first, and shoulder movements are restricted until the pain eventually settles. Ultimately this injury causes little pain or functional disability, even in people involved in contact sports, but the swelling remains unsightly.

EXAMINATION
The dislocation is readily observed as the patient stands with arms by the sides and may be made more obvious by holding a weight in the hand on the affected side. Diagnosis is confirmed on radiographs which show an increased distance between the acromion and the clavicle on the affected side. The outer end of the clavicle is elevated so that its inferior border lies level with or above the superior surface of the acromion. A radiograph with traction on both shoulders may be taken and used for comparison but is of little value unless surgery is contemplated.

MANAGEMENT OF LIGAMENT INJURIES
There is little controversy about management of first and second degrees of injuries. Conservative methods are successful and surgery is never indicated. Although considerable controversy exists as to whether conservative or surgical reduction is to be preferred for third degree injuries, conservative treatment is indicated for most injuries, including those in body contact sports [3,5–14]. Such treatment, aimed at reducing and immobilizing the dislocation, may be difficult to attain but even if it does not produce a perfect reduction, functional results

are often satisfactory [5,7,8,10,12]. The outer end of the clavicle must be forced downwards and the scapula with its acromion upwards by elevating the scapula via the elbow. Numerous methods have been described including strapping, slings, braces, harnesses and a plaster cast. A Kenny–Howard splint applied over the clavicle and under the elbow until pain settles provides relief in most cases [3,4]. Currently, conservative methods should be used for at least 6 weeks before assessment of the need for surgery.

Surgical repair that is designed to restore the complex anatomy and joint function is not always successful nor necessary. Factors to be taken into account include:

1 The type and degree of activity to be undertaken. Heavy manual workers and sports that involve throwing may need to be considered for surgery whereas a sedentary worker probably need not be. A cosmetic result without an unsightly lump could be more important to a model than to a manual worker.
2 Whether the dominant or non-dominant shoulder is involved.
3 The age of the patient.

Surgical procedures for the acromioclavicular joint with screws, pins, wires and fascial transplants usually produce an unsatisfactory end result. Coracoclavicular stabilization has been achieved with Bosworth screws, pins and wire loops, fascial or Dacron repair. Removal of the outer end of the clavicle and fixation of the remaining distal end of the clavicle to the coracoid, combined with a repair of the origins of the deltoid and trapezius, has been advocated with recurrent dislocation [3,15].

Intra-articular meniscus

Injury to the articular cartilage and meniscus in young athletes may rarely cause recurrent attacks of a painful catching sensation on shoulder movements [4,15]. These can be reproduced on testing passive physiological or accessory joint movements. If symptoms recur surgery to remove the disc and outer end of the clavicle may be indicated.

Osteolysis

Osteolysis of the outer end of the clavicle may occur in athletes. Its cause is unknown but it may follow trauma. Radiographs or especially a nuclear bone scan are necessary for diagnosis [16,17].

Arthritis

Osteoarthritis in this joint is common, more so than in the sternoclavicular joint, as it occurs at an earlier age and is more liable to limit activity. It may result from previous trauma [3] or may follow rupture of the rotator cuff, which allows the head of the humerus to sublux upwards (see p. 51). It may present with a large synovial swelling over the joint.

Osteoarthritis may be asymptomatic and pain then usually develops after excessive use of the joint in the middle-aged patient (Figure 6.8). Pain may occur after playing golf or from movements which involve use of the shoulder with the arm above the head. Pain may be reproduced by passive movement of the joint or horizontal flexion of the shoulder. Accessory movements are restricted and painful. Crepitus is often palpable over the joint. The diagnosis may be confirmed from radiography.

MANAGEMENT

1 Rest from those shoulder movements that aggravate pain.
2 Anti-inflammatory agents.
3 Local corticosteroid injections, as described above.
4 Mobilization techniques. Treatment by mobilization techniques uses accessory joint movements within the limits of pain. Pain and stiffness in the acromioclavicular joint are often associated with disorders of the glenohumeral joint and pain is reproduced on shoulder movements. Both joints then require treatment by passive movements and treating the glenohumeral joint also moves the acromioclavicular joint. The usual treatment technique is posteroanterior and anteroposterior movements of the humeral head plus accessory movements of the acromioclavicular joint.
5 Conservative treatment is highly successful and surgery, with arthroplasty of the joint, is only rarely indicated.

Sternoclavicular joint

The sternoclavicular joint functions as a ball and socket joint as the inner end of the clavicle rotates on its long axis during most shoulder movements (Figure 6.9). For example, during abduction of the

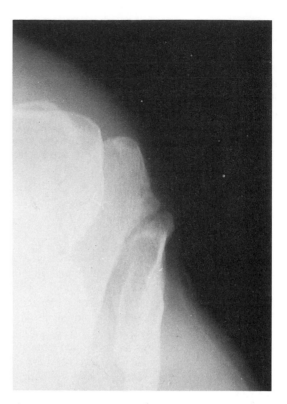

Figure 6.8 Osteoarthritis of the acromioclavicular joint

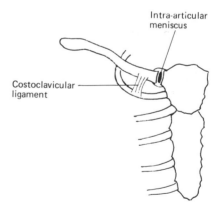

Figure 6.9 Sternoclavicular joint

shoulder, scapular rotation with movement in the clavicle and sternoclavicular joint also occur. On abduction or flexion of the shoulder the clavicle rolls upwards and backwards rotating about its longitudinal axis. When the shoulder is returned to the neutral position, opposite movements take place in the clavicle. The total range of axial rotation is approximately 30 degrees. Sternoclavicular pain is well localized to the area of the joint or first rib and is usually made worse by shoulder movements such as abduction or flexion that entail rotation of the inner end of the clavicle. Pain may radiate into the chest wall and so cause confusion with heart or lung diseases. It may also need to be differentiated from disorders affecting the costochondral cartilage of the first rib. Pain may also be referred to the sternoclavicular area from the cervical spine or shoulder region.

Clinical examination

1 Inspection, observe:
  (a) Swelling.
  (b) Subluxation.
2 Movements.
  (a) Active.
  (b) Passive.
  (c) Accessory.
3 Palpation.

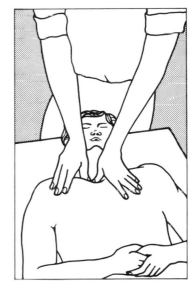

Figure 6.10 Anteroposterior accessory movement of the sternoclavicular joint

Inspection

The sternoclavicular joint lies subcutaneously and is easy to inspect and palpate. Synovitis is usually evident as a rounded soft tissue swelling localized over the joint or just lateral to the joint line, filling in the angle between the clavicle and the first rib.

Subluxation of the joint usually occurs in an anterosuperior direction that is best appreciated if the examiner stands behind the seated patient and looks down onto both joints.

Movements

The sternoclavicular joint moves with movements of the shoulder, especially flexion, horizontal flexion, and scapular movements. In general, movement of the glenohumeral joint beyond 60 degrees will produce sternoclavicular pain.

Accessory movements

There are seven accessory movements in the sternoclavicular joint:

1 Anteroposterior movement produced by pressure over the sternal end of the clavicle (Figure 6.10).
2 Posteroanterior movement is produced by hooking the fingers and thumb around the posterior surface of the clavicle to pull it forwards.

3 Longitudinal caudad movement is produced by pressure against the superior border of the clavicle adjacent to the joint.
4 Longitudinal cephalad movement is produced by pressure against the inferior border of the clavicle.
5 Transverse medial movement is produced by compression along the clavicle from the acromion.
6 Transverse lateral movement distracts the joint by pulling the humerus laterally.
7 Rotation is produced at the limit of the ranges of shoulder and scapular movements.

Palpation

This joint is easy to palpate. An anterior subluxation can be seen and felt, and is easily repositioned.

Lesions of the sternoclavicular joint are:

1 Arthritis.
  (a) Degenerative.
  (b) Inflammatory.
  (c) Infective.
2 Injuries.
  (a) Subluxation.
  (b) Dislocation.

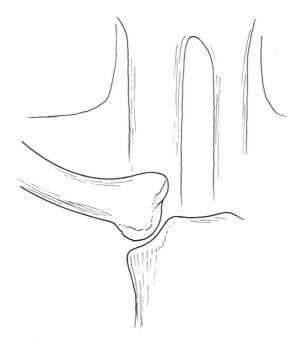

Figure 6.11 Osteoarthritis of the sternoclavicular joint with subluxation

Arthritis

Osteoarthritis is not as common in the sternoclavicular joints as in the acromioclavicular joints and may follow trauma (Figure 6.11). It is usually unilateral and produces an anterior subluxation of the joint that is easily recognizable on inspection. This may be of concern to the patient as it may be noticed to be gradually increasing in size. Pain may be present on shoulder movement; tenderness and thickening are localized over the sternoclavicular joint. Inflammatory changes usually occur in spondyloarthropathies [18].

Injuries

The sternoclavicular capsular ligament may be sprained as a result of an injury that usually results from a fall or blow during which the shoulder joint is thrust medially. Minor degrees of asymptomatic subluxation are common.

A third-degree sprain with disruption of the costoclavicular and sternoclavicular ligaments results in dislocation of the joint. In the usual type of injury, the inner end of the clavicle dislocates upwards and outwards. Posterior dislocation of the clavicle behind the sternum is rare but potentially much more serious because of damage to the superior mediastinal contents.

MANAGEMENT

The principles of management, including rest, local steroid injection and mobilization techniques, are similar to those described for the acromioclavicular joint.

References

1 Cahill, B.R. (1985) Understanding shoulder pain. *American Academy of Orthopedic Surgeons.* **34**, 332–336
2 Wilk, V. (1990) The acromioclavicular joint: Pathophysiology and management. *Australian Association of Manipulative Medicine Bulletin*, **6**, 20–26
3 Taft, J.N., Wilson, F.C. and Oglesby, J.W. (1987) Dislocation of the acromioclavicle joint. *Journal of Bone and Joint Surgery*, **69A**, 1045–1051
4 Cox, J.S. (1981) The fate of the acromioclavicular joint in athletic injuries. *American Journal of Sports Medicine*, **9**, 50–53
5 Bannister, G.C., Wallace, W.A., Stableforth, P.G. *et al.* (1989) Management of acute acromioclavicular dislocation. *Journal of Bone and Joint Surgery*, **71B**, 848–850
6 Carr, J.A. and Broughton, N.S. (1989) Acromioclavicular dislocation associated with fracture of the coracoid process. *Journal of Trauma*, **29**, 125–126
7 Cook, D.A. and Heiner, J.P. (1990) Acromioclavicular joint injuries. *Orthopaedic Reviews*, **19**, 510–516
8 Dias, J.J., Steingold, R.F., Richardson, R.A. *et al.* (1987) The conservative treatment of acromioclavicular dislocation. *Journal of Bone and Joint Surgery*, **69B**, 719–722
9 Fullerton, L.R. Jr. (1990) Recurrent third degree acromioclavicular joint separation after failure of a dacron ligament prosthesis. *American Journal of Sports Medicine*, **18**, 106–107
10 Larsen, E., Bjerg-Nielson, A. and Christensen, P. (1986) Conservative or surgical treatment of acromioclavical dislocation. *Journal of Bone and Joint Surgery*, **68A**, 552–555
11 Tsou, P.M. (1989) Percutaneous cannulated screw coracoclavicular fixation for acute acromioclavicular dislocations. *Clinics in Orthopaedics*, **8**, 112–121
12 Walsh, W.M., Peterson, D.A., Shelton, G. and Newmann, R.D. (1985) Shoulder strength following acromioclavicular injury. *American Journal of Sports Medicine*, **13**, 153–158
13 Warren-Smith, D.D. and Ward, M.W. (1987) Operation for acromioclavicular dislocation. *Journal of Bone and Joint Surgery*, **59B**, 715–718
14 Wilson, K. and Colwill, J.C. (1989) Combined A-C dislocation with coracoclavicular ligament disruption and coracoid process fracture. *American Journal of Sports Medicine*, **17**, 697–698
15 Wickiewicz, T.L. (1983) Acromio clavicular and sterno clavicular joint injuries. *Clinics in Sports Medicine*, **2**, 429–438
16 Kaplan, P.A. and Resnick, D. (1986) Stress-induced osteolysis of the clavicle. *Radiology*, **158**, 139–140
17 Quinn, S.F. and Glass, T.A. (1983) Post traumatic osteolysis of the clavicle. *South Medical Journal*, **76**, 307–308
18 Kofold, H., Thomsen, P. and Lindenberg, S. (1985) Serous synovitis of the sternoclavicular joint. Differential diagnostic aspects. *Scandinavian Journal of Rheumatology*, **14**, 61–64

7 Elbow

The elbow is made up of two primary joints, humero-ulnar and superior radioulnar, and one secondary joint, radiohumeral. They function as a unit within a single synovial cavity (Figures 7.1 and 7.2), the major function being to allow the hand to be positioned, e.g. by lifting it to the face while eating. The elbow forms a link between the shoulder and the hand so that the range of motion in the hand also depends upon the position of the elbow. With the elbow flexed to 90 degrees and the arm placed by the side, the total range of supination and pronation in the hand is approximately 180 degrees; if the arm hangs by the side, the total range of supination and pronation of the hand is 360 degrees, as the shoulder, by rotating laterally and medially, can also participate in this movement. If the range of elbow movement is restricted, compensatory movements at the shoulder can then help to maintain function.

Marked disturbance of function follows loss of the range of movement in both the shoulder and elbow.

During flexion of the elbow, the trochlear notch of the ulna glides around the trochlea of the humerus until blocked by approximation of the muscles and the bony prominence of the coronoid process engaging in the coronoid fossa of the humerus. During extension, the trochlear notch of the ulna glides round the trochlea until the bony prominence of the olecranon process engages the olecranon fossa. Simultaneously with flexion and extension, the head of the radius glides backwards and forwards on the capitulum. Rotation of the forearm producing supination or pronation occurs as the concave radial head moves around the lateral side of the stable ulna. Moving from supination to pronation the head of the radius tilts distally and medially and glides on the capitulum.

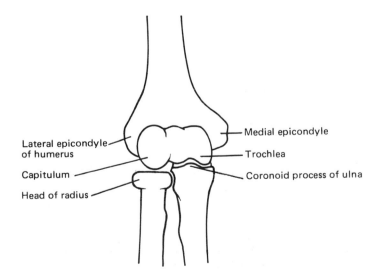

Lateral epicondyle of humerus

Capitulum

Head of radius

Medial epicondyle

Trochlea

Coronoid process of ulna

Figure 7.1 Elbow joint

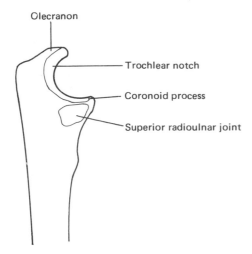

Figure 7.2 Upper end of right ulna viewed from lateral side

On passive abduction and adduction, the radio-humeral joint surfaces close and open with superior and inferior gliding of the superior radioulnar joint. These same movements occur with full abduction and adduction of the wrist.

Elbow pain

Pain in the elbow is usually due to local musculoskeletal disorders. It may also be produced by lesions of the cervical spine or less commonly as a referred pain from lesions in other areas in the arm. Pain from shoulder lesions may radiate down the arm but rarely as far as the elbow and is made worse by shoulder and not elbow movements. Occasionally pain may be felt in the elbow from an entrapment neuropathy of the median nerve in the carpal tunnel.

Soft tissue lesions are the most common cause of elbow pain and the patient may be aware that pain is related to certain movements of the elbow or wrist. Sporting injuries may be classified into (1) lateral compression, (2) medial stress, and (3) forced extension injuries [1]. Of the soft tissue lesions, epicondylitis is the most common but considerable controversy still exists about its basic nature and correct nomenclature. However, epicondylitis is probably the best term to describe this multifactorial condition that may involve the lateral or medial epicondyle. Loss of the normal elbow accessory movements and neural mobility are often overlooked as a cause of painful disability.

Examination

Examination of a patient with elbow pain commences by first examining the cervical spine pain or restriction of movement and whether pain can be reproduced by neck movements. It also includes an examination of the whole upper limb.

Examination of the elbow

1. Inspection.
    (a) Deformities.
    (b) Swellings.
    (c) Colour changes.
2. Movements.
    (a) Active.
    (b) Passive.
    (c) Accessory.
    (d) Isometric.
3. Palpation.

Inspection

In the anatomical position, with the elbow fully extended and the forearm supinated with the palm facing forwards, the forearm normally forms a slight degree of valgus at the elbow. This so-called carrying angle is usually about 5 degrees in males but may be greater in females. It disappears when the arm is placed in full pronation. The carrying angle is of advantage when an object is being carried by allowing the elbow to be tucked in above the iliac crest.

Deformities

Three types of deformity may be present. An alteration in the normal carrying angle of the elbow may be increased, cubitus valgus, or decreased, cubitus varus. Cubitus valgus may be a sign in Turner's syndrome but more commonly occurs as the result of a previous elbow fracture and may then produce an entrapment neuropathy of the ulnar nerve behind the medial epicondyle. Cubitus varus, a decrease in the carrying angle of the elbow, called the 'gunstock deformity' because of its shape, may occur as the late result of a fracture. Flexion deformity of the elbow with loss of full extension is common in patients with arthritis. Hyperextension of the elbow, or cubitus recurvatus, may occur as part of a hypermobility syndrome.

Swellings around the elbow joint

A synovial effusion bulges into the lateral paraolecranon groove (Figure 7.3), best seen with the elbow flexed to less than a right angle. Rheumatoid synovitis

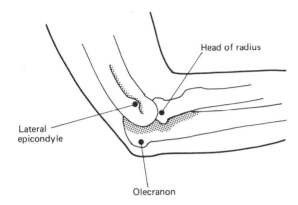

Head of radius

Lateral
epicondyle

Olecranon

Figure 7.3 Bony landmarks around the elbow. Shading
indicates position of the lateral paraolecranon groove

may track down into the forearm or up around the
triceps insertion to produce a cystic synovial swelling.

Rheumatoid nodules are found in the subcutaneous tissue over the olecranon and extensor surface
of the elbow in up to 25% of rheumatoid patients.
They feel firm, often rubbery, may be multiple, vary
up to 3 cm in size and a small necrotic area may be
found in the overlying skin. They are caused by a
combination of an underlying vasculitis and local
pressure or friction.

The elbow is also a common site for tophaceous
deposits to develop in patients with gout. They can
clinically resemble rheumatoid nodules and, for a
correct diagnosis, should be aspirated to confirm
urate crystals.

Olecranon bursitis presents as a swelling localized
to the bursa over the olecranon process. This common
condition may result from trauma, infection or arthritis. Traumatic bursitis may be caused by a direct injury
to the elbow or follow chronic friction and pressure. A
synovial effusion, which tends to be recurrent, develops in the bursa and may at times be haemorrhagic.
Olecranon bursitis, 'beat elbow', is common in miners,
caused by the repetitive nature of their work and may
lead to an infected bursitis. Two common conditions,
rheumatoid arthritis and gout, may be associated with
olecranon bursitis. Swelling may occur as part of the
acute inflammatory synovitis in both these conditions
or the bursa may be chronically involved, with rheumatoid nodules or gouty tophaceous deposits.

Movements

Active movements

Active movements tested at the elbow are flexion,
extension, pronation and supination.

The patient is first asked to extend the elbow by
straightening out the arm and then to flex it fully.
The active range of extension is normally designated
as 0 degrees and is blocked by bony apposition. The
active range of flexion, approximately 140 degrees,
is blocked by the bulk of the arm muscles.

The active range of supination and pronation is
tested in two different positions: first, with the elbow
in full extension, and then with the elbow held at 90
degrees of flexion.

When performing active movements, the patient
is requested to move the arm to the limit of each
range and then to bounce the arm three or four
times into this position. The range of these
movements and whether they reproduce the
patient's pain should be noted.

Passive movements

The passive range of each of the four elbow
movements is usually a few degrees more than the
active range. The range is noted and over-pressure
is then applied at the limit of range to assess the
end-feel of each movement.

Accessory movements

The accessory movements in the three separate
joints of the elbow are tested separately.

HUMEROULNAR JOINT
The two important accessory movements tested in
this joint are:

1   The range of adduction and abduction of the
    elbow throughout its last 5 degrees of extension.
2   The longitudinal caudad movement in the line of
    the humerus.

With the elbow fully extended, the range of lateral
accessory movement can be felt by passive movement
of the elbow into adduction and abduction. This may
be represented diagrammatically by a straight line X_1,
Y_1: where X_1 represents the limit of adduction and Y_1
the limit of abduction. If the elbow is now passively
flexed by 10 degrees the range between adduction and
abduction is increased and may be represented
diagrammatically by a line X_2, Y_2 (Figure 7.4).

In practice this test is carried out by holding the
fully extended elbow firmly in adduction (Figure 7.5)
and then moving it from full extension to a position
of 10 degrees of flexion (i.e. from X_1 to X_2). During
this movement the elbow is felt to move not in a
straight line but in a slight curve.

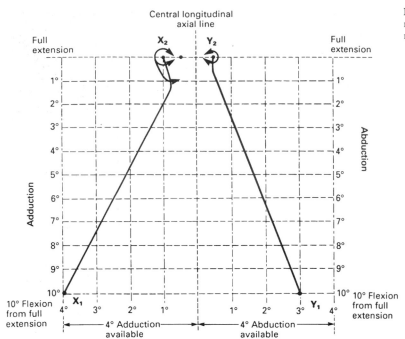

Central longitudinal axial line

Figure 7.4 Diagrammatic representation of accessory movements in elbow extension

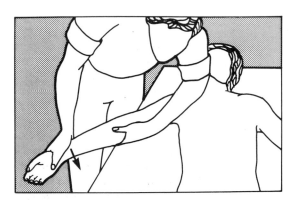

Figure 7.5 Elbow: extension–adduction

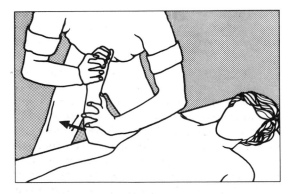

Figure 7.6 Humeroulnar joint; longitudinal caudad accessory movement

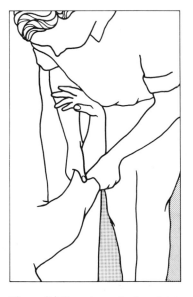

Figure 7.7 Superior radioulnar joint: anteroposterior accessory movement

A similar movement is made with the extended elbow held in passive abduction and moving it from full extension to a position of 5 degrees of flexion (from Y_1 to Y_2). This movement also follows a slight curve, less marked than when the arm is moved in adduction (Figure 7.4).

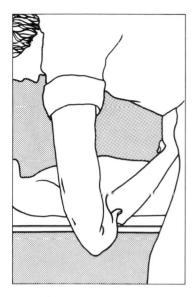

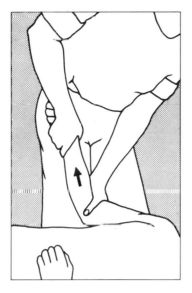

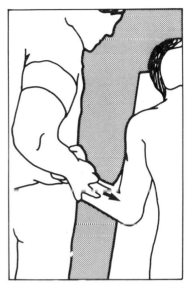

Figure 7.8 Superior radioulnar joint: posteroanterior accessory movement

Figure 7.9 Superior radioulnar joint: longitudinal caudad accessory movement

Figure 7.10 Superior radioulnar joint: longitudinal cephalad accessory movement

Longitudinal caudad movement is produced by pressure along the forearm to distract the humeroulnar joint (Figure 7.6).

SUPERIOR RADIOULNAR JOINT
There are four accessory movements in this joint:

1　Anteroposterior movement, produced by pressure over the anterior surface of the head of the radius, placed either in supination (Figure 7.7) or in pronation.
2　Posteroanterior movement is produced by pressure over the posterior surface of the radial head (Figure 7.8).
3　Longitudinal caudad movement is produced by pulling along the radius to distract the joint (Figure 7.9).
4　Longitudinal cephalad movement is produced by compressing the joint margins (Figure 7.10).

RADIOHUMERAL JOINT
Four accessory movements are tested in this joint:

1　Anteroposterior movement, a gliding movement applied to the head of the radius.
2　Posteroanterior movement is also a gliding movement applied to the head of the radius in an opposite direction.

3　Longitudinal cephalad movement is produced by compression along the radial shaft.
4　Longitudinal caudad movement is produced by pulling on the patient's hand to apply a longitudinal movement to the radius.

Isometric tests

Isometric tests should be first assessed at the wrist and then at the elbow. To test resisted movements at the wrist the patient is asked to grip the examiner's hand and squeeze strongly. If elbow pain is reproduced, additional isometric contractions of the wrist are examined. With pain over the lateral compartment of the elbow, the isometric movements tested are wrist extension, radial deviation of the wrist and finger extension. With pain over the medial elbow compartment, the isometric movements tested are wrist flexion, ulnar deviation of the wrist and finger flexion.

The four elbow movements of flexion, extension, supination and pronation are then tested using isometric contraction. Flexion is tested with the patient supine with the elbow flexed to a right angle and the forearm supinated. The examiner fully resists the patient's attempt to lift the hand towards the mouth. A painful weakness of elbow flexion may be present in bicipital tendinitis. A painless weakness may occur in C5 and C6 nerve root lesions.

Extension is also tested with the patient lying with the elbow flexed to a right angle and the forearm supinated. The examiner places one hand over the extensor aspect of the patient's wrist, who then attempts to extend the hand towards the floor. A painful weakness of this movement may occur in triceps tendinitis. A painless weakness usually indicates the presence of a C7 nerve root lesion and may be associated with a loss or diminution of the triceps reflex.

Supination is tested with the patient lying supine and the elbow flexed to a right angle with the forearm in the midposition. The examiner holds the hand of the patient who attempts to turn the palm to face upwards. Pain on resisted supination of the forearm may occur with a bicipital tendinitis.

Pronation is also tested with the patient lying supine and the elbow flexed to right angles with the forearm in the midposition. The examiner grips the hand of the patient, who then attempts to turn the palm face downwards. Pain on pronation may occur in medial epicondylitis.

Palpation

The elbow is best palpated with the patient lying supine and the elbow held in a position of approximately 70 degrees of flexion. If the right elbow is being palpated, the examiner supports the patient's forearm with his left hand and uses the right thumb and fingers to palpate. The olecranon process of the ulna lies subcutaneously and may be easily palpated, as can the triceps tendon which is inserted into it. In front of the olecranon, on the lower end of the humerus, the two small bony protuberances of the medial and lateral epicondyles of humerus are also easily palpable (Figure 7.1). When the elbow is fully extended these three bony landmarks can be felt to lie in a straight line but when the elbow is flexed to 90 degrees these three bony prominences form an isosceles triangle with its apex over the olecranon and its base between the two epicondyles. The area around both epicondyles should be tested for tenderness.

Above the epicondyles run the medial and lateral supracondylar ridges of the humerus. This ridge is easily felt on the medial side but needs deep palpation on the lateral side. The median nerve runs anteriorly to the medial supracondylar ridge. From the anterior aspect of the lateral epicondyle arise the musculotendinous origins of the wrist extensors and from the medial epicondyle arise the wrist flexors and pronators. They can be felt to contract by

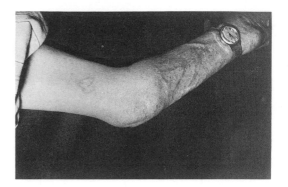

Figure 7.11 Synovial swelling in the elbow joint

palpating distally to the epicondyles while the patient clenches his fist.

A finger-breadth below the lateral epicondyle, the head of the radius can easily be felt as it moves while the forearm is rotated. The line of the radiohumeral joint can be palpated just above the radial head. The biceps tendon is easily palpated as it inserts into the radius in the middle of the cubital fossa on the anterior aspect of the elbow joint.

The space between the olecranon and the epicondyle is known as the paraolecranon groove. The synovial membrane lies close to the surface in the lateral paraolecranon groove (Figure 7.11) and synovitis can be easily palpated here as a slightly tender, soft swelling that bulges against the examining thumb as the elbow is slowly flexed and extended. The medial paraolecranon groove contains the ulnar nerve which can be rolled in its groove on the back of the medial humeral epicondyle; the nerve is palpated for any tenderness, swelling or thickening. The supratrochlear lymph nodes should be palpated just above the medial epicondyle.

Classification of elbow lesions

1   Soft tissue injuries.
    (a) Musculotendinous lesions.
        (i)   Lateral epicondylitis.
        (ii) Medial epicondylitis.
        (iii) Bicipital tendinitis.
        (iv) Triceps tendinitis.
    (b) Ligament sprains.
2   Joint lesions.
    (a) Pulled elbow.
    (b) Elbow stiffness.
    (c) Loose bodies.

3 Nerve entrapments.
   (a) Ulnar nerve.
   (b) Median nerve.
   (c) Radial nerve.

Soft tissue lesions

Musculotendinous lesions

Lateral epicondylitis

This condition occurs most often in the dominant arm of middle-aged patients, in females more commonly than males and is occasionally bilateral [2]. It occurs in patients whose occupation or sport involves excessive use of the wrist or supination or pronation of the forearm. Its onset may be gradual with an intermittent mild ache in the elbow. It can be sudden and in tennis players may follow either a mis-hit or a change in action. It may also follow a direct blow to the epicondylar region. Pain is felt originally over the lateral aspect of the elbow but when severe may radiate down the forearm into the dorsum of the hand and the middle and ring fingers. Pain is made worse especially on movements of the wrist, e.g. gripping and shaking hands may be particularly difficult. When severe, pain may disturb sleep.

Pain in the lateral aspect of the elbow and forearm may also be caused by C7 nerve root irritation but is usually associated then with paraesthesiae or other neurological signs, thus helping to differentiate it clinically

MAJOR SIGNS
Isometric contractions at the wrist reproduce elbow pain and several tests are available:
1 The patient with the elbow extended grips the examiner's index finger and attempts to lift his hand upwards. Pain is reproduced and the movement cannot be sustained because of painful weakness in the elbow (Figure 7.12).
2 The patient lies supine with elbow fully extended and the forearm pronated; the movement of wrist extension is then actively resisted.

OTHER SIGNS
Pain may also be reproduced by resisted radial deviation of the wrist or finger extension or on stretching the extensor muscles of the forearm by passively flexing the wrist and fingers with the elbow extended. Resisted movements of the elbow joint itself do not reproduce pain.

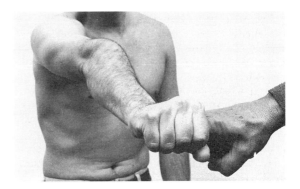

Figure 7.12 Test for lateral epicondylitis. The patient grips the examiner's fingers with the elbow extended and attempts to lift his arm

Loss of the last few degrees of passive extension is almost always present in the affected elbow compared with the normal side. The pain response and the end-feel of extension also indicate the loss of normal movement. Accessory movements, especially adduction in the fully extended position, usually show some restriction of movement and these tests may also reproduce the patient's pain. Palpation localizes the site of tenderness directly over the anterior aspect of the lateral epicondyle but it may occur more distally over the tendon or at the musculotendinous junction. Rarely, the site of tenderness may be in the muscle belly itself, over the annular ligament of the superior radioulnar joint or over the articular cartilage of the head of the radius.

Radiographs of the elbow usually are normal for the patient's age but small areas of calcification may at times be seen in the extensor origin [2].

AETIOLOGY
Many causes have been suggested and a single lesion evidently cannot adequately explain the aetiology in all cases [3]. The fibrous origin of the common extensor tendons from the lateral epicondyle is the usual site involved and this condition may be looked on as a form of enthesitis. The most likely explanation appears to be that an area of soft tissue degeneration develops at this site in the origin of the extensor carpi radialis brevis and that this area develops a tear, an inflammatory change or both. Degenerative changes commonly occur in this area probably as a result of ageing, repeated loading, or microtrauma [4], and are also the basis for the calcification that may ultimately develop. As the blood supply to this area is relatively poor in middle age, healing is slow and the lesion tends to become chronic.

Muscles that span two joints, such as the hamstrings, are commonly torn as a result of uncoordinated movements. The extensor of the wrist also spans two joints, the elbow and wrist, and uncoordinated movement is even more likely as the extensor arises partly from the surrounding mobile ligaments and aponeuroses. Should a tear occur, the lack of blood supply would again make healing extremely difficult.

Inflammatory changes may arise from overuse after repetitive wrist movements, either occupational or during sporting activity, and involve especially the tenoperiosteal origin from the lateral epicondyle.

Chondromalacia of the radial head may follow repeated pronation and supination with compression of the posteromedial aspect of the radial head. Other causes described include an entrapment neuropathy, known as the radial tunnel syndrome [3] and stenosis of the annular ligament. The role of cervical spine degenerative changes in the causation of epicondylitis has always been controversial. Many reports rely on radiographic changes in the cervical spine alone for confirmatory evidence and in this age group such changes are a common and often asymptomatic finding. Treatment to the neck only rarely produces any alteration to the symptoms.

MANAGEMENT

This condition tends to run a protracted course, with exacerbations and remissions often lasting up to 2 years, before most cases undergo natural remission [5].

1   Rest. The patient needs to rest from those activities associated with this condition. These usually involve prolonged gripping with the wrist, such as tennis. Resting is often difficult for the patient, who should be reassured that the condition tends to be self-limiting over a long period of time and that other treatments will not often be helpful unless activity is curtailed. Immobilization of the forearm and wrist in a cock-up splint is not recommended as it is most inconvenient and symptoms usually return after the wrist has been taken out of plaster.
2   Medication. Anti-inflammatory drugs are given as there is an inflammatory component to this disorder and they help to relieve pain.
3   Injections. An injection of corticosteroid is usually the quickest and most effective method of treatment but it must be accurately placed. The patient sits with the elbow flexed to a right angle and the site of maximal tenderness is found by

careful palpation with the examiner's thumb. He then places the left thumb over the patient's lateral epicondyle and the fingers are spread out around the elbow to steady it. A 25-gauge needle is used for the injection and so local anaesthetic need not be infiltrated into the overlying skin. An injection of 1 ml of corticosteroid solution and 1 ml of local anaesthetic is injected into and around the tender area. In the tenoperiosteal variety of epicondylitis it is necessary to direct the needle against the epicondyle and inject a small volume of solution into this area.

The patient is advised to rest the wrist and elbow for a week and is warned that there may be exacerbation of pain for a day or two after the injection, which may require analgesics. If after a week the pain is not fully relieved the injection may be repeated at intervals varying from 7 to 14 days. The injection may be repeated several times but if only transient relief is being obtained this treatment should not continue. If after a week, one injection has sufficed and the elbow is pain free, the management of the patient is similar to that discussed below for aftercare.

4   Physical methods. Ice, heat and deep-pressure massage have been advocated but are rarely successful in long-term management and ultrasound may be more effective.
5   Mobilization techniques. These are helpful especially when, as is usual, examination has demonstrated loss of full passive elbow extension and loss of the normal accessory movements with a painful limitation in the range of extension–adduction.

If the passive range of extension is limited, mobilization techniques using large-amplitude extension movements at the limit of the range should be used first for 20–40 s. On the first day of treatment this technique should be repeated only once but on subsequent days treatment may be increased gradually lest it cause an exacerbation of symptoms. Treatment is performed daily for about 10 days and then on alternate days until full extension is possible.

If the accessory movement of extension–adduction is painfully limited treatment consists of small amplitude stretching movements at the limit of the range by:
(a)   Rocking the elbow medially from the abducted to the adducted position while holding the elbow just short of full extension.
(b)   Holding the elbow adducted and moving it in an arc through the last 5 degrees of extension and then back into 5 degrees of flexion.

(c) Moving the elbow in an arc from extension–abduction into extension–adduction, followed by a movement into 10 degrees of flexion while holding the elbow in adduction and then releasing the adduction strain (Figure 7.4).

6 Manipulation is performed using the Mill's technique but it does not often produce lasting benefits. The usual reason given for any success is that it stretches the extensor origin at the lateral epicondyle to separate the edges of any tear or scar tissue present. This may not be correct and it may work by restoring normal accessory movements to the elbow joint. This manipulation must never be performed if the elbow lacks extension.

Starting position. The patient is seated with the shoulder abducted and the arm medially rotated so that the lateral epicondyle is facing forwards. Stand behind the patient's shoulder and passively move the forearm into full pronation and the wrist into flexion with his right hand. The thumb is placed over the patient's palm with the fingers spread over the dorsum of the hand. The heel of the left hand is placed over the lower end of the patient's humerus (Figure 7.13a).

Method. The elbow is suddenly forced into full extension with the examiner's left hand while maintaining full flexion at the patient's wrist. The lower end of the humerus is pushed forward and this movement is not produced by pulling the forearm forwards (Figure 7.13b).

7 Aftercare

(a) The extensor muscles in the forearm should be passively stretched and strengthening exercises given before return to full activity [6]. It is important to ensure that the return to active sport is gradual [4].

(b) Correction of any provoking cause, such as poor technique [7], in consultation with a coach, and a double-handed back hand style may be preferred.

(c) This lesion may follow an alteration in the type of racquet used and its balance may need adjusting.

(d) The grip on the racquet handle may need to be altered. Experiments should be carried out to discover whether the grip should be enlarged [8].

(e) A brace for the forearm is useful to alter the leverage on the forearm muscles and relieve strain on the elbow [9]. The support made of calico is kept tightly in place with Velcro straps. It should only be worn during activities involving use of the forearm.

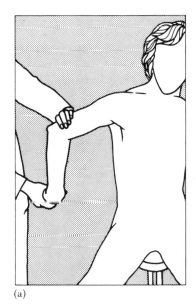

(a)

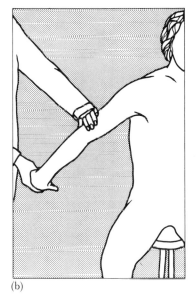

(b)

Figure 7.13 (a) and (b) Mill's manipulation

8 Surgery. Surgery for patients resistant to conservative therapy or who have recurrent problems [10] is only rarely indicated. Several operations have been described. The most common is a tenotomy and stripping of the common extensor origin and is usually combined with debridement of any chronic granulation tissue. Active rehabilitation and an early return to sport after the operation are essential. A tenotomy may also be performed as a closed procedure under local

anaesthesia, using either a beaver-eye blade, a tenotome or even a wide-bore needle. The tenoperiosteal origin is detached by a series of sweeping incisions [11,12]. An acute tear may be successfully repaired.

Medial epicondylitis

A similar but less common condition occurs over the medial epicondyle, the site of origin of the wrist flexors and the pronator of the forearm. It is also known as golfer's elbow but often occurs in people who have never played golf. It occurs in middle-aged patients, often involved in sporting or occupational activities that require a strong hand grip and an adduction movement of the elbow. Pain is experienced over the medial compartment of the elbow and may radiate distally. It is made worse by wrist movements, especially gripping or repeated wrist flexion.

MAJOR SIGNS

Pain is reproduced by an isometric contraction of the wrist flexors, which is tested by having the patient lie with the elbow extended and supinated, and gripping the examiner's finger. Alternatively, fully resisting flexion of the wrist may reproduce the elbow pain.

OTHER SIGNS

Pain may also be reproduced by fully resisting pronation of the forearm or stretching the flexor muscle group by fully extending the supine forearm and then passively hyperextending the wrist. Tenderness on palpation is usually felt under the medial epicondyle.

MANAGEMENT

This is similar to that outlined for lateral epicondylitis: rest, medication, local corticosteroid injections and mobilization techniques. A forced manipulation, as with the Mill's technique, is not indicated.

Bicipital tendinitis

This is uncommon. Pain, usually well localized to the middle of the cubital fossa, is reproduced by fully resisting either elbow flexion or supination or by stretching the tendon, best achieved by extending the elbow and then applying full passive pronation to the forearm. Accessory movements in the superior radioulnar joint are commonly restricted. An area of tenderness may be palpated with the elbow flexed to 90 degrees, over the insertion of the biceps tendon into the bicipital tuberosity of the radius [13].

MANAGEMENT INCLUDES:

1 Injection. The tender area in the tendon insertion is injected using a 25-gauge needle carefully inserted alongside the insertion, so as not to inject into the tendon.
2 Deep-friction massage. This may be used across the tendon insertion as an alternative method of treatment.
3 Accessory movements in the superior radioulnar joint. If these are limited and painful, passive movement techniques using large amplitude pronation movements in the pain-free range. The patient lies supine with the elbow flexed to a right angle and the forearm pronated. The therapist places the left hand over the dorsum of the patient's wrist and supports under the elbow with the right hand. As movement improves and pain subsides, small-amplitude stretching movements are used at the limit of the range of pronation and compression may be added.

Triceps tendinitis

This is rare. It follows the sudden severe strain to the triceps tendon, e.g. in javelin throwers, as the arm is fully extended. Pain is reproduced on fully resisting extension of the elbow while the patient stands with the elbow flexed and forearm fully supinated. An area of tenderness may be palpated over the insertion of the triceps tendon into the olecranon.

Ligament sprains

The elbow joint is stabilized by medial, lateral and collateral ligaments such as thickenings in the dense capsule, and the annular ligament. Ligaments are damaged, particularly by hyperextension and lateral motion injuries. A third-degree sprain may avulse a fragment of bone.

Assessment of collateral ligament instability is performed with the elbow flexed approximately by 15 degrees. Valgus instability is tested with the arm in lateral rotation; varus instability with the arm in medial rotation.

Joint lesions

Pulled elbow

This common, dramatic condition occurs in young children who present with a painful inability to use

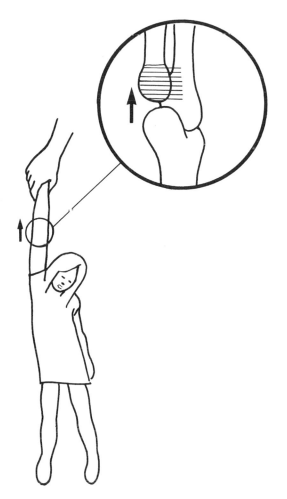

Figure 7.14 Pulled elbow: mechanism of production

lifting the child out of the bath or up from the floor, lifting the child's arm as the adult goes up a step or if the child is being swung by the arms in play. Occasionally the child will trip or fall and is grabbed by the arm, which is jerked upwards.

The onset of pain may be accompanied by an audible or palpable click in the elbow. The child cries and refuses to use the arm. As the pain may be poorly localized, diagnosis can be difficult; either the neck, shoulder, elbow or wrist may be considered as the site of the problem and the differential diagnosis may include a brachial plexus injury. Even in the absence of a classical history, subluxation of the radial head should be suspected in any child who complains of arm pain with restricted elbow movements.

Examination usually shows a crying child who carries the affected arm limply by the side or supported on the lap. There is no obvious elbow swelling, which is held slightly flexed with the forearm held pronated or in the midposition. A useful manoeuvre is to stand on the child's painful side and offer him a sweet. The child does not use the nearby, painful arm to take it but reaches across with the other, painless arm. With suitable encouragement normal shoulder and wrist movements may be demonstrated but there may be a small loss in the range of passive elbow flexion and extension. However, any attempt at producing supination beyond the midposition produces tearful and often violent resistance from the child. Radiographs are usually normal but some subtle changes have been described [19,23].

the arm [14]. It is caused by subluxation of the head of the radius after a traction injury, and is completely and rapidly cured by manipulation.

Clinical features

It occurs in young children before the age of 8 years, with a peak incidence between 2 and 3 years [15] and has been reported under the age of 6 months [16]. The youngest child we have seen was aged 10 months. It is at least twice as common in the left elbow as the right and girls are affected twice as commonly [15–22] and may be hypermobile [22].

The history is of sudden traction applied to the child's arm while held in an extended and pronated position above the head by an adult, who then lifts the child's hand suddenly upwards (Figure 7.14). This may occur in many different situations, e.g.

Mechanism

Because the lesion occurs only in young children, anatomical factors are considered to be responsible with the head of the radius pulled through the normally restraining fibres of the annular radioulnar ligament. Salter and Zahn [17] applied traction at post mortem to the elbow while it was held extended in supination and could not produce this subluxation. However, when traction was applied, as in the clinical setting, to the extended elbow held in pronation, a transverse tear could easily be produced in the distal attachment of the annular ligament to the neck of the radius. The head of the radius can then readily slip through the tear, the annular ligament becomes detached and is interposed between the head of the radius and the capitulum (Figure 7.15). Button-holing of the ligament would then produce a painful block to active supination. The ligament is released after manipulation and can heal when

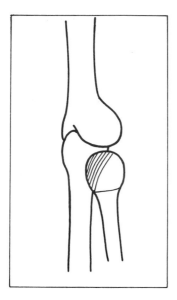

Figure 7.15 Annular ligament displaced over the head of the radius in pulled elbow

repositioned in its normal anatomical relationship. The age incidence is related to the fact that until about the age of 5 years the attachments of the ligament are thin and easily disrupted whereas above this age the attachments become increasingly thicker.

Recurrent attacks may occur [15,21] and cause diagnostic confusion with child abuse [16].

Management

Manipulation is simple, effective and usually produces a dramatic cure. The child's confidence is first gained by gently supporting the injured arm. The left hand is placed around the child's elbow to support it with the thumb placed over the head of the radius. The child's hand is held in the therapist's right hand and the forearm is suddenly and firmly forced into full supination. A palpable and often audible click can usually be detected in the region of the radial head as the subluxation is reduced. The child usually stops crying and starts to use the arm again, although this may be delayed for several hours if it has been present for some time. This manipulative reduction is sometimes achieved by a radiographer when the forearm is forcibly supinated to obtain a true anteroposterior radiograph. Only in a very small percentage of patients does the manipulation fail at the first attempt [24] and it is then

necessary to put the arm in a sling [17] and repeat the manipulation the next day.

The child needs no active treatment after the pulled elbow is reduced but the parents are carefully instructed on the mechanism of the injury to prevent the possibility of a recurrence.

Elbow stiffness

A fall onto the outstretched hand may damage the articular cartilage of the radiohumeral joint, e.g. after a Colles' fracture, elbow stiffness may develop leading ultimately to osteoarthritis. With myositis ossificans, which follows a haemorrhage into the capsule or the brachialis muscle, elbow movements become severely limited and the ossified mass is usually easily palpable.

Treatment of elbow stiffness

Mobilization techniques with physiological and accessory movements are used. If the range of flexion is limited, the elbow is flexed to the limit of its range, and small-amplitude oscillatory movements are performed slowly for about 1 min to stretch the joint. This is followed by small-amplitude accessory movements performed at the limit of flexion: distraction, flexion–adduction and flexion–abduction. The physiological and accessory movements are repeated three times and the range of passive flexion again measured. The patient is then reassessed to find whether there has been any painful reaction. If so, the strength and amount of treatment must be reduced; if not, treatment is repeated more strongly. Over the next few days this routine is repeated and if the patient is improving active movements are added to increase the range and increase muscle strength. If there is no improvement it is most unlikely that passive movement techniques will be successful.

If the range of extension is limited, the principles of treatment are similar but the physiological movement of extension and the three accessory movements of distraction, extension–adduction and extension–abduction are used.

Treatment of painful, stiff elbow

If the elbow movements are limited more by pain than by stiffness, large-amplitude flexion movements within the pain-free range are used as the mobilization technique. These are continued for 1 min and the physiological movements reassessed. If pain has not been exacerbated, this treatment is repeated four times. On the following days, the range of movement and behaviour of pain throughout this range are reassessed. If they have improved, treatment is continued; if not, the movement should be carried out in the painful range. If it causes an exacerbation of pain, treatment should be discontinued and the treatment outlined above for the stiff elbow substituted.

Loose bodies

Aetiology

1 Loose bony foreign bodies may arise as the result of previous trauma to the joint, especially in rugby players and wrestlers who often fall onto the elbow.
2 Osteoarthritis may produce either a loose cartilaginous or bony foreign body.
3 Osteochondritis dissecans occurs usually in young males [25] involving the capitulum of the right humerus. At times there may be no history of direct trauma and the patient presents with a gradual onset of pain and stiffness in the elbow.
4 Synovial osteochondromatosis with multiple loose bodies occasionally occurs in the elbow (Figure 7.16).

Patients present with varying degrees of pain, locking, stiffness and swelling of the elbow. Pain usually comes in sudden attacks associated with locking of the joint. In the usual pattern, there is a

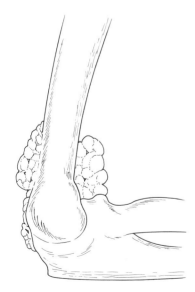

Figure 7.16 Osteochondromatosis

block to full extension but flexion remains full and painless. Synovial swelling is usually present.

Management

The elbow is usually locked in extension and manipulation is used to attempt to free the joint. The elbow is extended to the limit of its range and then rocked backwards and forwards through the full range of abduction to adduction, at the same time easing the elbow into extension. If the loose body is freed the elbow suddenly moves into full extension.

Arthroscopy is indicated for diagnosis and removal of loose bodies, assessment of any degenerative changes [26–30] or trapped synovial fringes [29].

Entrapment neuropathies

Ulnar nerve

The ulnar nerve passes behind the medial epicondyle in a groove converted into a fibro-osseous canal, the cubital tunnel, by the arcuate ligament that runs from the medial epicondyle to the olecranon. This ligament is taut at 90 degrees of flexion. The bony floor of this tunnel, formed by the humerus, is lined by the medial ligament of the elbow, which also bulges in flexion. An entrapment neuropathy of the ulnar nerve in the cubital tunnel is common [31,32] especially after prolonged flexion of the elbow. The ulnar nerve enters the forearm by passing between the two heads of the flexor carpi ulnaris where it is covered by an aponeurosis and may also be the site of entrapment [33].

Aetiology

1 Acute trauma. The nerve lies superficially in its groove and may be damaged by a single traumatic episode.
2 Repeated trauma usually occurs from occupations that involve leaning on the elbow.
3 Previous trauma to the elbow may result in a cubitus valgus deformity that gradually stretches the nerve. The deformity and symptoms take some time to develop (tardy ulnar palsy).
4 Cubitus valgus may also result from arthritis.
5 As the nerve is tethered in its groove, overuse of the elbow can also produce an entrapment neuropathy.
6 The nerve may sometimes sublux in and out of the groove on elbow movements.

Clinical features

Symptoms are mainly sensory with pain and/or paraesthesiae, hyperaesthesia or numbness in the sensory distribution of the nerve in the medial one and a half fingers. Clumsiness of the hand may result from weakness of the intrinsic muscles.

On examination, there may be weakness and wasting of the hypothenar eminence and the intrinsic muscles of the hand, often best seen in the first dorsal interosseous space. The typical hand deformity is hyperextension at the metacarpophalangeal joints owing to intrinsic muscle weakness, and the ulnar two fingers are cocked up because of weakness of their flexor digitorum profundus tendons. Sensation may be disturbed on the palmar or dorsal aspects of the ulnar one and a half fingers and/or on the ulnar side of the palm of the hand.

The sensory symptoms may be reproduced by pressure over the ulnar nerve behind the medial epicondyle where tenderness or thickening of the nerve may be palpable when compared with the nerve in the other elbow. Tinel's sign may also be positive and symptoms may be reproduced on sustained full passive flexion of the elbow and wrist for 3 min [34]. Palpation over the ulnar nerve while the elbow is flexed and extended may demonstrate that the nerve subluxes in and out of its groove.

Diagnosis needs to be confirmed by nerve conduction tests because similar symptoms may arise from lesions in the neck, such as thoracic outlet syndrome or an entrapment neuropathy of the C8 nerve root.

Management

1 Avoid local trauma by use of foam-rubber elbow pads worn continuously.
2 Extra rest to the elbow, especially by avoiding repeated or excessive flexion.
3 Injections. An injection of corticosteroid may be given along the groove behind the medial epicondyle. If the site of entrapment is between the two heads of the flexor carpi ulnaris, palpation may reveal a localized area of tenderness which can be injected.
4 Surgery. Anterior transposition of the nerve may be combined with excision of the medial epicondyle or division of the tendinous origin of the flexor carpi ulnaris [31]. Surgery needs to be performed early [35] as late operations may produce poor results [33,36].

Median nerve

The median nerve crosses the medial side of the lower end of the humerus above the elbow. In this area a vestigial ligament may persist. The nerve runs under this ligament in a fibro-osseous canal. Below the elbow, the nerve passes through the two heads of origin of the pronator teres muscle. An entrapment neuropathy is rare but may occur in one of these two sites, either above or below the elbow.

Sensory symptoms are similar to those produced by a carpal tunnel syndrome as the nerve innervates the lateral three and a half fingers. However, motor symptoms are different and may include weakness of pronation of the forearm, flexion of the wrist, opposition of the thumb or flexion of the index and middle fingers. If the site of entrapment is in the pronator teres, symptoms may be aggravated by pronation of the forearm as occurs when using a screwdriver.

Radial nerve

The radial nerve at the elbow divides into two branches: one superficial and mainly sensory, the other deep and mainly motor [37]. The latter, also known as the posterior interosseous nerve, passes under the fibrous origin of the extensor carpi radialis brevis, then pierces the supinator muscles to pass along the interosseous membrane, where it supplies the extensor muscles in the forearm, to reach the wrist [38].

The radial tunnel syndrome [3,39,40] produces lateral or anterolateral elbow pain, and may be labelled as a lateral epicondylitis. It may follow repetitive rotary movements and be reproduced on resisted supination or resisted extension of the middle finger [3]. Treatment is by local injection into the tender area or surgery [39].

Entrapment of the superficial branch may cause pain and altered sensation over the radial aspect of the wrist or thumb.

References

1 Andrews, J.R. and Carson, W.G. (1985) Arthroscopy of the elbow. *Arthroscopy*, **1**, 97–107
2 Wadsworth, T.G. (1987) Tennis elbow: conservative, surgical and manipulative treatment. *British Medical Journal*, **294**, 621–624
3 Watrous, B.G. and Ho, G. Jr. (1988) Elbow pain. *Primary Care*, **15**, 725–735
4 Nirschl, R.P. (1988) Prevention and treatment of elbow and shoulder injuries in the tennis player. *Clinics in Sports Medicine*, **7**, 289–308
5 Gerberich, S.G. and Priest, J.D. (1985) Treatment for lateral epicondylitis: Variables related to recovery. *British Journal of Sports Medicine*, **19**, 224–227
6 Wilkerson, G.B. (1984) Preventing epicondylitis. *Physician and Sportsmedicine*, **12**, 194–197

7 Legwold, G. (1984) Tennis elbow: joint resolution by conservative treatment and improved technique. *Physician and Sportsmedicine*, **12**, 168–182

8 Kamien, M. (1988) Tennis elbow in long-time tennis players. *Australian Journal of Science and Medicine in Sport*, June, 19–27

9 Burton, A.K. (1985) Grip strength and forearm straps in tennis elbow. *British Journal of Sports Medicine*, **19**, 37–38

10 Goldberg, E.J., Abraham, E. and Siegel, I. (1988) The surgical treatment of chronic lateral humeral epicondylitis by common extensor release. *Clinical Orthopaedics*, **233**, 208–212 ⌐

11 Baumgard, S.H. and Schwartz, D.R. (1982) Percutaneous release of the epicondylar muscles for humeral epicondylitis. *American Journal of Sports Medicine*, **10**, 233–236

12 Murtagh, J. (1988) Tennis elbow. *Australian Family Physician*, **17**, 90–95

13 Nielsen, K. (1987) Partial rupture of the distal biceps brachii tendon. A case report. *Acta Orthopaedica Scandinavica*, **58**, 287–288

14 Jongschaap, H.A., Youngson, G.G. and Beattie, T.F. (1990) The epidemiology of radial head subluxation ('pulled elbow') in the Aberdeen city area. *Health Bulletin Edinburgh*, **48**, 58–61

15 Quan, L. and Marcuse, E.K. (1985) The epidemiology and treatment of radial head subluxation. *American Journal of Diseases of Children*, **139**, 1194–1197

16 Newman, J. (1985) Nursemaid's elbow in infants six months and under. *Journal of Emergency Medicine*, **2**, 403–404

17 Salter, R.B. and Zahn, C. (1971) Anatomic investigation of the mechanism of injury and pathologic anatomy of 'pulled elbow' in young children. *Clinical Orthopaedics and Related Research*, **77**, 134–143

18 David, M.L. (1987) Radial head subluxation. *American Family Physician*, **35**, 143–146

19 Frumkin, K. (1985) Nursemaid's elbow: a radiographic demonstration. *Annals of Emergency Medicine*, **14**, 690–693

20 Corrigan, A.B. (1965) The pulled elbow. *Medical Journal of Australia*, **11**, 187–189

21 Illingworth, C.M. (1975) Pulled elbow: A study of 100 patients. *British Medical Journal*, **11**, 672–674

22 Amir, D., Frankl, U. and Pogrund, H. (1990) Pulled elbow and hypermobility of joints. *Clinical Orthopaedics*, **257**, 94–99

23 Snyder, H.S. (1990) Radiographic changes with radial head subluxation in children. *Journal of Emergency Medicine*, **8**, 265–269

24 Schunk, J.E. (1990) Radial head subluxation: epidemiology and treatment of 87 episodes. *Annals of Emergency Medicine*, **19**, 1019–1023

25 Jackson, D.W., Silvino, N. and Reimann, P. (1989) Osteochondritis in the female gymnast's elbow. *Arthroscopy*, **5**, 129–136

26 Guhl, J.F. (1985) Arthroscopy and arthroscopic surgery of the elbow. *Orthopaedics*, **8**, 1290–1296

27 Boe, S. (1986) Arthroscopy of the elbow. Diagnosis and extraction of loose bodies. *Acta Orthopaedica Scandinavica*, **57**, 52–53

28 Morrey, B.F. (1986) Arthroscopy of the elbow. *Instrument Course Lecture*, **35**, 102–107

29 Clarke, R.P. (1988) Symptomatic lateral synovial fringe (plica) of the elbow joint. *Arthroscopy*, **4**, 112–116

30 Poehling, G.G., Whipple, T.L., Sisco, L. and Goldman, B. (1989) Elbow arthroscopy: A new technique. *Arthroscopy*, **5**, 222–224.

31 Hirsch, L.F. and Thanki, A. (1985) Ulnar nerve entrapment at the elbow. Tailoring the treatment to the cause. *Postgraduate Medicine*, **77**, 211–215

32 Dellon, A.L. and Mackinnon, S.E. (1988) Human ulnar neuropathy at the elbow: clinical, electrical, and morphometric correlations. *Journal of Reconstruction Microsurgery*, **4**, 179–184

33 Amadio, P.C. (1986) Anatomical basis for a technique of ulnar nerve transposition. *Surgical and Radiologic Anatomy*, **8**, 155–161

34 Buchler, M.J. and Thayer, D.T. (1988) The elbow flexion test. A clinical test for the cubital tunnel syndrome. *Clinical Orthopaedics*, **233**, 213–216

35 Friedman, R.J. and Cochran, T.P. (1986) Anterior transposition for advanced ulnar neuropathy at the elbow. *Surgical Neurology*, **25**, 446–448

36 Friedman, R.J. and Cochran, T.P. (1987) A clinical and electrophysiological investigation of anterior transposition for ulnar neuropathy at the elbow. *Archives of Orthopedic and Trauma Surgery*, **106**, 375–380

37 Kaplan, P.E. (1984) Posterior interosseous neuropathies: natural history. *Archives of Physical and Medical Rehabilitation*, **65**, 399–400

38 Papilion, J.D., Neff, R.S. and Shall, L.M. (1988) Compression neuropathy of the radial nerve as a complication of elbow arthroscopy: A case report and review of the literature. *Arthroscopy*, **4**, 284–286

39 Moss, S.H. and Switzer, H.E. (1983) Radial tunnel syndrome: a spectrum of clinical presentations. *Journal of Hand Surgery*, **8**, 414–420

40 Rosen, I. and Werner, C.O. (1980) Neurophysiological investigation of posterior interosseous nerve entrapment causing lateral elbow pain. *Electroencephalography and Clinical Neurophysiology*, **50**, 125–133

8 Wrist and hand

The wrist is a functional unit made up of the joints between the distal ends of the radius and ulna with the carpal bones. The three joints so formed are:

1 Inferior radioulnar joint: movements produce supination and pronation as the radius rotates around the head of the ulna.
2 Radiocarpal joint: between the distal end of the radius and three bones in the proximal row of the carpus (the scaphoid, lunate and triquetrum; Figure 8.1).
3 Midcarpal joint: formed between the proximal and the distal rows of the carpal bones (Figure 8.2).

Function

The function of the wrist is to position the hand in space and to transmit forces from or to the hand.

This requires a great degree of mobility and stability.

Active wrist movements produce flexion, extension, radial deviation, ulnar deviation and a combined movement of circumduction. This large range of movement takes place in a compound joint, the radiocarpal and midcarpal joints (Figure 8.1).

Flexion–extension or adduction–abduction are rarely pure movements and the usual plane of movement is from extension–radial deviation to flexion–ulnar deviation.

Radiocarpal movements are accompanied by alterations in the shape and direction of the proximal carpal row mainly. The proximal row of carpal bones acts as an intercalated segment in a mechanical linkage system made up of three longitudinal carpal chains. These bones change shape as they are displaced during movement [1–3].

Flexion of the wrist is a combined movement that takes place mostly at the midcarpal joints and is of greater range than extension (Figure 8.3a).

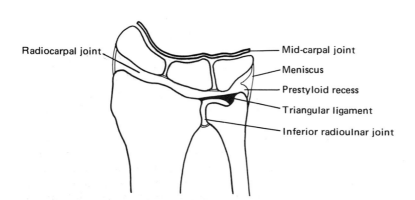

Radiocarpal joint — Mid-carpal joint
— Meniscus
— Prestyloid recess
— Triangular ligament
— Inferior radioulnar joint

Figure 8.1 The wrist

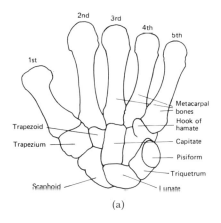

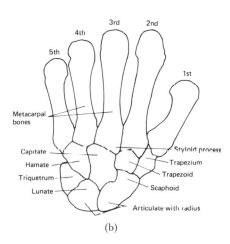

Figure 8.2 Carpal and metacarpal bones of the left hand.
(a) Palmar aspect; (b) dorsal aspect

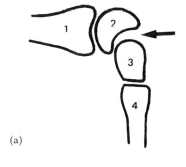

(a)

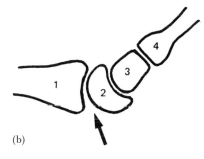

(b)

Figure 8.3 Wrist, showing: 1, radius; 2, lunate; 3, capitate; 4, metacarpal. Flexion (a) takes place mainly in the midcarpal joint. Extension (b) takes place mainly in the radiocarpal joint

Extension of the wrist (Figure 8.3b) is also a combined movement but the range is greater at the radiocarpal than at the midcarpal joint [2]. During flexion and extension the lunate and capitate bones rotate synchronously; on flexion the space between the dorsal surfaces of the two bones widens and on extension the space between their palmar surfaces widens.

In radial deviation the proximal row of carpal bones and midcarpal joint slide reciprocally in an ulnar direction, the lunate flexes and moves to a position under the inferior radioulnar joint. The distal end of the scaphoid also flexes and volar rotates [4]. The space between the lunate and triquetrum becomes slightly wider and the capitate slides in an ulnar and proximal direction to become tight-packed. Ulnar deviation of the radiocarpal joint causes the proximal row of carpal bones and the midcarpal joint to glide reciprocally in a radial direction. In this position the scaphoid becomes elongated and the space between it and lunate is slightly widened. The proximal row extends and the lunate rotates into the palm.

Movements of the carpometacarpal joint

The joint surfaces of the carpometacarpal joint of the thumb are quite different from those of the second to fifth fingers and permit flexion, extension, abduction, adduction, rotation and circumduction. The joints of digits two to five have a small rotary movement of horizontal flexion and extension. The movement is obvious during opposition of the head of the first metacarpal towards that of the fifth metacarpal. If the movement from horizontal flexion (cupping the palm) to horizontal extension (flattening the palm) is viewed from the back of the hand, the fifth and fourth metacarpals move much more than the third and second metacarpals.

Active movements of the metacarpophalangeal joint

Movements of the metacarpophalangeal joint are flexion, extension, adduction and abduction. The metacarpophalangeal joint, involved in nearly all hand function, is subject to great stress from surrounding muscles. Their movements are not a simple hinge type and functionally a pure flexion–extension movement only occurs in the hook grip, as used in carrying a bag. Flexion is usually combined with a degree of ulnar deviation and rotation in most functional movements, e.g. when the finger is opposed to the thumb in precision grips or to the thenar eminence in palmar grips. Abduction and adduction are accompanied by a gliding movement of the proximal phalanx on the metacarpal head, limited by tightening of the collateral ligaments. Stability is supplied by the joint capsule and its collateral ligaments as the bony joint surfaces are incongruous. This provides more strength at the expense of stability and the joint readily becomes unstable when ligament stretching and muscle imbalance occur as in rheumatoid arthritis.

Interphalangeal joints

The proximal joint formed between the concave articular head of the proximal phalanx and the convex base of the middle phalanx is a hinge joint and the movements of flexion and extension take place by gliding.

The terminal joints have a similar anatomical arrangement and the only active movements in these hinge joints are flexion and extension.

Hand function

The hand has many functions; it may be used as a tactile organ, a means of expression and a weapon. Its major musculoskeletal function lies in its ability to grip objects. As the hand is required to function as a unit, grip can never be fully measured in terms of movement of the individual joints. The word grip implies the final static phase of the necessary movements involved; prehension, which implies a taking hold or grasping, is also used. Grip is divided into (1) precision or (2) power grip [5].

Precision grip

The object has to be picked up and manipulated by the fingers and thumb. This dynamic movement is mainly a radial-sided movement as the pad of the thumb is manipulated mainly against the next two fingers. Three types of grip, according to the area of contact, are:

1 Tip pinch, in which the pad of the thumb is opposed to the tip of the index finger.
2 Lateral or key pinch, in which the pad of the thumb is opposed to the side of the index finger.
3 Palmar pinch, in which the pad of the thumb is opposed to the pad of one or, more commonly, two pads of the fingers, used for picking up and holding an object.

Power grip

The object is picked up and held tightly as in a clamp. The ulnar two fingers flex across towards the thenar eminence. In the final posture the thenar and hypothenar eminence are used as buttresses and the fingers flex around the object to be grasped. The thumb is used either with its pulp pressed against an object or else wrapped over a heavy object. The crude form of this grip is used while gripping a heavy object such as a hammer and the thumb is used to provide stability and power. A more refined power grip, or ulnar grip, is used when a lighter object lying across the palm is gripped mainly by the two ulnar fingers and the thumb is used only for control. With all power grips the hand is kept stable and the power movements are produced by either ulnar and radial deviation of the wrist, as in the action of hammering, or by supination and pronation of the hand, or by flexion and extension of the elbow.

Examination of the hand and wrist

1 Inspection.
   (a) Posture.
   (b) Swelling.

(c) Deformities.
(d) Muscle wasting.
(e) Skin changes.
2 Movements.
  (a) Active.
  (b) Passive.
  (c) Accessory.
  (d) Isometric.
3 Palpation.
  (a) Warmth.
  (b) Swelling.
  (c) Crepitus.
  (d) Tenderness.

Inspection

Posture

The hand and wrist are inspected for any abnormalities in posture, which should begin as the patient is first met. The normal hand posture is derived from its three arches, one longitudinal and two transverse, and the hand is normally held slightly flexed. A painful or stiff hand may restrict the normal swinging movement of the arm, as the hand is held stiffly by the side. A patient may be unwilling to use the hand or it may be held splinted across the chest. The hand may also provide a clue to the clinical diagnosis of numerous systemic disease processes.

Swelling

Swelling may be either intra- or extra-articular. Intra-articular swelling may either affect bone, and is then usually caused by osteoarthritis, or affect the soft tissues, when it is usually the result of a synovial effusion with inflamed and thickened synovium (Figure 8.4).

Synovitis of the wrist usually presents as a diffuse swelling, commonly on the dorsum of the wrist. It is easily confused with tenosynovitis of the surrounding extensor tendon sheaths which may also be clinically involved. Synovitis of the metacarpophalangeal and proximal interphalangeal joints bulges onto the looser tissues on the extensor surface of the hand; its shape is determined by the synovial attachments around the joints so that it is limited distally and spreads more proximally on either side of the extensor tendon. This gives it a characteristic fusiform or spindle-shaped appearance. The effusion is usually evident on inspection but in the early stages of metacarpophalangeal synovitis the hand should be

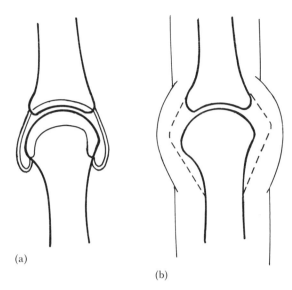

(a)

(b)

Figure 8.4 (a) Reflection of the synovium in MCP and IP joints; (b) this accounts for the spindle-shape of the synovial swelling bulging on the extensor surface

inspected with the fingers clenched into a fist, when the effusion may become apparent by filling in of the normal valley between the metacarpal heads. Synovitis produces a diffuse swelling within the synovial joint and can be easily differentiated from traumatic swellings of the articular structures, which usually form a localized swelling on one side of the joint.

Extra-articular swelling may be either diffuse or localized. Diffuse swelling of the hand is usually due to oedema which may result from venous or lymphatic obstruction but also occurs in the early stages of rheumatoid arthritis, scleroderma, the shoulder–hand syndrome or Sudeck's atrophy. Diffuse swelling of a digit produces a sausage-shaped deformity which may be caued by psoriatic arthritis or Reiter's disease with synovitis in the proximal interphalangeal joints and the tendon sheaths.

Localized swellings may involve the soft tissues around a joint and tendon sheaths. Tenosynovitis of the wrist may occur in the extensor, flexor or ulnar tendon sheaths. In the palm and fingers it usually involves the flexor tendon sheath and may then be associated with nodule formation and triggering of the finger or thumb. Swelling over the radial styloid occurs in de Quervain's disease. Localized swellings may be rheumatoid nodules, tophi, ganglia, granuloma annulare, calcinosis, Garrod's pads, Dupuytren's contracture or cystic swellings associated with

Heberden's nodes. A localized bony swelling over the carpus may arise from a dislocated lunate bone.

Deformities

Deformity of the inferior radioulnar joint results in a dorsal subluxation of the head of the ulna and this prominence may be accentuated by synovitis in the overlying soft tissues.

The wrist is normally held in a position midway between flexion–extension and adduction–abduction. Three deformities that result from inflammatory arthritis are: (1) a fixed flexion deformity occurs when the wrist cannot be actively and passively extended to the neutral position, (2) palmar subluxation of the carpal bones on the radius results in a bayonet-shaped deformity, and (3) radial deviation of the wrist carries the hand in a radial direction so that the radial styloid approximates the base of the thumb with undue prominence of the ulnar-sided carpal bones.

Thumb

The three linked joints of the thumb – the carpometacarpal, metacarpophalangeal and interphalangeal joints – may be deformed by rheumatoid arthritis, producing either a flexion deformity of the metacarpophalangeal joint usually associated with a hyperextension deformity of the interphalangeal joint, or an adduction deformity of the carpometacarpal joint associated with either a hyperextension deformity of the metacarpophalangeal joint or a hyperextension deformity of the interphalangeal joint.

Deformity from osteoarthritis of the carpometacarpal joint is usually evidenced by a square-shaped prominence of the base of the metacarpal and adduction deformity of the thumb (see p. 105).

Metacarpophalangeal joints

A flexion deformity of the metacarpophalangeal joints is evidenced by an inability to extend the fingers to the neutral position. In rheumatoid arthritis the most common deformity is a palmar subluxation of the proximal phalanx on the metacarpal bone or an ulnar deviation (medial subluxation) of the fingers.

Proximal interphalangeal joints

In rheumatoid arthritis either a hyperextension swan-neck deformity or a flexion button-hole deformity may occur.

Terminal interphalangeal joint

The common deformity in this joint is a flexion deformity of the terminal phalanx caused by rupture of the extensor tendon (p. 101).

Muscle wasting

Wasting may be evident in the intrinsic muscles in the hand either between the metacarpals or over the thenar or hypothenar eminences. Small muscle wasting may follow inflammatory arthritis or neurological diseases such as peripheral neuropathy, motor neurone disease or T1 nerve root lesions. Weakness and wasting of the thenar eminence may occur in median nerve lesions, e.g. compression in the carpal tunnel.

Skin

The hand should also be inspected for any rashes, colour changes, vascular disturbances or nail changes.

Movements

The active and passive movements are tested in all joints of the wrist and hand.

Inferior radioulnar joint

Two active movements are tested, supination and pronation, and their range is usually 90 degrees in either direction. The patient is first asked to turn the palm face upwards and then downwards and the examiner then repeats these movements passively.

Radiocarpal joint

Five movements are tested: flexion, extension, radial deviation, ulnar deviation and a small passive range of supination and pronation. The active range of wrist extension is approximately 70 degrees, flexion 80–90 degrees and the passive range of both these movements is normally a few degrees greater. While the passive range is tested, the lower arm should be stabilized by gripping over the dorsal aspect of the lower forearm. A quick practical demonstration of the passive range is to have the patient adopt two attitudes. First (Figure 8.5), the wrists are extended

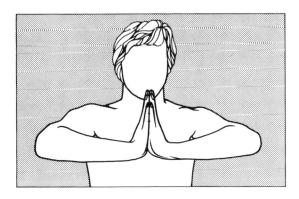

Figure 8.5 Passive dorsiflexion

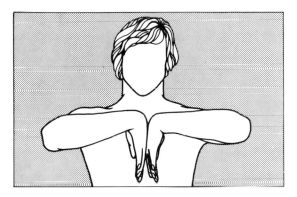

Figure 8.6 Passive palmar flexion

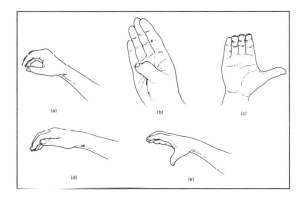

Figure 8.7 Testing thumb movements. (a) First place the thumb in the position of rest. Active movements follow logically; (b) Flexion; (c) Extension; (d) Adduction; (e) Abduction. Note that full extension and full abduction obtain the same angle.

with the elbow flexed and the forearms pronated. The palms of the hands are approximated into a praying position with both wrists passively extended. Second (Figure 8.6), the wrists are passively flexed by having the hands placed back to back. The range

of ulnar deviation is approximately 60 degrees and of radial deviation approximately 20 degrees.

Thumb

Five active movements are tested: flexion, extension, adduction, abduction and opposition. The thumb movements are tested with the patient's hand in the position of function and the thumb in neutral position (Figure 8.7).

Active flexion is tested by a combined flexion of the interphalangeal joint by asking the patient to carry the thumb across the palm to touch the tip of the thumb against the fat pad at the base of the little finger.

Active extension is tested by having the patient carry the dorsum of the thumb away from the palm in the palmar plane. It is more practical to compare the angle formed at the web of the thumb, normally about 90 degrees, in the two hands than to measure the actual range of this movement.

Adduction of the thumb is tested actively by moving the thumb into line with the fingers so that it rests against the second metacarpal.

Abduction of the thumb is tested actively by moving the thumb away from the palmar surface of the hand. It normally forms an angle of about 90 degrees with the web of the thumb.

Opposition of the thumb is tested by rotating the pad of the thumb to touch the pad of the little finger.

Finger joints

Two movements, flexion and extension, are tested while the patient's lower forearm is stabilized by gripping over it.

1 The active range of metacarpophalangeal movements is 90 degrees of flexion and up to 40 degrees of extension. The fingers should be tested together and then individually.
2 The active range of flexion at the proximal interphalangeal joint is 100 degrees and the range of extension is 0 degrees.
3 The range of flexion at the terminal interphalangeal joint is to approximately 80 degrees and a few degrees of extension are possible.

Hand and wrist lesions

Joint changes are summarized as follows:

Terminal interphalangeal joint

1 Swelling. Soft tissue swelling may occur in psoriatic arthritis and occasionally in rheumatoid

arthritis or tophaceous gout. Bony swelling may be due to Heberden's nodes or an erosive osteoarthritis.

2 Deformity. The common deformity is a flexion deformity producing a mallet finger.

3 Instability. Instability may occur in psoriatic arthritis or rheumatoid arthritis and may then form part of the opera-glass hand, or in osteoarthritis.

4 Ankylosis. Ankylosis usually occurs in psoriatic arthritis but may rarely occur in rheumatoid arthritis or gout.

Proximal interphalangeal joint

1 Swelling. Soft tissue swelling most commonly occurs in rheumatoid arthritis, producing a spindle-shaped swelling. Bony swelling may be due to Bouchard's nodes or an erosive osteoarthritis.

2 Deformity is common. Rheumatoid arthritis may produce a flexion deformity, swan-neck deformity or boutonnière deformity. Flexion deformity of the little finger may be congenital.

3 Instability. Lateral instability may occur in ligament rupture, rheumatoid arthritis or psoriatic arthritis.

4 Ankylosis is uncommon but may occur in an erosive osteoarthritis.

Metacarpophalangeal joint

1 Swelling. Soft tissue swelling is common in rheumatoid arthritis and other forms of arthritis. Bony swelling due to osteoarthritis is rare but may occur with chondrocalcinosis or after trauma.

2 Deformity. The common deformity of rheumatoid arthritis is a palmar and/or ulnar subluxation. Flexion deformity may result from rupture of the extensor tendon.

3 Instability. Marked instability may occur in the opera-glass hand.

Carpometacarpal joint of the thumb

1 Swelling. Soft tissue swelling may be caused by rheumatoid arthritis; bony swelling is more common and is the result of osteoarthritis.

2 Deformity. Deformity is common in osteoarthritis. In rheumatoid arthritis the common deformity is an adduction deformity of the thumb.

3 Instability. Lateral instability occurs as the result of osteoarthritis or inflammatory arthritis.

Wrist and carpus

1 Swelling. Soft tissue swelling may be due to an inflammatory or infective arthritis, tenosynovitis, de Quervain's syndrome or a ganglion. Bony swelling of the radiocarpal joint is rare and usually post-traumatic. In the inferior radioulnar joint it may be due to dorsal subluxation of the ulnar head.

2 Deformity. Deformity may be traumatic as in Colles' fracture or Smith's fracture. A flexion deformity occurs in any form of inflammatory arthritis and rheumatoid arthritis may also result in a volar subluxation or radial deviation of the wrist.

3 Ankylosis may follow inflammatory arthritis.

4 Instability of the inferior radioulnar joint may follow rupture of the triangular ligament.

Accessory movements

Inferior radioulnar joint

There are five accessory movements routinely tested in this joint:

1 Posteroanterior movement, produced by pressure on the posterior surface of the ulna (Figure 8.8).

2 Anteroposterior movement, produced by pressure over the anterior surface of the ulna.

3 Compression, produced by approximating the joint surface (Figure 8.9).

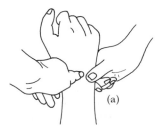

(a)

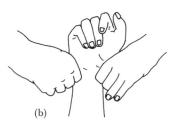

(b)

Figure 8.8 Inferior radioulnar joint; posteroanterior accessory movement; (a) posterior view; (b) anterior view

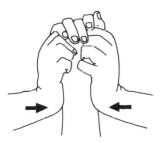

Figure 8.9 Inferior radioulnar joint: compression

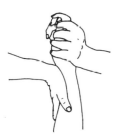

Figure 8.10 Radiocarpal joint: posteroanterior movement

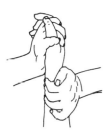

Figure 8.11 Radiocarpal joint: anteroposterior movement

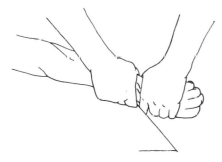

Figure 8.12 Radiocarpal joint: lateral transverse movement

4 Longitudinal cephalad movement, produced on radial deviation of the wrist.
5 Longitudinal caudad movement, produced on ulnar deviation of the wrist.

Radiocarpal joint

There are eight accessory movements in the radiocarpal joint:

1 Posteroanterior movement, produced by pressure over the posterior surface of the carpus (Figure 8.10).
2 Anteroposterior movement, produced by pressure over the anterior surface of the carpus (Figure 8.11).
3 Lateral transverse movement, produced by moving the carpus in a lateral direction (Figure 8.12).
4 Medial transverse movement, produced by moving the carpus medially (Figure 8.13).
5 Supination, produced by pressure over the anterior surface of the proximal carpus (Figure 8.14).
6 Pronation, produced by pressure over the posterior surface of the proximal carpus (Figure 8.15).
7 and 8 Longitudinal caudad and longitudinal cephalad movements.

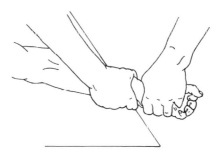

Figure 8.13 Radiocarpal joint: medial transverse movement

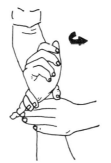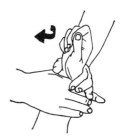

Figure 8.14
Radiocarpal joint: supination

Figure 8.15
Radiocarpal joint: pronation

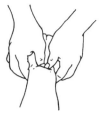

Figure 8.16 Intercarpal joints: posteroanterior movement

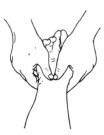

Figure 8.17 Intercarpal joints: anteroposterior movement

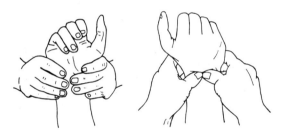

Figure 8.18 Intercarpal joints: horizontal extension

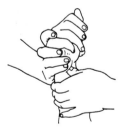

Figure 8.19 Intercarpal movements: horizontal flexion

Intercarpal joints

There are six accessory intercarpal movements. Their range of movement is small and considerable practice is needed for their assessment; nevertheless, their importance cannot be too highly stressed. They are:

1   Posteroanterior movement of one carpal bone on another by pressure over the dorsal surface (Figure 8.16).
2   Anteroposterior movement, produced by pressure over the palmar surface (Figure 8.17).
3   Horizontal extension, produced by pressure over the dorsal surface of one carpal bone as a fulcrum and extending the other carpal bones around it (Figure 8.18).
4   Horizontal flexion, produced by pressure over the palmar surface of one carpal bone and cupping the other carpal bones around it (Figure 8.19).
5   Longitudinal caudad movement, produced by distraction along the metacarpal.
6   Longitudinal cephalad movement, produced by compression along the metacarpals.

Carpometacarpal joints

There are eight accessory movements in the medial four carpometacarpal joints: medial rotation, lateral rotation, anteroposterior, posteroanterior, medial gliding, lateral gliding, longitudinal caudad and longitudinal cephalad.

Metacarpophalangeal joints

There are eight accessory movements in the metacarpophalangeal joints:

1 and 2 Medial and lateral rotation, produced by rotating the proximal phalanx (Figures 8.20 and 8.21).
3   Longitudinal caudad movement, produced by distracting the joint surfaces (Figure 8.22).
4   Longitudinal cephalad movement, produced by compressing the joint surfaces (Figure 8.23).
5   Posteroanterior movement, produced by pressure over the posterior surface of the proximal phalanx (Figure 8.24).
6   Anteroposterior movement, produced by pressure over the anterior surface of the proximal phalanx.
7   Abduction, produced by movement of the proximal phalanx away from the middle finger (Figure 8.25).
8   Adduction, produced by movement of the proximal phalanx towards the middle finger.

Isometric tests

Four isometric contractions are tested at the wrist, three at the thumb, four at the metacarpophalangeal joints and two at the interphalangeal joints.

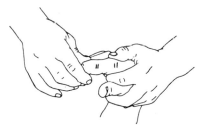

Figure 8.20 Metacarpophalangeal joints: medial rotation

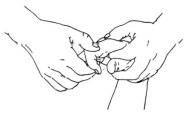

Figure 8.21 Metacarpophalangeal joints: lateral rotation

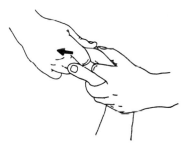

Figure 8.22 Metacarpophalangeal joints: longitudinal caudad movement

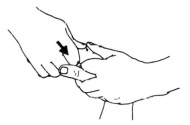

Figure 8.23 Metacarpophalangeal joints: longitudinal cephalad movement

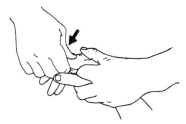

Figure 8.24 Metacarpophalangeal joint: posteroanterior movement

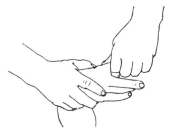

Figure 8.25 Metacarpophalangeal joint: abduction

Wrist

The four isometric contractions tested are flexion, extension, radial deviation and ulnar deviation.

Pain on resisted flexion may occur in tendinitis of the flexor carpi radialis or of the flexor carpi ulnaris. Pain on resisted extension may occur in tendinitis of the extensor carpi radialis or of the extensor carpi ulnaris. Pain on resisted radial deviation may occur in tendinitis of the flexor carpi radialis or of the extensor carpi radialis. Pain on resisted ulnar deviation may occur in tendinitis of the flexor carpi ulnaris or of the extensor carpi ulnaris.

Thus pain may be reproduced either on wrist flexion or on extension; and with either of these, pain may also be reproduced either on radial or on ulnar deviation of the wrist. From the pattern of movements then built up, the site of tendinitis can be accurately located, as indicated in Table 8.1. A painless weakness of any of these four movements usually indicates the presence of a neurological lesion as rupture of the musculotendinous structures controlling these movements at the wrist is extremely rare.

Table 8.1 Isometric tests in the wrist and hand

Tendon	Flexion	Extension	Radial deviation	Ulnar deviation
Flexor carpi ulnaris	+	–	–	+
Flexor carpi radialis	+	–	+	–
Extensor carpi ulnaris	–	+	–	+
Extensor carpi radialis	–	+	+	–

+ = Painful; – = No pain.

Thumb

Pain on resisted flexion of the thumb may occur in flexor tenosynovitis which may be associated with nodule formation in the tendon. A painless weakness may occur in rupture of the flexor tendon or in C6 nerve root lesions.

Pain on resisted extension of the thumb may occur with a tenosynovitis of the extensor tendon in the forearm or with a de Quervain's syndrome over the radial styloid. A painless weakness of thumb extension may occur in rupture of the thumb extensor or a C7 nerve root lesion.

Weakness on resisted abduction of the thumb is usually associated with wasting of the thenar eminence owing to a severe degree of compression of the median nerve in the carpal tunnel.

Fingers

The four finger isometric tests are flexion, extension, adduction and abduction. Finger flexion is tested with all fingers flexed at the proximal interphalangeal and terminal interphalangeal joints and attempting to pull them into extension. Normal strength should render this impossible. To differentiate between weakness of the flexor digitorum profundus and the flexor digitorum superficialis, the hand is laid flat on the desk, palm upwards. To test the profundus tendon, the examiner supports the middle phalanx. The terminal interphalangeal joint is flexed without bending the other joints of that finger. To test the superficialis tendon, with the hand in the same position, the proximal phalanx is supported and the proximal interphalangeal joint is flexed without bending the metacarpophalangeal or terminal interphalangeal joints of the same finger.

To test finger extension, the wrist is held supported and the metacarpophalangeal joint is extended with the proximal interphalangeal joint held flexed to prevent the use of intrinsic muscles. The examiner then pushes with his hand over the dorsum of the proximal phalanx and this movement is fully resisted.

Abduction and adduction of the fingers, controlled by the intrinsic muscles, are best tested with the hand facing palm down, the metacarpophalangeal and interphalangeal joints fully extended. The examiner then fully resists the attempt to push each finger either towards or away from the middle finger to test the intrinsic muscles. The strength of these movements in the two hands is compared.

Palpation

Three bony prominences on the dorsum of the wrist are easily identifiable: the radial styloid, the ulnar styloid and Lister's tubercle on the radius, about midway between the two styloids. The line of the radiocarpal joint lies just distal to Lister's tubercle. The radiocarpal joint is best palpated with two hands so that the thumbs palpate the dorsum of the wrist while the index and middle finger support and palpate its flexor surface. The patient should be relaxed and the wrist held palm down in the neutral position. The inferior radioulnar joint is palpated by the thumb and index finger of one hand with the wrist in the same position.

The carpometacarpal compartments of the thumb and fingers should be palpated next with the hand and wrist in the same position. The metacarpophalangeal joints are easily palpable over the dorsal surface of the patient's extended finger by the thumb and index finger of the examiner's hand. The finger is kept stable by the ulnar three fingers of the examiner's hand.

The wrist and hand should be palpated for the presence of any warmth, crepitus, swelling or tenderness.

1　The presence of any warmth is detected most easily in the wrist and may be due to inflammatory or infective arthritis.
2　Coarse crepitus due to osteoarthritis may be felt, e.g. in the carpometacarpal joint of the thumb. A fine crepitus occurs in tenosynovitis and a peculiar leathery crepitus is felt over the wrist tendons in scleroderma.
3　Palpation may be also used to confirm the presence of synovitis which is, as in other areas, often better appreciated by inspection than palpation. Synovitis of the metacarpophalangeal joint is felt as a soft tissue swelling that bulges on either side of the extensor tendon and may be ballotted from side to side. The interphalangeal joints are also examined with the finger extended and supported, and the finger and thumb are used to palpate any synovial soft tissue or bony swelling.
4　Tenderness is also sought over the insertions of ligaments and tendons into the carpus and in their course in the hand while flexing and extending the fingers.

Classification of musculoskeletal disorders

1　Soft tissue lesions.
　(a)　Tendon lesions.
　　　Tendinitis.

Tenosynovitis.
de Quervain's disease.
Tendon rupture.
Trigger finger.
(b) Ligament injuries.
(c) Dupuytren's contracture.
(d) Ganglion.
(e) Volkmann's ischaemic contracture.
2 Joint diseases: arthritis.
3 Bone.
(a) Kienböck's disease of the lunate.
(b) Fractured hook of hamate.
4 Nerve entrapments.
(a) Median nerve.
(b) Ulnar nerve.
(c) Bowler's thumb.

Soft tissue lesions

Tendon lesions

Tendinitis usually involves one of four tendons at the wrist, two on the extensor surface and two on the flexor surface. They are common sporting injuries [6] following trauma, such as a fall on the outstretched hand, overuse as in racquet sports or repetitive work loads. It usually occurs just proximal to their insertion or as a tenoperiosteal lesion at their insertion and is also commonly associated with a loss of intercarpal accessory movements.

Extensor carpi radialis

Two tendons are involved in radial extension of the wrist: the extensor carpi radialis longus, inserted into the base of the second metacarpal bone, and the extensor carpi radialis brevis, inserted into the base of the third metacarpal.

Pain is reproduced by an isometric contraction that fully resists: (1) radiation deviation of the wrist with the wrist first passively stretched into ulnar deviation and the movement back into radial deviation fully resisted, and (2) wrist extension (see Table 8.1).

Localized tenderness over the tendon insertion is usually best appreciated if the hand is held clenched with the wrist extended.

Extensor carpi ulnaris

This tendon runs over the ulnar styloid and inserts into the extensor surface of the base of the fifth metacarpal. Pain is reproduced by fully resisting: (1) ulnar deviation of the wrist, made more pronounced if the wrist is first passively stretched into full radial deviation and the movement back into ulnar deviation is fully resisted, and (2) wrist extension.

Tenderness, usually well localized over the tendon insertion, is best appreciated if the hand is clenched into a fist with the wrist held in extension.

Flexor carpi ulnaris

Tendinitis usually occurs as a tenoperiosteal lesion at the insertion of the tendon into the palmar surface of the pisiform bone. Pain is reproduced by fully resisting: (1) ulnar deviation of the wrist, made more pronounced if the wrist is first held in full passive radial deviation and the movement back into ulnar deviation of the wrist is fully resisted, and (2) wrist flexion.

Localized tenderness over the insertion of this tendon is usually best felt with the wrist held in full extension.

Flexor carpi radialis

Tendinitis of the flexor carpi radialis is the least common tendon lesion [6]. It is usually a tenoperiosteal injury at its insertion into the palmar surface of the base of the second metacarpal bone.

MANAGEMENT OF TENDINITIS

1 Rest from those activities that produce pain is usually necessary.
2 Non-steroidal anti-inflammatory drugs are given.
3 Physical methods, such as ultrasound or deep pressure massage.
4 Injections. The tender area in the tendon is identified by palpation and the wrist is positioned to stretch the tendon. A 25-gauge needle is used and 1 ml of local anaesthetic and corticosteroid is injected around the tender area.
5 Stretching and exercises are taught once movement is painless.
6 Mobilization techniques. Many patients with tendinitis have a restriction in the range of carpal accessory movements. Treatment by mobilization should ease pain and restore normal joint movement. Careful examination is essential to determine which joint is restricted and treatment techniques are localized to that joint using the movement that provokes pain most readily.

When pain is dominant, large amplitude movements, performed painlessly at first and then

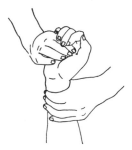

Figure 8.26 Treatment of tendinitis using radiocarpal extension

into the most painful direction, are used. For example, if wrist extension is painful, treatment is started first with the wrist fully flexed and is then rocked back and forth into extension using large amplitude grade II movements without provoking pain (Figure 8.26). If pain-free range of active movement increases, treatment is taken further into the range until it produces some discomfort.

When stiffness is dominant, treatment uses the restricted physiological movement. Strong stretching movements, using small amplitude oscillatory movements at the end of that range, are necessary. Accessory carpal movements with anteroposterior or posteroanterior pressures on adjacent carpal bones are then added.

When pain and stiffness are present, treatment consists of three stages: (1) pain is first treated as above. (2) Movements are next taken into a degree of stiffness and discomfort, taking care not to provoke an exacerbation. If not, treatment is taken further into the most restricted range, using smaller amplitude movements more strongly. (3) If there is no response, treatment is modified using movements that reproduce pain carried slowly further into the range, until pain suddenly becomes exacerbated. Small amplitude oscillatory movements are used at this point and then eased off into the less painful range, where accessory and physiological movements are used.

Tenosynovitis

Extensor tenosynovitis at the wrist presents as a swelling localized within the anatomical confines of the synovium over the extensor tendons to the fingers which terminates in the middle of the dorsum of the hand. Pain over the dorsal aspect of the hand and the swelling is made more obvious by resisted extension of the fingers throughout their full range. It may be difficult to differentiate this swelling clinically from synovitis of the wrist. Crepitus may be present.

Tenosynovitis of the ulnar tendons is common in rheumatoid arthritis, when it may be the first manifestation of this disease and is usually bilateral. Pain may be produced by resisting ulnar deviation of the wrist.

Tenosynovitis of the flexor tendons in the wrist usually occurs as the result of overuse or in inflammatory diseases such as rheumatoid arthritis. It may cause swelling in or proximal to the carpal tunnel, or else present as a compound palmar ganglion.

COMPOUND PALMAR GANGLION

This is a chronic inflammatory synovitis of the flexor tendon sheath at the wrist with visible and palpable swelling proximal to the flexor retinaculum in the forearm and distal to it in the palm. Cross-fluctuation between these two sites may be obtained by compressing over one or the other part of the swelling. Formerly most commonly tuberculous in origin, the most common cause now is rheumatoid arthritis. The inflamed synovial membrane is thickened and may contain deposits of fibrin formed into rice bodies.

De Quervain's disease

This form of stenosing tendovaginitis involves two thumb tendons at the wrist, the abductor pollicis longus and the extensor pollicis brevis, which run in a bony groove across the styloid process of the radius invested in a common synovial sheath which is exposed to repeated friction [6,7]. Overuse and inflammation of the tendon sheath result in thickening that ultimately causes a constriction of the two tendons. The patient is usually a middle-aged female with pain over the radial surface of the wrist, often severe and made worse by movements of either the thumb or wrist. Pain usually occurs in a pinch grip during which the abductor pollicis stabilizes the base of the thumb. Pain on wrist movements occurs particularly on supination of the wrist with the hand clenched, as in wringing out clothes. The patient may be conscious of a tender swelling over the radial styloid.

MAJOR SIGN

Pain is reproduced by ulnar deviation of the wrist with the thumb held flexed and adducted and then grasped by the other fingers into the palm of the hand (Figure 8.27). Pain on this movement is also reproduced with osteoarthritis of the carpometacarpal joint of the thumb.

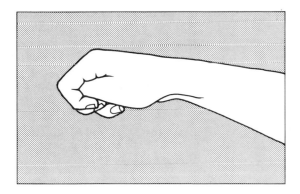

Figure 8.27 De Quervain's disease: major sign. The patient's thumb is grasped in his fingers; passive ulnar deviation then reproduces the patient's pain

OTHER SIGNS

Swelling localized over the radial styloid process is usually obvious on inspection. It is associated with tenderness, at times extreme, over the swelling itself or over the nearby radial styloid.

MANAGEMENT

1   Rest from those movements that aggravate pain is usually difficult to achieve and splints are usually impractical.
2   Anti-inflammatory drugs and physical methods usually provide little or temporary benefit.
3   A local injection of corticosteroid is the treatment of choice as one or two injections usually produce complete relief of symptoms. The patient sits with the wrist in ulnar deviation and the thumb flexed to stretch the tendon. A 25-gauge needle is inserted distal to the tender swelling and directed proximally under the tendon sheath. Then 1 ml of corticosteroid solution is injected, and may be repeated in a few weeks if symptoms have not completely resolved. Care must be taken not to inject directly into the tendon itself.
4   Surgery is indicated in those patients whose symptoms fail to resolve or are recurrent. The thickened tendon sheath is split longitudinally to decompress the tendon. It is important to determine whether the extensor pollicis brevis lies within the same sheath and not in a separate sheath or that anatomical variations are not present. If these are not corrected the operation will fail.

Tendon rupture

Rupture of the finger tendons is common and usually involves the extensor tendons of the ring or little fingers. The affected digit is held in a position of flexion, active extension is impossible, passive movement is normal and resisted extension is weak and painless.

Flexor tendon rupture may occur in rheumatoid arthritis [8] but occurs mainly in football players as the flexor digitorum profundus tendon of the ring finger is avulsed from its insertion into the distal phalanx [9,10] when the jumper is grasped. The player cannot actively flex the distal phalanx but the diagnosis is often missed as there is no obvious deformity. Surgery is required if seen early enough [9].

Mallet finger

This common condition [11] is the result of rupture of the long extensor of the finger at its insertion into the base of the distal phalanx. Two implements that may produce it are a mallet or a baseball, and a fragment of bone may be avulsed with the tendon from the distal phalanx. The usual mechanism of injury is a direct blow to the end of the finger while the terminal joint is held extended.

A flexion deformity of the terminal joint of the involved finger is present. Active extension of the flexed terminal interphalangeal joint is impossible and is associated with a painless weakness of resisted extension but passive movement of the joint can straighten the terminal phalanx. The area of the tendon insertion is tender and swollen and a radiograph may reveal an avulsed fragment of bone [12].

MANAGEMENT

The terminal interphalangeal joint may be splinted in slight hyperextension by a dorsal splint that does not immobilize the proximal joint [13]. The splint needs to be maintained in position undisturbed for approximately 6 weeks and may then be applied intermittently over the next few weeks to protect the joint [12,14–18]. Operation [12,15,16,19] with fixation by a Kirschner wire inserted through the terminal phalanx across the terminal interphalangeal joint is rarely indicated. If a large fragment of bone has been avulsed open reduction should be carried out.

Trigger finger

Triggering of the fingers or thumb occurs as a result of nodule formation within a flexor tendon. This may occur as a complication of either a simple tenosynovitis, usually from overuse, or in rheumatoid arthritis. The nodule formed within the synovial sheath is usually small, so that on flexion it moves with its tendon under the ligament that binds the flexor tendon. The finger is locked in flexion and active extension is impossible. To unlock the finger the patient may have to extend it passively, producing a sudden snapping (triggering) of the digit. This manoeuvre occurs repeatedly, producing a traumatic tenosynovitis in the flexor sheath so that movement becomes even more easily impeded. At times, there may be a painful restriction of finger flexion or the nodule may be so large that it will not pass under the flexor ligament and active flexion of the finger is impossible.

A similar type of triggering may occur in the thumb as the result of nodule formation preventing free movement of the flexor pollicis tendon. This occurs also in children, who usually present with a flexion deformity of the thumb.

MANAGEMENT

Injection of corticosteroid usually relieves symptoms for a prolonged period of time, presumably by decreasing the swelling around the sheath and so relieving the obstruction.

A 25-gauge needle inserted distal to the nodular swelling is directed proximally under the tendon sheath. Then 1 ml of corticosteroid solution is injected and may be repeated after a few weeks if symptoms are not completely relieved. If the patient has other evidence of flexor tenosynovitis, with swelling over the proximal phalanx, this area should also be injected.

If injections fail, surgery to incise the thickened tendon sheath usually gives permanent relief and it is not necessary to remove the nodule.

Ligament injuries

Inferior radioulnar joint

A tear of the triangular ligament in the inferior radioulnar joint usually follows an indirect injury in which the forearm is suddenly forcefully pronated or supinated, e.g. in tennis players. Pain and clicking over the distal end of the ulna, with a sensation of weakness in the wrist, may be reproduced on circumduction and ulnar or radial deviation of the wrist. It needs to be differentiated from chronic instability of the inferior radioulnar joint by passive movements of the ulnar head.

Diagnosis is confirmed by arthrography [20–22], CT scan [23–28], arthroscopy [29,30] or MRI [30].

MANAGEMENT

The inferior radioulnar joint forms an integral part of wrist function and significant loads are transmitted from the hand to the forearm via the triangular ligament [31–33]. All efforts then should be made to conserve the ligament [34]. Cast immobilization is used to attempt to promote healing. In younger patients, surgery may be considered [35] with simple excision of the free flap at the site of the tear [36,37] but may result in pain and instability [38] with the patient unable to resume his sport. Arthroscopic debridement of the ligament may be possible [39,40].

Wrist ligaments

Wrist ligament injuries [41] are common in sport but are often labelled as a wrist 'strain' which is not only a vague diagnosis but also results in a wrong or missed diagnosis, including a fractured scaphoid. Intercarpal sprains also follow trauma and the scaphoid lunate ligament is most commonly involved.

First or second degree sprains of radiocarpal and intercarpal joints can usually be localized clinically by stretching the involved ligament on movement of the wrist.

Investigations include radiography [4,42,43], stress views [44], arthrography [45,46], arthrotomography [47], MRI [30,48,49] and arthroscopy [50–52].

MANAGEMENT

Management consists of:

1   Rest from activities that aggravate pain and protective splinting [9] may be required.
2   Physical methods, such as ultrasound or deep pressure massage.
3   Mobilization techniques used are: (a) pain-free passive physiological movements in the direction of the injury, and (b) accessory movements to ease pain and restore normal joint movement.
4   Injections of corticosteroid into locally tender areas.

Carpal instability

The individual proximal carpal bones act as intercalated segments that are formed into three functionally independent longitudinal chains:

1 The scaphoid forms part of the radial chain and bridges across the two carpal rows to provide stability.
2 The central chain of capitate–lunate–radius allows flexion and extension.
3 The ulnar chain of triquetrum and hamate allows rotation.

This system allows great mobility with stability supplied by contact between the surfaces of the individual carpal bones and the integrity of surrounding ventral, dorsal and interosseous ligaments.

Third degree sprains associated with ligament rupture and carpal instability can result from injury to any of the wrist ligaments. Common patterns are dependent on the underlying mechanisms. Instability may be volar or dorsal according to the site of ligament rupture [53].

Rupture of the scaphoid–lunate ligament

The scaphoid is the key to normal carpal stability and when ligaments connecting it to the lunate are ruptured, the carpus collapses with a rotary subluxation of the scaphoid and a dorsal subluxation of the lunate [53].

The patient presents, usually following a fall on the outstretched hand, with diffuse pain, clicking and restricted wrist movements. With the wrist in ulnar deviation, movements directed against the volar tubercle of the scaphoid in a dorsal direction with one hand, while the other stabilizes the lower radius, can produce a painful clicking instability. Tenderness is felt diffusely over the wrist and the diagnosis is often missed. If suspected, stress radiographs should be taken with the hand in full supination, ulnar deviation or by making a fist [41] and compared with the other wrist [54]. A separation of the scaphoid–lunate joint by more than 2 mm is diagnostic and has been given the felicitous title of the Terry Thomas sign as it is likened to the gap present in that comedian's front teeth. Arthrography [4] or cineradiography [4,55] may be used for diagnosis.

MANAGEMENT
Optimal treatment would be a primary repair of the ruptured ligament but this is rarely possible and most cases are seen late [56]. Ligamentous reconstruction does not produce consistently good results [56,57]. Initial therapy is best in a padded protective cast worn for at least 6 weeks [34,58]. Arthrodesis may be necessary to allow the scaphoid to regain its stabilizing function [7,59–61] as a bridge between the proximal and distal carpal rows. Fusion of the scaphoid and lunate markedly disturbs hand movements and so a triscaphe fusion to the trapezoid and trapezium is the treatment of choice.

Skier's thumb

A complete rupture of the ulnar collateral ligament of the metacarpophalangeal joint of the thumb follows a fall onto the hand with the stick held firmly clenched by the thumb [62]. It is also known as gamekeeper's thumb [63] because he used his thumb to break a rabbit's neck. The distal attachment of the ligament is usually avulsed and displaced proximally.

The rupture is diagnosed with the patient's thumb fully extended and an abduction strain applied to the metacarpophalangeal joint to demonstrate any lateral instability. A radiograph may show a flake of bone avulsed with the ligament.

MANAGEMENT
Complete rupture either as an acute [64,65,66] or late injury [67] should be treated surgically as conservative management gives unsatisfactory results.

Partial tears (breakdancer's thumb [68]), are also common and are best treated with removable cast immobilization [65] in an over-corrected position.

Finger injuries

The proximal interphalangeal joint is commonly injured (Figure 8.28) in sport or work [69–71]. Collateral ligaments lying on either side of the joint are continuous with the fibrocartilaginous volar plate so forming a three-sided protection to the joint which resists all movement except flexion and extension. The main function of the thick volar plate is to prevent hyperextension. Partial tears of this complex usually involve the radial sided ligament [69] with pain, swelling, loss of movement and localized tenderness. Complete rupture is evidenced by lateral instability.

Injuries of the volar plate may avulse a piece of bone from the base of the middle phalanx [53]; the finger is then held in a position of slight flexion and all proximal interphalangeal movements are painful.

Immediate care of proximal interphalangeal injuries needs ice and padded splinting with the joint in 20 degrees of flexion [72,73]. Surgery is the treatment of choice for complete ligament ruptures [70,72].

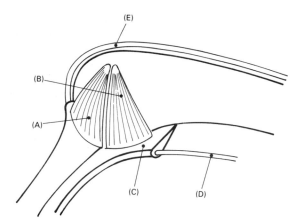

Figure 8.28 PIP joint. (A) and (B) Collateral ligament; (C) volar plate; (D) flexor tendon; (E) extensor tendon

Dupuytren's contracture

This fibrous proliferation in the palmar fascia of the hand [74] gradually results in a flexion deformity of the metacarpophalangeal and proximal interphalangeal joints. The palmar fascia is an expansion of connective tissue covering the palm with elongations passing distally into the fingers and thumb. Beginning as a small, fibrous nodular thickening about the distal palmar skin crease, it increases in size to form a thickened longitudinal fibrous cord-like band. The skin, firmly attached by fasciculi, becomes dimpled and puckered and the fingers develop a flexion contraction. The thickening does not directly involve the joints but they may develop a secondary fibrous capsular contracture with loss of function. It occurs mainly in elderly white males of European descent, usually in the ring and little fingers of either hand, and is present bilaterally in approximately half of the patients. Its aetiology is unknown.

Ganglion

A ganglion is a small, pea-shaped, soft tissue swelling found most commonly over the dorsum of the carpal bones, especially the capitate, and less commonly on the flexor surface. It is made up of myxoid degeneration of collagen fibres [75] and is usually soft and cystic or may be tense, when it is confused with a bony swelling [76]. A ganglion arises from a joint capsule or a tendon sheath and may follow trauma. The patient, usually a young adult, presents with a

lump which may be associated with some degree of pain usually related to movement. The well-defined swelling may be slightly tender or may be occult [77–79] and may at times spontaneously disappear.

If symptomatic, the swelling may be repeatedly punctured with a 22-gauge needle [80–83] and injected with 1 ml corticosteroid. Alternatively, sustained thumb pressure may be used. If this fails, or readily recurs and is troublesome, operation to remove the sac may be required. This often requires quite an extensive dissection and a pedicle that connects to a tendon or carpal joint should be sought and closed off [84]. The recurrence rate may be up to 50% [85].

Volkmann's ischaemic contracture

Volkmann's contracture results from ischaemia and fibrosis of flexor muscles of the forearm after a lesion of the brachial artery which may be damaged in elbow injuries. It starts with pain in the forearm with associated neurological symptoms and an absent radial pulse. The forearm becomes wasted and the fingers are held flexed, to produce a claw hand. Extension of the fingers is possible only if the wrist is held flexed.

Arthritis

The hand and wrist are involved during the course of most forms of arthritis and the differential diagnosis of the more common forms has been considered above. Osteoarthritis commonly involves the interphalangeal joints of the fingers and the carpometacarpal joint of the thumb. Degenerative changes produce bony swellings around the margins of the joint known as Heberden's nodes in the terminal joint and Bouchard's nodes in the proximal joints. They occur commonly in middle-aged females as part of a primary generalized osteoarthritis. The joint becomes enlarged and tender, and pain may be related to overuse of the joint. Heberden's nodes may begin insidiously with little pain or discomfort then gradually increase in size or may develop rapidly with pain, redness and tenderness around the joint. A cystic swelling containing gelatinous mucoid material may present over the joint margin or over the extensor surface of the distal phalanx and cause nail damage.

Primary osteoarthritis in the metacarpophalangeal joints is uncommon but may occur secondary to chondrocalcinosis, haemochromatosis or repeated trauma as in boxing.

Osteoarthritis of the carpometacarpal joint of the thumb

This joint is most important for normal hand function as it plays a major role in positioning the thumb [86]. It has two biconcave saddle-shaped surfaces which allow flexion, extension, abduction, adduction and rotation; combined movements produce opposition and circumduction of the thumb [87]. As the thumb rotates around the long axis of its metacarpal bone, stability is maintained by the strong but lax joint capsule [86] and the joint has a tendency to sublux dorsally and radially.

Osteoarthritis occurs most commonly in middle-aged females, may be bilateral and occur as part of a primary generalized osteoarthritis. It may also occur in a young male patient after previous trauma, such as Bennett's fracture. The patient presents with pain around the base of the thumb, made worse by use, especially pinch grip, with axial compression of the thumb such as opening a car door, or rotational movements such as wringing out clothes. In the early stages, active and passive movements may be restricted. Pain may be reproduced by compressing the metacarpal shaft proximally and into adduction. Crepitus and instability of the joint may be felt with the thumb placed over the joint. Subsequently, deformities develop with the thumb in a position of adduction. Hyperextension deformity of the metacarpophalangeal or interphalangeal joint of the thumb may develop, possibly in an attempt to increase the range of the grasp. The carpometacarpal joint develops a bony, square enlargement owing to the degenerative changes and dorsal subluxation.

It may be associated with tenosynovitis, carpal tunnel syndrome and de Quervain's syndrome [88] and also needs to be differentiated from these conditions. It may also be associated with degenerative changes in the trapezium–scaphoid joint, especially in hypermobile patients who have practised repetitive trick movements with their thumb.

Diagnosis needs to be confirmed by radiography, including oblique views.

MANAGEMENT

1 Rest from movements that aggravate pain is important but difficult as this joint is involved in many functional hand movements. Various forms of splints have been described but may be difficult for the patient to manage.
2 Anti-inflammatory drugs and analgesics are given as necessary.
3 Physical methods are only of limited value.
4 Passive movements: large-amplitude movements are given without provoking discomfort. As pain settles, these movements can be increased further into the range and so may provoke some discomfort. Small-amplitude physiological and accessory movements that provoke pain are used next.
5 Injections of local anaesthetic and corticosteroid into the joint may be given using a 25-gauge needle but rarely provide any lasting relief.
6 Surgery is indicated if pain and disability are severe [89]. The choice of operation [89] lies between arthrodesis [90], removal of the trapezium [91], or a Silastic implant [92].

Bone disorders

Kienböck's disease

In this condition (Figure 8.29), a progressive disruption of the lunate follows vascular compromise [93,94] owing to an avascular necrosis, fracture or external

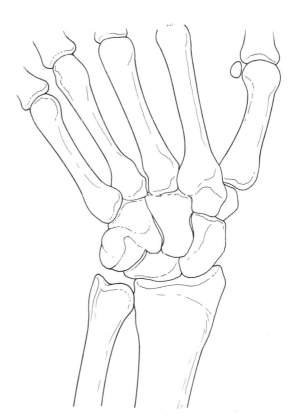

Figure 8.29 Kienbock's disease of the lunate

compression forces [95]. It usually occurs in the right wrist of males over the age of 15 years. Pain and stiffness in the wrist are made worse by use and usually a gradually progressive swelling may be present. Tenderness is usually well localized over the lunate. Radiographic changes may take some time to develop and CT or MRI give better imaging [96] but the bone becomes sclerotic at first and later fragmented, irregular and altered in shape [97]. Ulnar variance is commonly present [97]. The disease usually runs a benign course over 2 years [98] but osteoarthritis of the wrist commonly develops in later life.

MANAGEMENT

Management of this condition is controversial [98], especially in young players of racquet sports. In the early stages the wrist should be immobilized in a cast for several months to allow pain to settle and attempt repair [98]. Protection may then be given by a reinforced wrist splint which can be worn when the patient attempts to return to sport. Surgery for persistent pain has included revascularization, radial shortening, ulnar lengthening, silicone replacement and intercarpal or wrist arthrodesis [63,93,95, 99–101].

Fractured hook of hamate

This sporting injury occurs especially when a golf club, tennis racquet, baseball bat or hockey stick abuts against the palm of the hand [102]. Pain in the palm is made worse by grasping and grip strength is weak [103]. Tenderness is localized over the bone. Diagnosis is confirmed by radiography [104] with special views [105,106], and tomography, bone scans or CT scanning [103,107,108] may be needed.

This injury is usually associated with non-union, so surgical excision is often the best management [102,103,109].

Nerve entrapments

Carpal tunnel syndrome

This entrapment neuropathy of the median nerve in the carpal tunnel of the wrist is very common. The convex anterior surface of the carpal bones is converted into a fibro-osseous tunnel by the transverse carpal ligament. The flexor tendons of the fingers and the median nerve run through this tunnel as they pass from the forearm into the hand (Figure 8.30) [110,111].

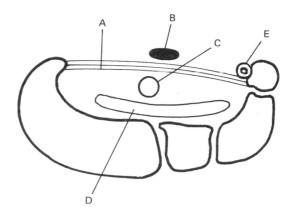

Figure 8.30 Carpal tunnel. (A), transverse carpal ligament running from the scaphoid to the pisiform; (B), palmaris longus tendon; (C), median nerve; (D), flexor tendons of the fingers; (E), ulnar nerve and artery

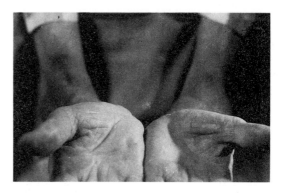

Figure 8.31 Bilateral carpal tunnel syndromes. Note wasting of thenar eminence and tenosynovial swelling in the carpal tunnel

The most common cause in females is idiopathic with no discernible underlying pathology (Figure 8.31). The most likely explanation is an overuse phenomenon of the hand as in process workers or housewives. Possibly a low-grade tenosynovitis is produced or the carpal tunnel is of small volume. In addition, alterations in any of the anatomical structures in the tunnel can result in a loss of volume or deformity of available space in the carpal tunnel and so produce median nerve irritation or compression. A common cause is swelling associated with a tenosynovitis in the flexor tendons [112]. This may follow overuse of the wrist, e.g. in occupational stresses which involve repeated wrist flexion or gripping movements with the wrist held extended [113,114]. It may also follow prolonged use of the wrist by arthritics who use a walking stick. Rheumatoid arthritis produces an inflammatory synovitis of the flexor tendons of the wrist joint (which may occur in the early stages) and the correct diagnosis may be overlooked as the hand pain is presumed to be from the rheumatoid disease alone. Carpal tunnel syndrome may also be associated with previous trauma, such as Colles' fracture or subluxation of the lunate, osteoarthritis of the wrist or ganglion formation. It may also occur during the last trimester of pregnancy or as part of the premenstrual syndrome, presumably from fluid retention. Various metabolic causes, including tophaceous gout, hypothyroidism, acromegaly or amyloidosis have also been described [115].

The patient is usually a middle-aged female. One or both hands, but more commonly the dominant hand, may be involved. The symptoms of pain and/or paraesthesias are usually characteristic. Pain is felt in the distribution of the median nerve in the hand and is most severe at night, when it commonly disturbs sleep. Pain may radiate up the arm and may be felt in the elbow or shoulder. Paraesthesias occur in the hands, especially at night, and are often relieved by moving the hands about or posturing them over the edge of the bed or above the shoulder. They are usually felt in the distribution of the median nerve in the hand but the patient often complains that they are present in all fingers. Careful questioning may then determine whether the little finger is spared. The patient may also complain of an unpleasant sensation of fullness or stiffness in the fingers, especially in the morning, or that the fingers feel clumsy or weak.

MAJOR SIGNS
The patient's symptoms may be reproduced by various manoeuvres designed to increase compression of the nerve in the carpal tunnel. This may be achieved by placing the thumb over the wrist and then fully flexing the hand for approximately 1 min. Alternatively, both wrists may be held fully flexed by compressing the dorsal surfaces of the hands together.

OTHER SIGNS
Tapping over the median nerve at the wrist (Tinel's sign) may reproduce the symptoms. A neurological examination must be undertaken to determine any loss of sensation in the fingers, wasting of the thenar prominence and any weakness in opposition or abduction of the thumb. Examination of the upper limb and neck is necessary to exclude a more proximal entrapment neuropathy. Carpal tunnel

syndrome may be confused with a cervical spondylosis, or the two conditions may occur together.

INVESTIGATIONS
Nerve conduction tests using sensory latencies and motor conduction velocity may be carried out [110,116]. Radiographs of the wrist should also include a carpal tunnel view [117]. Underlying metabolic disorders or space-occupying lesions of the carpal tunnel are excluded using appropriate investigations [112,116,117].

MANAGEMENT

1 Rest to the wrist. This may require a volar splint that includes the flexed fingers, with the wrist held in the neutral position. It may be worn at night only.
2 Anti-inflammatory drugs rarely provide any relief.
3 Injections. An injection of corticosteroid into the carpal tunnel is a simple procedure [7] that usually produces significant symptomatic relief within a day; 1 ml of corticosteroid solution is injected using a 25-gauge needle without any local anaesthetic as it may anaesthetize the nerve. This injection usually produces such symptomatic relief that it may also be used as a diagnostic test.
4 Physical methods, i.e. heat, exercise or massage, have no role in treatment.
5 Mobilization. Passive movements to attempt stretching the flexor retinaculum and improving the posteroanterior range of the intercarpal joints are useful in idiopathic cases.
6 Surgery is indicated if conservative methods fail or repeated injections are necessary at frequent intervals. Wasting in the muscles of the thenar eminence requires urgent decompression, and division of the transverse carpal ligament may be combined with a synovectomy of the flexor tendons.

Ulnar nerve compression

The ulnar nerve crosses the wrist with the ulnar artery. In the hand it passes through the tunnel of Guyon, bounded on its ulnar side by the pisiform bone and on its radial side by the hook of the hamate; it lies anterior and medial to the transverse carpal ligament [82] (see Figure 8.30). Near the pisiform the nerve divides into a superficial and deep branch. The superficial, mainly sensory, nerve supplies the skin over the hypothenar eminence, the little finger and half of the ring finger. The deep branch supplies the muscles of the hypothenar eminence and most of the intrinsic muscles of the hand.

The ulnar nerve may be compressed in the wrist after trauma, such as a Colles' fracture, or from tendinitis of the flexor carpi ulnaris at its insertion into the pisiform. It occurs especially in cyclists as handle bar palsy [6]. It may also occur as an acute injury after a blow to the open hand, as in attempting to push upwards a jammed window, or by compression after repeated occupational trauma to the palmar surface of the wrist. The nerve may also be entrapped in the tunnel of Guyon by a ganglion or after repeated overuse of the wrist, such as using a walking stick.

If the superficial division of the nerve is involved pain and/or paraesthesias in the sensory distribution of the ulnar nerve to the ring and little fingers are present. Pressure and percussion over the nerve near the pisiform bone should reproduce symptoms.

If the deep branch is entrapped, patients complain of a deep aching pain in the palm of the hand but no sensory disturbances. Weakness and wasting develop in the hypothenar, interossei and adductor pollicis brevis muscles [119].

MANAGEMENT

The same principles of managing carpal tunnel compression apply to this condition.

Bowler's thumb

Bowlers use their thumb and index finger inserted into the holes in the bowl for control. This may cause a traumatic neuroma of the digital nerve on the ulnar side of the thumb with pain in the distribution of the nerve with hyperaesthesia and atrophy of the overlying skin [120]. If conservative management, including a protective shell for the thumb, fails to improve symptoms, surgery to relieve the nerve compression produces good results [120].

References

1 Fisk, G.R. (1984) The wrist. *Journal of Bone and Joint Surgery*, **66B**, 396–407
2 Linscheid, R.L. (1986) Kinematic considerations of the wrist. *Clinical Orthopaedics*, **202**, 27–39
3 Kauer, J.M. and de Lange, A. (1987) The carpal joint. Anatomy and function. *Hand Clinics*, **3**, 23–29
4 Belsole, R.J. (1986) Radiography of the wrist. *Clinical Orthopaedics*, **202**, 50–56

5 Mayer, V. and Gieck, J.H. (1986) Rehabilitation of hand injuries in athletes. *Clinics in Sports Medicine*, **5**, 783–794
6 Wood, M.B. and Dobyns, J.H. (1986) Sports-related extraarticular wrist syndromes. *Clinical Orthopaedics*, **202**, 93–102
7 Watson, H.K. and Black, D.M. (1987) Instabilities of the wrist. *Hand Clinics*, **3**, 103–111
8 Ertel, A.N., Millender, L.H., Nalebuff, E. *et al.* (1988) Flexor tendon ruptures in patients with rheumatoid arthritis. *Journal of Hand Surgery (Am.)*, **13**, 860–866
9 Mosher, J.F. (1985) Current concepts in the diagnosis and treatment of hand and wrist injuries in sport. *Medicine and Science in Sports and Exercise*, **17**, 48–55.
10 Bynum, D.K. Jr. and Gilbert, J.A. (1988) Avulsion of the flexor digitorum profundus: anatomic and biomechanical considerations. *Journal of Hand Surgery (Am)*, **13**, 222–227
11 Thayer, D.T. (1988) Distal interphalangeal joint injuries. *Hand Clinics*, **4**, 1–4
12 Wehble, M.A. and Schneider, L.H. (1984) Mallet fractures. *Journal of Bone and Joint Surgery (Am)*, **66**, 658–669
13 Evans, D. and Weightman, B. (1988) The pipflex splint for treatment of mallet finger. *Journal of Hand Surgery*, **13**, 156–158
14 Hovoaard, C. and Klareskov, B. (1988) Alternative conservative treatment of mallet finger injuries by elastic double finger bandage. *Journal of Hand Surgery*, **13**, 154–155
15 Niechajev, I.A. (1985) Conservative and operative treatment of mallet finger. *Plastic Reconstructive Surgery*, **76**, 580–585
16 Stern, P.J. and Kaastrup, J.J. (1988) Complications and prognosis of treatment of mallet finger. *Journal of Hand Surgery*, **13**, 329–334
17 Ludahn, J.D. (1989) Mallet finger fractures: a comparison of open and closed technique. *Journal of Hand Surgery*, **14**, 394–398
18 Warren, R.A., Norris, S.H. and Ferguson, D.G. (1988) Mallet finger: atrial of two splints. *Journal of Hand Surgery*, **13**, 151–153
19 Warren, R.A., Kay, N.R. and Ferguson, D.G. (1988) Mallet finger: comparison between operative and conservative management in those cases failing to be cured by splintage. *Journal of Hand Surgery*, **13**, 159–160
20 Reinus, W.R., Hardy, D.C., Totty, W.G. *et al.* (1987) Arthrographic evaluation of the carpal triangular fibrocartilage complex. *Journal of Hand Surgery*, **12**, 495–503
21 Green, D.P. (1985) The sore wrist without a fracture. *Instructional Course Lecturers*, **34**, 300–313
22 Herbert, T.J., Faithfull, R.G., McCann, D.J. *et al.* (1990) Bilateral arthrography of the wrist. *Journal of Hand Surgery*, **15B**, 233–235
23 Mino, D.E., Palmer, A.K. and Levinsohn, E.M. (1985) Radiography and computerized tomography in the diagnosis of incongruity of the distal radio-ulnar joint. A prospective study. *Journal of Bone and Joint Surgery (Am)*, **67**, 247–252
24 Scheffler, R., Armstrong, D. and Hutton, L. (1984) Computed tomographic diagnosis of the distal radioulnar joint disruption. *Journal of the Canadian Association of Radiologists*, **35**, 212–213

25 King, G.L., McMurtry, R.Y., Rubenstein, J.D. *et al.* (1986) Computerized tomography of the distal radioulnar joint. *Journal of Hand Surgery*, **11**, 711–717

26 Wechsler, R.J., Webbe, M.A., Rifkin, M.D. *et al.* (1987) Computed tomography: diagnosis of distal radioulnar subluxation. *Skeletal Radiology*, **16**, 1–5

27 Space, T.C., Louis, D.S., Francis, I. *et al.* (1986) CT findings in distal radioulnar dislocation. *Journal of Computer Assisted Tomography*, **10**, 689–690

28 Quinn, S.F., Belsole, R.J., Greene, T.L. *et al.* (1989) CT of the wrist for the evaluation of traumatic injuries. *Critical Review of Diagnostic Imaging*, **29**, 357–380

29 Drewniany, J.J. and Palmer, A.K. (1986) Injuries to the distal radioulnar joint. *Orthopedic Clinics of North America*, **17**, 451–459

30 Zlatkin, M.B., Chao, P.C, Osterman, A.L. *et al.* (1989) Chronic wrist pain: evaluation with high-resolution MR imaging. *Radiology*, **173**, 723–729

31 Palmer, A.K. (1987) The distal radioulnar joint. Anatomy, biomechanics, and triangular fibrocartilage complex abnormalities. *Hand Clinics*, **3**, 31–40

32 Palmer, A.K. and Werner, F.W. (1987) Biomechanics of the distal radioulnar joint. *Clinical Orthopaedics*, **187**, 26–35

33 Boulas, H.J. and Milek, M.A. (1990) Ulnar shortening for tears of the triangular fibrocartilaginous complex. *Journal of Hand Surgery*, **15A**, 415–420

34 Gieck, J.H. and Mayer, V. (1986) Protective splinting for the hand and wrist. *Clinics in Sports Medicine*, **5**, 795–807

35 Van der Linden, A.J. (1986) Disk lesion of the wrist joint. *Journal of Hand Surgery (Am)*, **11**, 490–497

36 Neviaser, R.J. and Palmer, A.K. (1984) Traumatic perforation of the articular disc of the triangular fibrocartilage complex of the wrist. *Bulletin of the Hospital for Joint Diseases Orthopaedic Institute*, **44**, 376–380

37 Menon, J., Wood, V.E., Schoene, H.R. *et al.* (1984) Isolated tears of the triangular fibrocartilage of the wrist: results of partial excision. *Journal of Hand Surgery (Am)*, **9**, 527–530

38 Palmer, A.K. and Werner, F.W. (1987) Biomechanics of the distal radioulnar joint. *Clinical Orthopaedics and Related Research*, **187**, 26–35

39 Osteman, A.L. (1990) Arthroscopic debridement of triangular fibrocartilage complex tears, *Arthroscopy*, **6**, 120–124

40 Palmer, A.K. (1990) Triangular fibrocartilage disorders: injury patterns and treatment. *Arthroscopy*, **6**, 125–132

41 Jones, W.A. (1988) Beware the sprained wrist. The incidence and diagnosis of scapholunate instability. *Journal of Bone and Joint Surgery (Br)*, **70**, 293–297

42 Yeager, B.A. and Dalinka, M.K. (1985) Radiology of trauma to the wrist: dislocations, fracture dislocations, and instability patterns. *Skeletal Radiology*, **13**, 120–130

43 Schernberg, F. (1990) Roentgenographic examination of the wrist: A systematic study of the normal, lax and injured wrist. Part 1: The standard and positional views. *Journal of Hand Surgery*, **15**, 210–211

44 Schernberg, F. (1990) Roentgenographic examination of the wrist: A systematic study of the normal, lax and injured wrist. Part 2: Stress views. *Journal of Hand Surgery*, **15**, 243–248

45 Mikic, Z.D. (1984) Arthrography of the wrist joint. An experimental study. *Journal of Bone and Joint Surgery (Am)*, **66**, 371–378

46 Frahm, R., Saul, O. and Mannerfelt, L. (1990) Diagnostic applications of wrist arthrography. *Archives of Orthopaedics and Trauma Surgery*, **109**, 39–42

47 Blair, W.F., Berger, R.A. and el-Khoury, G.Y. (1985) Arthrotomography of the wrist: an experimental and preliminary clinical study. *Journal of Hand Surgery (Am)*, **10**, 350–359

48 Baker, L.L., Hajek, P.C., Bjorkengren, A. *et al.* (1987) High-resolution magnetic resonance imaging of the wrist: normal anatomy. *Skeletal Radiology*, **16**, 128–132

49 Linn, M.R., Mann, F.A. and Gilulua, L.A. (1990) Imaging the symptomatic wrist. *Orthopedic Clinics of North America*, **21**, 515–543

50 Roth, J.H. and Haddad, R.G. (1986) Radiocarpal arthroscopy and arthrography in the diagnosis of ulnar wrist pain. *Arthroscopy*, **2**, 234–243

51 Kelly, E.P. and Stanley, J.K. (1990) Arthroscopy of the wrist. *Journal of Hand Surgery*, **15**, 236–242

52 Koman, L.A., Poehling, G.G., Toby, E.B. *et al.* (1990) Chronic wrist pain: Indications for wrist arthroscopy. *Arthroscopy*, **6**, 116–119

53 Recht, M.P., Burk, D., Lawrence, D. *et al.* (1987) Radiology of wrist and hand injuries in athletes. *Clinics in Sports Medicine*, **6**, 811–828

54 Nielsen, P.T. and Heaeboe, J. (1984) Post-traumatic scapholunate dissociation detected by wrist cineradiography. *Journal of Hand Surgery (Am)*, **9A**, 135–138

55 Nielsen, P.T. and Heaeboe, J. (1984) Post-traumatic scapholunate dissociation detected by wrist cineradiography. *Journal of Hand Surgery (Am)*, **9A**, 135–138

56 Glickel, S.Z. and Millender, L.H. (1984) Ligamentous reconstruction for chronic intercarpal instability. *Journal of Hand Surgery (Am)*, **9**, 514–527

57 Linscheid, R.L. and Dobyns, J.H. (1985) Athletic injuries of the wrist. *Clinical Orthopaedics and Related Research*, **198**, 141–151

58 Linscheid, R.L. (1985) Kienbock's disease. *Journal of Hand Surgery (Am)*, **10**, 1–3

59 Kleinman, W.B. (1987) Management of chronic rotary subluxation of the scaphoid by scapho-trapezoid arthrodesis. Rationale for the technique, postoperative changes in biomechanics, and results. *Hand Clinics*, **3**, 113–133

60 Hastings, D.E. and Silver, R.L. (1984) Intercarpal arthrodesis in the management of chronic carpal instability after trauma. *Journal of Hand Surgery (Am)*, **9**, 834–840

61 Trumble, T., Bour, C.J., Smith, R.J. *et al.* (1988) Intercarpal arthrodesis for static and dynamic volar intercalated segment instability. *Journal of Hand Surgery (Am)*, **13**, 384–390

62 Fairclough, J.A. and Mintowt-Czyz, W.J. (1986) Skier's thumb – a method of prevention. *Injury*, **17**, 203–204

63 Sternbach, G. and Campbell, C.S. (1984) Gamekeeper's thumb. *Journal of Emergency Medicine*, **1**, 345–347

64 Derkash, R.S., Matyas, J.R., Weaver, J.K. *et al.* (1987) Acute surgical repair of the skier's thumb. *Clinical Orthopaedics*, **216**, 29–33

65 Hankin, F.M. and Wylie, R.J. (1988) Gamekeeper's thumb. *American Family Physician*, **38**, 127–130

66 Derkash, R.S., Matyas, J.R., Weaver, J.K. *et al.* (1987) Acute surgical rupture of the skier's thumb. *Clinical Orthopaedics and Related Research*, **216**, 29–33

67 Lamb, D.W. and Angarita, G. (1985) Ulnar instability of the metacarpophalangeal joint of the thumb. *Journal of Hand Surgery*, **10**, 113–114

68 Winslet, M.C., Clarke, N.M. and Mulligan, P.J. (1986) Breakdancer's thumb. Partial rupture of the ulnar collateral ligament with a fracture of the proximal phalanx of the thumb. *Injury*, **17**, 201–202

69 Wray, R.C., Young, V.L. and Holtman, B. (1984) Proximal interphalangeal joint sprains. *Plastic and Reconstructive Surgery*, **74**, 101–107

70 Ali, M.S. (1984) Complete disruption of collateral mechanism of proximal interphalangeal joint of fingers. *Journal of Hand Surgery (Br)*, **9**, 191–193

71 Bowers, W.H. (1986) Sprains and joint injuries in the hand. *Hand Clinical*, **2**, 93–98

72 Isani, A. and Melone, C.P. Jr. (1986) Ligamentous injuries of the hand in athletes. *Clinical Sports Medicine*, **5**, 757–772

73 Bittinger, S. (1986) Sprains and joint injuries: therapists' management. *Hand Clinics*, **2**, 99–105

74 Hill, N.A. (1985) Dupuytren's contracture. *Journal of Bone and Joint Surgery*, **67**, 1439–1443

75 Soren, A. (1982) Pathogenesis, clinic and treatment of ganglion. *Archives of Orthopaedic and Trauma Surgery*, **99**, 247–252

76 Goldenstein, C., McCauley, R., Troy, M. *et al.* (1989) Ultrasonography in the evaluation of wrist swelling in children. *Journal of Rheumatology*, **16**, 1079–1087

77 Gunther, S.F. (1985) Dorsal wrist pain and the occult scapholunate ganglion. *Journal of Hand Surgery (Am)*, **10**, 697–703

78 Sanders, W.E. (1985) The occult dorsal carpal ganglion. *Journal of Hand Surgery (Br)*, **10**, 257–260

79 Hollister, A.M., Sanders, R.A. and McCann, S. (1989) The use of MRI in the diagnosis of an occult wrist ganglion cyst. *Orthopaedic Review*, **18**, 1210–1212

80 Richman, J.A., Gelberman, R.H., Engber, W.D. *et al.* (1987) Ganglions of the wrist and digits: results of treatment by aspiration and cyst wall puncture. *Journal of Hand Surgery (Am)*, **12**, 1041–1043

81 Zubowicz, V.N. and Ishii, C.H. (1987) Management of ganglion cysts of the hand by simple aspiration. *Journal of Hand Surgery (Am)*, **12**, 618–620

82 Nield, D.V. and Evans, D.M. (1986) Aspiration of ganglia. *Journal of Hand Surgery (Br)*, **11**, 264

83 Estaban, J.M., Oertel, Y.C., Menddza, M. *et al.* (1986) Fine needle aspiration in the treatment of ganglion cysts. *South Medical Journal*, **79**, 691–693

84 Clay, N.R. and Clement, D.A. (1988) The treatment of dorsal wrist ganglia by radical excision. *Journal of Hand Surgery (Br)*, **13**, 187–191

85 Duncan, K.H. and Lewis, R.C. Jr. (1988) Scapholunate instability following ganglion cyst excision. A case report. *Clinical Orthopedics*, **228**, 250–253

86 Kauer, J.M. (1987) Functional anatomy of the carpometacarpal joint of the thumb. *Clinical Orthopaedics*, **220**, 7–13

87 Zancolli, E.A., Ziadenberg, C. and Zancolli, E. Jr. (1987) Biomechanics of the trapeziometacarpal joint. *Clinical Orthopaedics*, **220**, 14–26

88 Melone, C.P. Jr., Beavers, B. and Isani, A. (1987) The basal joint pain syndrome. *Clinical Orthopaedics*, **220**, 58–67

89 Burton, R.I. (1986) Basal joint arthritis. Fusion, implant, or soft tissue reconstruction? *Orthopedic Clinics of North America*, **17**, 493–503

90 Carroll, R.E. (1987) Arthrodesis of the carpometacarpal joint of the thumb. A review of patients with a long postoperative period. *Clinical Orthopaedics*, **220**, 106–110

91 Deil, P.C. and Muniz, R.B. (1987) Interposition arthroplasty of the trapeziometacarpal joint for osteoarthritis. *Clinical Orthopaedics*, **220**, 27–34

92 Herndon, J.H. (1987) Trapeziometacarpal arthroplasty. A clinical review. *Clinical Orthopaedics*, **220**, 99–105

93 Alexander, A.H. and Lichtman, D.M. (1986) Kienbock's disease. *Orthopedic Clinics of North America*, **17**, 461–472

94 Linscheid, R.L. (1985) Kienbock's disease. *Journal of Hand Surgery*, **10**, 1–3

95 Almquist, E.E. (1987) Kienbock's disease. *Hand Clinics*, **3**, 141–148

96 Kursunoglu-Brahme, S., Gundry, C.R. and Resnick, D. (1990) Advanced imaging of the wrist. *Radiologic Clinics of North America*, **28**, 307–309

97 Mirabello, S.C., Rosenthal, D.I. and Smith, R.J. (1987) Correlation of clinical and radiographic findings in Kienbock's disease. *Journal of Hand Surgery (Am)*, **12**, 1049–1054

98 Kristensen, S.S., Thomassen, E. and Christensen, F. (1986) Kienbock's disease: late results by non-surgical treatment. A follow-up study. *Journal of Hand Surgery (Br)*, **11**, 422–425

99 Evans, G., Burke, F.D. and Barton, N.J. (1986) A comparison of conservative treatment and silicone replacement arthroplasty in Kienbock's disease. *Journal of Hand Surgery (Br)*, **11**, 98–102

100 Trumble, T., Glisson, R.R. and Seaber, A.V. *et al.* (1986) A biochemical comparison of the methods for treating Kienbock's disease. *Journal of Hand Surgery American*, **11**, 88–93

101 Watson, H.K., Ryu, J. and DiBella, A. (1985) An approach to Kienbock's disease: triscaphe arthrodesis. *Journal of Hand Surgery*, **10**, 179–187

102 Schlosser, H. and Murray, J.F. (1984) Fracture of the hook of the hamate. *Canadian Journal of Surgery*, **27**, 587–589

103 Bishop, A.T. and Beckenbaugh, R.D. (1988) Fracture of the hamate hook. *Journal of Hand Surgery (Am)*, **13**, 135–139

104 Norman, A., Nelson, J. and Green, S. (1985) Fractures of the hook of the hamate: radiographic signs. *Radiology*, **154**, 49–53

105 Papilion, J.D., DuPuy, T.E., Aulcno, P.L. *et al.* (1988) Radiographic evaluation of the hook of the hamate: a new technique. *Journal of Hand Surgery (Am)*, **13**, 437–439

106 Bray, T.J., Swafford, A.R. and Brown, R.L. (1985) Bilateral fracture of the hook of the hamate. *Journal of Trauma*, **25**, 174–175

107 Polivy, K.D., Millender, L.H., Newberg, A. *et al.* (1985) Fractures of the hook of the hamate. A failure of clinical diagnosis. *Journal of Hand Surgery (Am)*, **10**, 101–104

108 Mizuseki, T., Ikuta, Y., Murakami, T. *et al.* (1986) Lateral approach to the hook of hamate for its fracture. *Journal of Hand Surgery*, **11**, 109–111

109 Parker, R.D., Berkowitz, M.S., Brahms, M.A. *et al.* (1986) Hook of the hamate fractures in athletes. *American Journal of Sports Medicine*, **14**, 517–523

110 Howard, F.M. (1986) Controversies in nerve entrapment syndromes in the forearm and wrist. *Orthopedic Clinics of North America*, **17**, 375–381

111 Dorwart, B.B. (1984) Carpal tunnel syndrome: a review. *Seminars in Arthritis and Rheumatism*, **14**, 134–140

112 Healy, C., Watson, J.D., Longstaff, A. *et al.* (1990) Magnetic resonance imaging of the carpal tunnel. *Journal of Hand Surgery*, **15**, 243–248

113 Rettig, A.C. and Wright, H.H. (1989) Skier's thumb. *Physician and Sports Medicine*, **17**, 65–75

114 Rojviroj, S., Sirichativapee, W., Kowsuwon, W. *et al.* (1990) Pressures in the carpal tunnel. A comparison between patients with carpal tunnel syndrome and normal subjects. *Journal of Bone and Joint Surgery*, **72B**, 516–518

115 Hodgkins, M.L. and Grady, D. (1988) Carpal tunnel syndrome. *Western Journal of Medicine*, **148**, 217–220

116 Gellman, H., Gelberman, R.H., Tan, A.M. *et al.* (1986) Carpal tunnel syndrome. An evaluation of the provocative diagnostic tests. *Journal of Bone and Joint Surgery (Am)*, **68**, 735–737

117 Fodor, J., Malott, J.C. and Merhar, G.L. (1987) Carpal tunnel syndrome: the role of radiography. *Radiological Technology*, **58**, 497–501

118 Gross, M.S. and Gelberman, R.H. (1985) The anatomy of the distal ulnar tunnel. *Clinical Orthopedics*, **196**, 238–247

119 Wu, J.S., Morris, J.D. and Hogan, G.R. (1985) Ulnar neuropathy at the wrist: case report and review of literature. *Archives of Physical and Medical Rehabilitation*, **66**, 785–787

120 Dobyns, J.H., O'Brien, E.T., Linscheid, R.L. *et al.* (1972) Bowler's thumb – diagnosis and treatment. *Journal of Bone and Joint Surgery*, **54A**, 751–755

9 Hip

The hip is a synovial ball and socket joint formed between the head of the femur, which normally constitutes two-thirds of a sphere, and the cup-shaped acetabular cavity, which constitutes only one-third of a sphere. These surfaces are incongruent and the hip becomes congruent only on heavy loading so that stress on the articular cartilage can then be distributed over a wider area. The hip combines great stability with considerable mobility, less than in the shoulder but enhanced by coordinated movements in the pelvis and lumbar spine.

The pelvis and hips are well adapted to their function of transferring body-weight from the trunk to the legs, while at the same time allowing the leg to adopt the numerous positions necessary for standing, walking and running [1,2]. The spinal column is wedged into the sacrum and the sacroiliac joints are tightly bound by strong ligaments. Weight is transferred through the bony ring of the pelvis to the two legs.

At rest, the hip is subjected to a constant pressure from surrounding muscles. When standing on two legs, the hips may be compared with a balance, the pelvis acting as a crossbar. Body-weight is transmitted equally to each femur, which acts as a supporting pillar (Figure 9.1). On one leg, weight distribution is altered and a different type of lever system applies (Figure 9.2). The fulcrum is now at the hip joint of the supporting limb and body-weight is carried on the inner arm of the lever. This must be counteracted by a muscle pull on the outer arm of the lever if the pelvis is not to overbalance and tip laterally to the unsupported side. This muscle pull is supplied mainly by the gluteus medius which runs from the ilium to the greater trochanter. The lengths of the lever arms are altered so that the ratio between the inner arm of the lever to the outer arm is increased by three to one. Thus, the hip joint reaction force is the sum of the body-weight plus three times the body-weight; a total force of four times the body-weight (Figure 9.3). The resultant of these forces normally passes in a line running obliquely downwards across the upper inner part of the roof of the acetabulum and the load is transmitted via the articular cartilage of the acetabular roof to the femoral head.

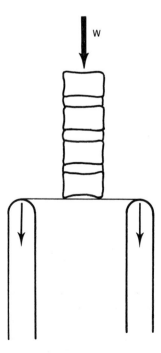

Figure 9.1 When standing on two legs, body-weight (W) is distributed equally through the hips

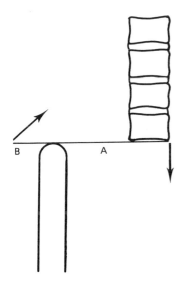

Figure 9.2 When standing on one leg, body-weight is redistributed. The ratio of the inner arm A to the outer arm B is now 3 : 1

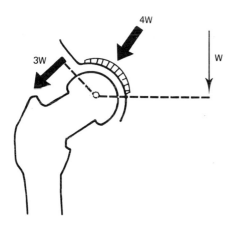

Figure 9.3 Total compressive force on the hip when standing on one leg is 1W + 3W = 4W. W, body-weight

Walking and running subject the hip to large intermittent loads as body-weight is taken alternately on each leg [1,2] and the joint must transfer forces equivalent to several times the body-weight at each step; obesity increases these forces. Theoretically, as body-weight is transferred, the pelvis should tilt away from the supporting leg. This is prevented by the gluteus medius which counterbalances this load and keeps the balanced pelvis steady by approximating the hip and the ilium.

Hip pain

Pain in the hip region may be referred from proximal structures in the spine and pelvis or from local causes in the hip [3]. As the site and nature of such pain are often similar, care must be taken during the examination to differentiate extrinsic from the intrinsic causes.

Extrinsic causes of hip pain

1 Intra-abdominal causes, e.g. appendicitis, intrapelvic diseases [4] or obturator hernia.
2 Disease of local structures, e.g. lymphadenopathy or femoral hernia.
3 Spinal diseases. Hip pain may be referred from the upper lumbar spine (L2), e.g. secondary deposits or psoas abscess. Radicular pain from L3 nerve root pressure may present as pain in the hip and usually pain radiates down the front of the thigh. It may be exacerbated by coughing, straining or bending and quadriceps weakness or wasting and/or a diminished knee jerk are usually present.
4 Sacroiliac arthritis usually presents as buttock pain and may rarely present as groin pain.

Intrinsic hip disorders

Pain arising from the hip joint [3,5] may be felt at several sites, most commonly in the groin or in the lateral aspects of the thigh. Pain is rarely felt deep in the buttock or the back of the thigh. Pain may also radiate down the leg and the greater the degree of underlying inflammation, the further the pain radiates to the knee or even the shin. Pain in the knee may arise from the hip and is usually felt just above the knee in the front of the thigh. This is not the usual distribution for pain arising from knee disorders but a similar pain pattern may occur with pain referred from the lumbar spine.

Pain brought on by walking or standing and relieved by rest suggests a mechanical derangement of the lumbar spine or hip. Pain that is constant and disturbs sleep usually indicates an inflammatory or a neoplastic lesion. Night pain is common in patients with osteoarthritis of the hip but may indicate an inflammatory component often caused by overuse of the hip during the day.

In adults, the most common cause of pain is osteoarthritis of the hip, but other causes of arthritis and soft tissue lesions involving the tendons and bursae are not uncommon. In the older age groups, polymyalgia rheumatica may commence with bilateral hip pain and stiffness. Hip fractures, sometimes incomplete, are common in the elderly. The hip region is commonly involved in metastatic deposits or primary tumours, e.g. multiple myeloma, and pain from these conditions may be present at night.

Examination

Examination begins with the lumbar spine to determine the presence of any restricted movement and whether movements reproduce hip pain. When the patient stands, extension of the spine will also extend the hip joint. So, if pain is reproduced, the pelvis is slightly flexed to extend the lumbar spine further so increasing pain. If the pain decreases, retest hip extension with the patient lying prone. Routine examination should include the abdomen, nervous system and peripheral pulses. The leg is examined for deformities and leg length is measured [6].

Examination of the hip joint

1 Inspection.
   (a) Deformities.
   (b) Gait.
   (c) Swelling.
   (d) Muscle spasm.
   (e) Muscle wasting.
   (f) Trendelenburg test.
2 Movements.
   (a) Active.
   (b) Passive.
   (c) Accessory.
   (d) Isometric.
3 Palpation.
   (a) Swelling.
   (b) Crepitus.
   (c) Tenderness.
4 Radiology.

Inspection

The hip and surrounding structures are examined with the patient standing, walking and lying down.

Deformities

With the patient standing, look for deformities in the hip, lower leg and lumbar spine from in front, the side and behind. Fixed deformities may occur with the hip held in either flexion, lateral rotation, adduction or abduction. An extension deformity of the hip does not occur clinically. The most common deformity is flexion and lateral rotation as the hip is usually more comfortable in this position.

Fixed flexion deformity

This may be apparent on inspection, or may be masked by compensatory movement in the lumbar spine and pelvis with an exaggerated lumbar lordosis and anterior rotation of the pelvis. It is best observed on standing, and the lumbar lordosis and anterior pelvic tilt become evident. With the patient supine the hip may appear straight but the underlying flexion deformity may be revealed by either loss of extension in the affected hip, or Thomas's test, described on p. 116.

Lateral rotation deformity

In this, the foot and patella are rotated laterally and the leg cannot be rotated to the neutral position. The angle short of the neutral position reached by the leg is a measure of the fixed rotational deformity.

Adduction or abduction hip deformity

These are best observed while standing in front of the patient but may be masked by a compensatory pelvic tilt. Adduction deformity may follow arthritis, leg shortening, or protrusio acetabuli. When severe, the heel of the affected leg may cross over the opposite leg. It is compensated by a pelvic tilt to the opposite side, resulting in an apparent leg lengthening. It is usually associated with a lateral rotation deformity and may occur in fracture of the femoral neck or anterior dislocation of the femoral head.

Gait

Gait is observed from the front, side and from behind with the patient walking backwards, forwards and sideways to assess stride length, the time spent on each foot and whether the abnormal gait is produced by pain, deformity, stiffness or altered posture.

1 Antalgic gait, caused by a painful hip as the patient stands for as short a time as possible on the affected limb and a correspondingly longer time on the normal limb, produces a jerky movement rhythm as the trunk lurches towards the painful side.

2 Trendelenburg gait is produced by an intrinsic disorder of the abductors owing to weakness or inability to function properly in an unstable hip. The abductors are unable to stabilize the hip when the body-weight is transferred to the affected side and so the pelvis tilts towards the opposite side.

3 A waddling, or duck gait occurs when the abductor muscles on both sides are weak with bilateral hip disease. As the patient walks the body-weight can be seen to shift laterally from side to side.

4 A swinging gait occurs in ankylosis of the hip when the whole of the lower limb needs to be swung forwards and backwards from the lumbar spine.

5 An adductor gait, in which the legs cannot be adequately separated, occurs with bilateral hip disease, e.g. osteoarthritis, with marked adductor spasm or as a scissors gait owing to spasticity.

6 An uneven gait may be produced by disparity in the leg lengths or because the lumbar spine needs to be extended during locomotion.

Synovial swelling

Synovial swelling in the hip is only rarely obvious on inspection because the synovium lies deep to surrounding muscles. It may occasionally become evident with the patient standing, as the effusion bulges anteriorly and the normal concave surface of the front of the thigh becomes convex. Rarely, a synovial cyst may present as a swelling in the front of the groin or thigh [7,8].

Muscle spasm

This may be obvious on inspection, especially in the adductors.

Muscle wasting

This occurs early in most hip diseases, especially in the glutei and quadriceps, and is best appreciated by standing at the foot of the couch to compare their development on either side.

Trendelenburg test

This tests the ability of the abductor mechanism to stabilize the pelvis with the patient standing on one leg. Standing on one leg, the abductor muscles on that side will contract to maintain pelvic stability. This can be observed by watching the posterior superior iliac spines and iliac crests, which should remain level or slightly rise on the opposite side (Figure 9.4a). The test is positive when the patient stands on one leg and the opposite side of the pelvis drops. It is performed by standing on the leg to be tested and raising the opposite knee to 90 degrees of flexion when the pelvic level and buttock fold on the side of the elevated leg will drop downwards under the influence of gravity (Figure 9.4b). A positive sign indicates that the hip abductors are unable to function properly, as a result of muscular weakness or an inadequate leverage owing to abnormalities of the upper femur, e.g. congenital dislocation of the hip, coxa vara, or non-union of a fractured femoral neck.

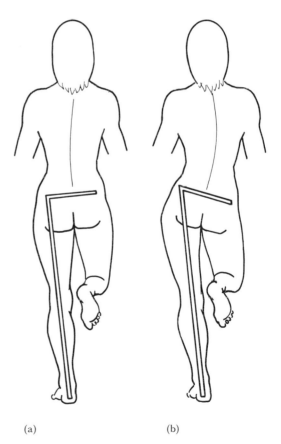

(a)   (b)

Figure 9.4 Trendelenburg test. (a) Normal; (b) positive test

Hip movements

Flexion, extension, abduction, adduction, medial and lateral rotation are tested by a series of active, passive, accessory and isometric movements. While carrying out active and passive movements, one hand is placed over the patient's iliac crest to detect any movement there rather than in the hip joint itself.

The examiner notes:

1   The range of motion.
2   Whether movements are painful or reproduce pain.
3   The presence of muscular spasm.
4   The behaviour of pain and spasm throughout the range of hip movement.
5   The end-feel of the movement.

With pain caused by underlying bone disease, e.g. osteomalacia or secondary deposits, testing hip movements may give confusing results, whereas in avascular necrosis of the hip the range of movement may remain full but painful.

Active movements

Active hip flexion and extension are best tested with the patient standing and the range of movement compared between the two sides. The active range of hip flexion is then tested with the patient supine with the knee flexed to 90 degrees. The normal range of active hip flexion in this position is to 120 degrees, with a wide individual variation.

Passive movements

In the hip, more information can usually be obtained by testing passive or combined movements. Flexion is best tested with the patient lying supine and the knee flexed. The range of passive hip flexion is normally greater than the active range and usually reaches 140 degrees before being limited by contact between the thigh and the anterior abdominal wall.

Thomas's test

This detects a fixed hip flexion deformity when a compensatory lumbar lordosis is developed that masks the hip flexion (Figure 9.5a). With the patient supine the contralateral hip is fully passively flexed which straightens out the lumbar lordosis and the pelvis will then tilt. The affected hip is then observed

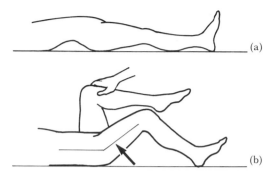

Figure 9.5 Thomas's test. (a) Hip flexion is masked by the lumbar lordosis; (b) flexion of the normal hip obliterates the lumbar lordosis

to develop a degree of flexion deformity (Figure 9.5b). The test may also be positive in bilateral hip disease.

EXTENSION
This is tested with the patient lying prone with the lower limb fully extended. The pelvis is steadied with one hand to prevent simultaneous movement in the hip and lumbar spine, and the hip is passively extended by holding under the anterior thigh and lifting the leg upwards. The normal range of hyper-extension is 15 degrees.

ABDUCTION
Abduction of one hip is normally accompanied by simultaneous rotation of the pelvis and side flexion of the lumbar spine. To test the true range of hip abduction, the pelvis must be fixed with one hand while the extended leg is passively abducted with the other hand. The normal range is 45 degrees.

ADDUCTION
Adduction is normally limited by one leg coming into contact with the other, so may be tested with the leg held in slight flexion to cross over the other leg. The normal range is 25 degrees.

ROTATION
Rotation is defined as rotation of the shaft of the femur and not of the head of the femur which rolls and slides in the acetabulum. Passive hip rotation may be tested by three methods.

1   The patient lies supine with the hip and knee flexed to 90 degrees. The patient's foot is then moved inwards so that the hip is laterally rotated (Figure 9.6a) and then outwards as the hip is

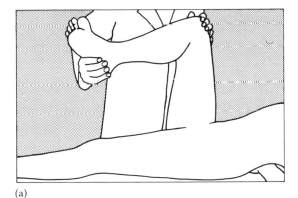

(a)

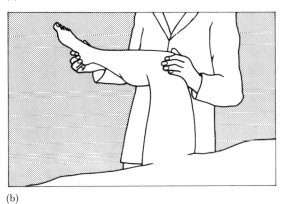

(b)

Figure 9.6 (a) Passive lateral rotation of the hip: supine;
(b) passive medial rotation of the hip: supine

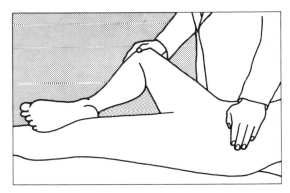

Figure 9.7 Faber test

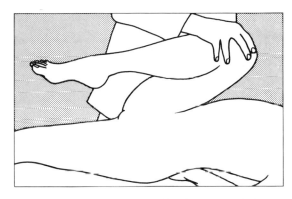

Figure 9.8 Combined flexion, adduction and medial
rotation of the hip

medially rotated (Figure 9.6b). The normal range
is approximately 60 degrees of lateral rotation
and 45 degrees of medial rotation.
2 The patient lies supine with hip and knee
extended and the leg is rapidly rotated inwards
and outwards. In the early stages of hip disease
the characteristic end-feel is an abrupt loss of the
normal fluid type of movement.
3 The patient lies prone with the hip extended and
the knee flexed to 90 degrees and the lower leg
is rotated inwards and outwards.

Combined movements

FABER TEST
This name is an acronym of Flexion, ABduction and
External Rotation, and is performed as a screening
test for hip disease but does not provide detailed
knowledge about loss of a specific hip movement.
The lower lumbar spinal joints, also moved during
this test, may produce pain.

The patient lies supine with the feet together.
The examiner passively flexes one hip and knee and
places the heel on the opposite knee. The knee is
then gently moved towards the floor, thus abducting and laterally rotating the hip (Figure 9.7). The
range of this movement, whether it reproduces or
is limited by pain, stiffness or muscle spasm, is
noted.

COMBINED FLEXION, ADDUCTION AND ROTATION
The patient lies supine. The examiner fully passively
flexes the hip, then adducts and medially rotates it
approximating the knee to the opposite side of the
chest (Figure 9.8). The distance of the knee from the
chest is then measured. It is a useful test for assessing the progress of hip disease. The range and pain
response to the adduction component of this test
should also be assessed with the hip in different
positions of flexion and rotation.

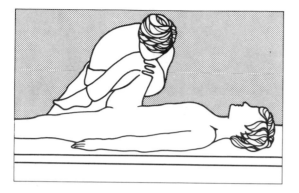

Figure 9.9 Flexion–adduction of the hip joint

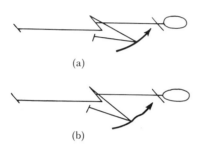

Figure 9.10 Diagrammatic representation of hip flexion–adduction

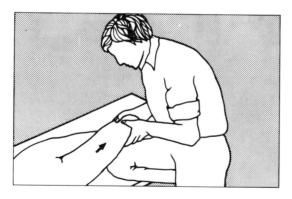

Figure 9.11 Longitudinal caudad accessory movement

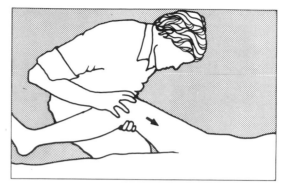

Figure 9.12 Longitudinal cephalad accessory movement

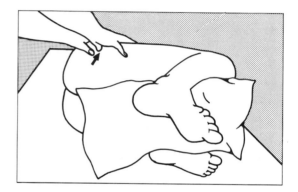

Figure 9.13 Posteroanterior accessory movement

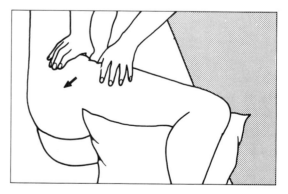

Figure 9.14 Anteroposterior accessory movement

BILATERAL HIP ABDUCTION

The patient lies supine and the examiner abducts both hips to measure the distance between the ankle malleoli. As bilateral movement cancels the effect of any unilateral pelvic rotation, the test provides a useful measure of any progression or improvement in the range of hip movement.

FLEXION–ADDUCTION

This is useful if other hip movements are normal.

The patient in the starting position lies supine near the edge of the couch with the hip flexed to 90 degrees. The examiner stands with fingers over the top of the patient's knee and adducts the hip until it starts to lift up (Figure 9.9).

The hip, while maintained in adduction, is moved in an arc from 90 to 140 degrees of flexion while pressure is maintained through the knee along the leg as the knee normally moves in a smooth arc of a circle (Figure 9.10a). An abnormality in movement is felt as a small hump on the arc which may reproduce pain (Figure 9.10b) [9].

Accessory movements

The five accessory movements in the hip are:

1 Longitudinal caudad. The patient lies supine and the examiner grasps the lower end of the femur applying an oscillatory pull along the femur (Figure 9.11).
2 Longitudinal cephalad. An oscillatory compression movement is applied to the femoral head into the acetabulum (Figure 9.12).
3 Posteroanterior. The patient lies on his side and a posteroanterior movement is applied from behind the greater trochanter (Figure 9.13).
4 Anteroposterior movement is felt by pressure over the greater trochanter (Figure 9.14).
5 Lateral. The patient lies supine with the hip flexed to 90 degrees. The femoral head is displaced laterally in the acetabulum (Figure 9.15).

Isometric tests

The six isometric tests of the hip are flexion, extension, abduction, adduction, medial and lateral rotation. Flexion may be tested in one of two positions with the patient lying supine. In the first position (Figure 9.16a) both the hip and knee are extended; in the second (Figure 9.16b) the hip and knee are flexed with the hip at 90 degrees. One hand is placed just above the knee and fully resists the patient's attempts to flex the thigh. A painful weakness of this movement usually indicates a psoas tendinitis; a painless weakness may be caused by rupture of the psoas tendon or an L2 nerve root lesion.

Extension of the hip is best tested with the patient supine and the extended leg is moved into approximately 20 degrees of flexion at the hip. The examiner places one hand under the patient's heel and resists the patient's attempt to push the leg downwards towards the couch (Figure 9.17). Pain in the upper part of the posterior thigh on this movement may be caused by a lesion of hamstring origin.

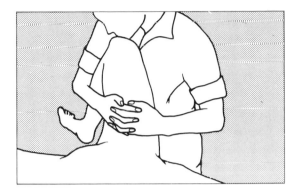

Figure 9.15 Lateral accessory movement

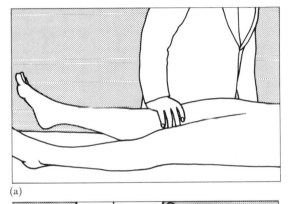

(a)

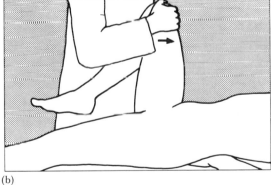

(b)

Figure 9.16 (a) and (b) Resisted flexion of the hip

Adduction is tested with the patient lying supine and the leg extended and fully abducted (Figure 9.18). The examiner places one hand above the medial malleolus of the patient's ankle and resists the patient's attempt to adduct the thigh.

Abduction is best tested with the patient lying on the side with the hip to be tested uppermost and in slight medial rotation and extension.

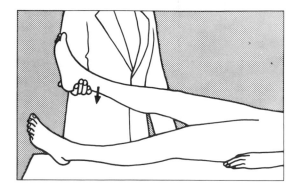

Figure 9.17 Resisted hip extension

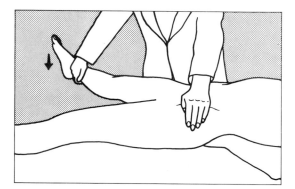

Figure 9.18 Resisted adduction of the hip

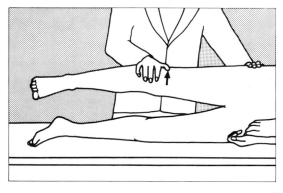

Figure 9.19 Resisted abduction of the hip

The examiner places one hand around the patient's knee and resists the attempt to abduct the thigh (Figure 9.19). A painful weakness of this movement is from a gluteus medius tendinitis. A painless weakness is unusual, but may follow an S1 nerve root lesion or a rupture of the gluteus medius tendon.

Rotation is best tested with the patient lying prone with the hip extended and the knee flexed to 90 degrees. The examiner places one hand above the ankle and first fully resists the patient's attempt to rotate the thigh medially and then laterally.

Palpation

Many of the bony landmarks and soft tissues around the hip are easily palpable. The subcutaneous iliac crest terminates anteriorly at the anterior superior iliac spine from which the tendon of the sartorius muscle arises. The greater trochanter of the femur is easily palpated about a palm's breadth below the iliac crest. Posteriorly the iliac crest terminates at the posterior superior iliac spine which lies under the dimple of Venus. The ischial tuberosity is easily palpable under the gluteal fold in the middle of the buttock, especially with the hip flexed. The sciatic nerve runs midway between the ischial tuberosity and the greater trochanter.

The hip joint itself is placed deeply under the thick muscles and synovial swelling is usually appreciated as a vague sensation of fullness or tenderness but may occasionally be detected by placing the thumb over the midpoint of the inguinal ligament with the four fingers placed posteriorly over the buttock opposite to the thumb. In the presence of synovial swelling the fingers may not be able to reach as far posteriorly as do the fingers on the normal side. A synovial cyst [8] may track anteriorly to present as a swelling in the groin and needs to be differentiated from a femoral hernia, a saphenous varix, arteriovenous fistula, psoas abscess, lymphadenopathy, iliopsoas bursitis, haematoma formation and synovial tumours.

Tenderness should be sought by deep palpation over the head of the femur just below the inguinal ligament lateral to the femoral artery. Tenderness over the greater trochanter is commonly found in trochanteric bursitis, over the adductor origin in adductor tendinitis or, in patients with psoas tendinitis, over the psoas insertion into the lesser trochanter.

Radiology

Standard radiographic views of the hip are usually taken in the anteroposterior (Figure 9.20) and lateral positions [10].

The normal relationship between the acetabulum and the head of the femur is determined by anteroposterior radiographs to measure several angles.

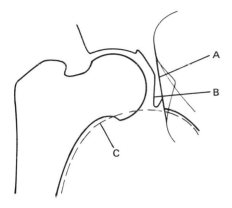

Figure 9.20 Tracing of a radiograph of the hip. (A) Ilioischial line; (B) acetabular U; (C) Shenton's Line (dotted) is continuous from the neck of the femur to the pubic ramus

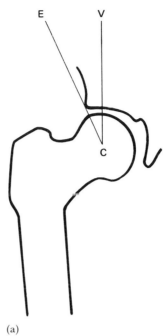

(a)

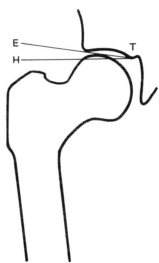

(b)

Figure 9.21 (a) Vertical angle VCE; (b) horizontal angle HTE

The vertical angle is measured from the centre of the femoral head (C) to the lateral edge of the acetabular roof (E) and a vertical line (V) from the centre of the head. The angle (VCE) measures the degree of envelopment of the femoral head by the acetabular roof and is approximately 25 degrees (Figure 9.21a). The horizontal angle is measured from the lateral edge of the acetabular roof (E) to where the acetabular roof meets the acetabular fossa (T) (Figure 9.21b). The angle HTE, normally less than 10 degrees, measures the obliquity of the acetabular roof. An increased obliquity is indicated by an increase in the angle HTE above 13 degrees.

Classification of diseases of the hip

1 Soft tissue lesions.
   (a) Tendinitis: gluteal, psoas, adductor, hamstring and rectus femoris tendons.
   (b) Bursitis: trochanteric, psoas and ischial.
   (c) Snapping hip.
   (d) Capsulitis of the hip.
2 Joint lesions.
   (a) Instability of the symphysis pubis.
   (b) Osteoarthritis.
   (c) Septic arthritis.
   (d) Monoarthritis of the hip.
3 Bone disorders.
   (a) Osteonecrosis.
   (b) Paget's disease.
   (c) Acute osteoporosis.
   (d) Stress fracture.
4 Entrapment neuropathy: lateral cutaneous nerve of the thigh.
5 Hip diseases in childhood.
   (a) Congenital dislocation, subluxation and acetabular dysplasia.
   (b) Juvenile chronic polyarthritis.

(c) Perthes' disease.
(d) Transient synovitis.
(e) Slipped femoral epiphysis.

Soft tissue lesions

Three bursae and five tendons around the hip are commonly involved: the trochanteric, psoas and ischial bursae; the tendinous insertions of the gluteus medius and psoas, and tendon origins of the adductor longus, hamstrings and rectus femoris muscles.

Tendinitis and bursitis

Gluteal tendinitis and trochanteric bursitis

These are the most common soft tissue lesions around the hip and usually occur together. The gluteus medius is a powerful hip abductor inserted via its tendon into the lateral aspect of the greater trochanter of the femur. The tendon is separated on its medial aspect from the greater trochanter and the gluteus minimus by a small bursa, and on its lateral aspect the large multilocular trochanteric bursa lies between the gluteus medius and the tensor fascia lata (Figure 9.22).

Pain is usually well localized over the outer aspect of the greater trochanter, but when severe may radiate down the lateral or posterolateral aspect of the thigh (Figure 9.23). It may follow direct trauma [11] but is usually brought on by hip movements, especially while walking, climbing stairs or crossing the leg. When severe, pain may disturb sleep, especially if the patient rolls onto the affected side. Pain tends to run an intermittent, protracted course, punctuated by exacerbations and remissions often related to activity. It occurs either in sporting activities that involve extensive running, or in middle-aged, usually female, often overweight, patients with associated degenerative changes in the lower lumbar spine [12] and may then be a form of referred pain. In most cases in athletes, bursitis is secondary to increased load on the tendon and associated biomechanical abnormalities [13] include leg length discrepancy, pronated feet, iliotibial band friction or local trauma. In elderly patients with lumbar spine

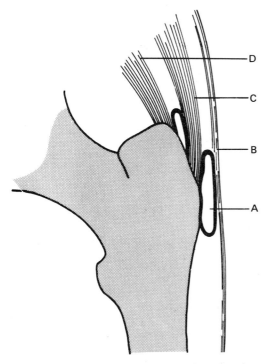

Figure 9.22 The trochanteric bursa (A) lies between the tensor fascia lata (B) and the gluteus medius tendon (C). Another small bursa lies between this tendon and the gluteus minimus (D)

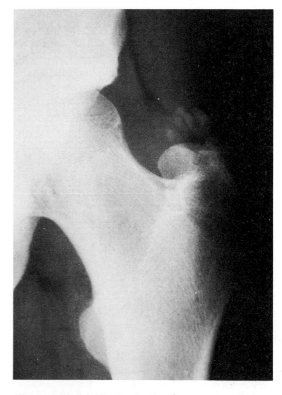

Figure 9.23 Calcification in the gluteus medius tendon

degeneration, tendinitis may follow increased muscle use in an attempt to stabilize the pelvis. It may also complicate arthritis in the hip [13–15].

MAJOR SIGNS

Pain is reproduced by stretching or contracting the gluteus medius. It is stretched with the hip and knee flexed to a right angle and the hip then fully laterally rotated (Figure 9.6a). Pain may be reproduced at its extreme range. Pain may also be reproduced on resisted contraction of the muscle. This is tested by resisting hip abduction as the patient lies on the unaffected side and attempts to lift the affected leg upwards in abduction (Figure 9.19).

CONFIRMATORY SIGNS

Tenderness, usually well localized over the upper lateral aspect of the trochanter, is palpated with the patient lying on the unaffected side. Radiographs are necessary to exclude any hip joint abnormality or calcification in the tendon or bursa [16].

MANAGEMENT

1 Rest from activities that produce pain.
2 Anti-inflammatory agents.
3 Physical methods including heat, ice, stretching of the tendon and deep-pressures are useful in relieving pain.
4 Low back, abdominal and pelvic tilting exercises are prescribed.
5 Mobilization techniques may be effective and are continued if the pain-free range improves.
6 Injections of local anaesthetic and corticosteroid are useful [13,17]. The patient lies on the unaffected side and the tender area around the tendon insertion and bursa is found by careful palpation. A 23-gauge needle is used to inject 5 ml of local anaesthetic and 1 ml of corticosteroid solution. Injections may need to be repeated several times at intervals of 2 weeks.

Adductor tendinitis

This common condition occurs most often in athletes but was previously described in horse riders as 'rider's strain'. Pain is usually well localized over the tendinous origin of the adductor longus from the pubis or a few centimetres distally at its musculotendinous junction. When it is associated with a tendinitis of the rectus abdominus, pelvic instability should be suspected. Occasionally, adductor tendinitis may be an early sign in spondyloarthritis.

MAJOR SIGN

Pain is reproduced by either stretching or contracting the adductor. It is stretched with the patient lying supine and the hip moved into full passive abduction and then fully resisting the patient's attempt to adduct the leg back towards the midline.

CONFIRMATORY SIGNS

Tenderness is usually well localized either over the tendon origin or its musculotendinous junction. Radiographs are usually normal but may occasionally reveal calcification, or even ossification, in the tendon origin. They are taken to exclude other, rare causes of pain in this area, e.g. osteochondritis, stress fracture of the pubis, or secondary metastases.

MANAGEMENT

This includes rest, anti-inflammatory drugs and physical methods. Stretching the tendon is essential and may also be undertaken in a warm pool. Deep-pressure applied to the tender area is often useful and mobilization techniques can be used to increase the pain-free range of hip abduction. Response is usually rapid. Injections of local anaesthetic and corticosteroid must never be given into the tendon but can be given around it or into the musculotendinous junction using a 25-gauge needle.

Psoas tendinitis and bursitis

The iliopsoas muscle is a powerful hip flexor inserted via its tendon into the lesser trochanter and separated from the anterior aspect of the hip capsule by the psoas bursa which may communicate with the hip joint [18].

Pain in the anterior aspect of the thigh tends to be made worse with activity such as weight training or sit-ups. In young athletes a traction injury occurs with separation of part of the lesser trochanter.

MAJOR SIGNS

Pain may be reproduced on contracting or stretching the tendon. The patient lies supine with hip flexed to 90 degrees and further flexion of the hip is resisted (Figure 9.16). Alternatively, the patient lies prone with knee flexed to 90 degrees and the hip is passively hyperextended, so stretching the tendon or compressing the bursa. Finally, pain may be reproduced if lateral rotation is resisted with the hip flexed.

CONFIRMATORY SIGNS

Effusions into the bursa rarely produce visible swelling [19] but if so may cause diagnostic confusion [8,9,18–21] and should be aspirated. Tenderness is felt deeply over the tendon insertion with the patient supine and the hip flexed to 90 degrees. The examiner places one finger just distal to the inguinal ligament over the lesser trochanter and passively abducts the hip with the other hand to palpate any localized tenderness. Radiographs are necessary to exclude underlying pathology [8].

MANAGEMENT
This condition is treated by rest, anti-inflammatory drugs, ice, and mobilization by oscillatory movements through an arc of the last 40 degrees of hip extension.

The bursa or tendinous insertion of the psoas into the lesser trochanter may be injected with local anaesthetic and corticosteroid, taking great care to avoid the femoral nerve. The patient lies supine with the knee flexed and the hip fully abducted and externally rotated. The tender area lateral to the femoral artery and nerve is injected with 1 ml of local anaesthetic and 1 ml of corticosteroid solution and may be repeated two or three times at intervals of 2 weeks.

Hamstring tendinitis

Tendinitis at the ischial origin of the hamstring muscle may occur in distance runners or milkmen, especially with running up hills. Pain is reproduced on resisting hip extension or by stretching the tendon origin by fully flexing the hip. Tenderness is well localized over the ischial tuberosity. Separation of part of the bony cortex may occur in young athletes owing to an avulsion of the hamstring origin from the ischial tuberosity. It is evident on radiographs and is called 'sprinter's fracture'. The young sprinter usually experiences sudden severe pain in the back of the thigh while starting from the blocks or while trying to increase speed, and often falls over.

Rectus femoris

Tendinitis may involve the origin of the rectus femoris from the anterior inferior iliac spine. In adolescents a traction injury with avulsion of the spine may follow sudden exertion in a patient with a previous tendinitis or a direct contusion injury to the thigh muscles. A similar avulsion injury may occur at the origin of the sartorius muscle from the anterior superior iliac spine.

Ischiogluteal bursitis

The ischiogluteal bursa can become chronically inflamed after prolonged sitting, a condition long recognized as 'weaver's bottom'. An acute bursitis may occur but is also rare. Pain over the ischial tuberosity is made worse by sitting and is relieved by standing. There are no specific signs but tenderness is localized over the ischial tuberosity and straight leg raising may reproduce pain.

Snapping hip

A loud snapping noise over the lateral aspect of the hip, sometimes painful, may occur on hip movements in athletes or ballet dancers [22,23]. It may be caused by: (1) intra-articular conditions, such as loose bodies, chondromatosis or exostoses; or (2) the most common cause is the iliotibial band as it slips over the greater trochanter. The iliopsoas tendon is rarely involved [22,24].

Diagnosis is facilitated by CT scan or MRI.

MANAGEMENT
No active therapy is required in most cases as the snapping hip is often merely inconvenient. The patient needs to be reassured about the benign nature of this condition and advised to limit activities that produce snapping. Through-range mobilization techniques may help pain. Symptoms may arise from an associated trochanteric bursitis and surgery may then be indicated [25].

Capsulitis of the hip

Capsulitis is rare in the hip and is found in the middle-aged and younger age groups. The patient presents with a relatively rapid onset of pain and stiffness, made worse by activity, and it may follow trauma [26].

MAJOR SIGNS
The major sign is a painful restriction of hip movement in all planes that usually becomes progressively worse. Routine hip radiography and ancillary tests, including blood studies, are normal. Arthrography demonstrates a reduction in joint capacity with loss of normal joint recesses [26].

MANAGEMENT

1 Analgesics and anti-inflammatory drugs are given.
2 Heat or ice is applied to the hip.
3 Passive stretching, especially extension, of the hip is necessary.

4 Passive mobilization techniques, flexion–adduction, extension, rotation and accessory movements at the limit of one or more of these movements are used.

5 As pain settles, active exercises are commenced and passive mobilization continued.

Joint lesions

Instability of the symphysis pubis

Instability of the symphysis pubis is a very common sporting injury especially in footballers and runners. The pelvis forms a bony ring with two posterior sacroiliac joints and anterior symphysis pubis. The symphysis pubis is a secondary cartilaginous joint formed between the bony surfaces of the pubis which are lined by hyaline cartilage and joined together by fibrocartilage [27]. It is protected by strong ligaments above and below [28]. It has a small normal physiological range of movement [29–31] in two different planes. In sports, the exact mechanism of its production is not known. The most likely explanation is that repetitive movement produces shear and tensile forces [27] resulting in disruption of the symphysis ligaments producing an increase in vertical symphysis mobility [30]. This abnormal movement may ultimately produce vascular changes which then result in osteitis pubis (Figure 9.24). Instability may also follow pregnancy [32], operations on the sacroiliac joints, direct trauma or inflammatory disorders such as spondyloarthritis [27,32,33].

The patient complains of pain in one or both groins which may radiate widely to the lower abdomen, adductor region of the thigh, hip, testis or perineum and may also cause low back pain when it is associated with a lesion of the sacroiliac joint. Pain is usually made worse by exercise, straining, or adopting certain postures, such as standing on one leg, walking upstairs, or thrusting the hip forward. Pain is usually severe, so that running, kicking or sidestepping is virtually impossible, and causes the patient to limp. A clicking sensation may also be present on certain movements such as walking over uneven ground or turning over in bed [32]. Gait is often wide-based or waddling. Back pain is common. It may be due to sacroiliac pain [29] which may be associated with radiographic evidence of osteitis condensans ilii. Ruz (personal communication) investigated 22 national team footballers with symphysis instability who complained of back pain and found an associated spondylolysis at L4–L5 in 14

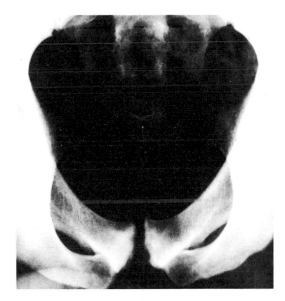

Figure 9.24 Pelvic instability

of them. The same mechanism of production of injury is common to both of them.

Pain may be reproduced by passively abducting the hip, by resisting the patient's attempt to sit up, by resisting adduction of the hip or by passive elevation of alternate legs. Pain and tenderness can be reproduced by pressure over or by springing the symphysis. Pain and tenderness also occur over the tendons of the adductor longus and the rectus abdominis near their attachments in the pubis and may represent an attempt by them to stabilize the pelvis. A loss of the range of medial rotation of the hip is found in about half of cases [34]. In the action of kicking this will then cause more force to be transmitted across the symphysis.

Diagnosis is confirmed by radiography, nuclide scan or CT scan. Radiography is performed while standing on alternate legs and comparing the heights of the two sides of the pubis [30]. Instability is present if the difference in their vertical height varies by more than 2 mm [29]. Other radiographic changes of the inflammatory non-infectious osteitis pubis include erosions and sclerosis of the bone ends, often with widening of the joint space (Figure 9.24). The lower margin is a better indicator than the upper [32].

MANAGEMENT
This is difficult:

1 Rest is essential, since pain is exacerbated by most weight bearing activities. All sporting activities

that involve running or walking must be avoided for several months, although swimming is usually possible.

2 Anti-inflammatory drugs and analgesics are given for pain relief.

3 Injections of local anaesthetic and corticosteroid may be given into painful, tender areas around the pelvis and may be repeated several times if they provide relief.

4 Pain-free passive and active stretching exercises are given when restriction of hip movement, usually medial rotation, is present.

5 In most patients the condition gradually settles over several months. The patient can then start to resume walking and functional activities. Stretching is still continued and abdominal and back exercises commenced. The return to sport needs to be gradual.

6 Various braces and sacroiliac belts have been tried.

7 Surgery with fusion may be necessary in some diseases [31,35] but is not practical in sportspeople [36].

Osteoarthritis of the hip

This is the most common form of hip disease and may be bilateral. It commences in patients of either sex, with any type of body build, usually after the age of 50 years. The hip is subjected to large mechanical forces and the presence of even a slight anomaly or incongruity on the joint surface can predispose to subsequent degenerative changes. In most cases diagnosed as primary osteoarthritis, an underlying abnormality of the joint surfaces can be found [37] including congenital anomalies, e.g. acetabular dysplasia or subluxation of the hip; or acquired defects after trauma, slipped epiphysis, joint disease, or infection.

Clinical features

The onset is insidious. Pain is the usual presenting symptom, but there is no strong correlation between the degree of pain and the radiological changes present. Pain is usually related to weight-bearing or movement and may appear first as attacks of hip or knee pain after prolonged or unaccustomed activities. It tends to become worse as the day goes on and is relieved by rest. Later, pain may be present at night and disturb sleep and may be related to the severity of the inflammatory or bony changes. The restricted hip movements in the early stages may be

considered by the patient to be part of the normal ageing process until the loss of function becomes more marked. This may be manifested by difficulty in putting on socks or stockings or in tying up shoelaces, especially in the morning when hip stiffness is more pronounced. Walking may become more difficult because of the loss of hip extension.

Subsequently, as hip pain and stiffness become more marked, walking distance is reduced and the patient develops a limp. Back pain may be a feature owing to the development of a compensatory lordosis and excessive use of the lumbar spine on walking. Deformity also increases as the patient tends to stand on the unaffected leg and the affected hip is often held in a position of flexion and lateral rotation, producing a characteristic deformity. There is difficulty both in sitting down and in standing up, going up or down stairs and sitting forwards in a chair. Disability produced by stiffness and deformity can ultimately become marked and the patient can only get about with difficulty by using sticks or crutches.

The most common site of radiological joint space narrowing is superolateral and the head of the femur tends to sublux upwards. The next is the superior aspect of the joint and, least commonly, the medial aspect of the joint cavity and the head of the femur then tends to migrate inwards, producing protrusio acetabuli. This classification has some prognostic significance as the superolateral narrowing tends to be more severe and progressive whereas the medial type can be more benign; clinical signs may also differ in these types.

CLINICAL EXAMINATION

Gait is usually disturbed, with either an antalgic gait; a swinging type of gait if the hip is stiff; a lurching of the trunk towards the affected side if there is any shortening of the limb; or a Trendelenburg gait with weakness of the abductors. Deformity is looked for first with the patient standing and viewed from in front and the side and then while lying supine. Muscle wasting is almost invariably present in the gluteal and the quadriceps group. Swelling as a result of synovitis of the hip is usually too deeply placed to become visible.

The first hip movements lost are flexion–adduction, medial rotation and extension, and so the hip is held in flexion and lateral rotation. Flexion deformity of the hip is usually compensated for by increased lumbar lordosis. When lying down, lordosis can mask the hip flexion unless it is revealed by a positive Thomas' test. An adduction deformity may also be present and results in apparent leg shortening on the affected side. The hip movements ultimately become restricted in all directions. The pattern of movement loss tends to vary according to the site of hip involvement. In the superolateral type there is a progressive loss of medial rotation, extension and abduction so that the common deformity of flexion, lateral rotation and adduction is produced. In the medial type the head of the femur is displaced into the deepened acetabular cavity, so that rotation in both directions and abduction tend to be most affected.

The leg length disparity is common and both legs should be measured to determine the presence of any true or apparent shortening [6], and the thighs are measured to chart any quadriceps wasting. The lumbar spine should be examined for any pain and/or restricted movement.

MANAGEMENT

The management of osteoarthritis has been revolutionized since the introduction of new surgical techniques and total hip replacement. In its earlier stages much can be achieved by conservative measures to relieve the patient's pain and stiffness, prevent deformity, and maintain functional capacity.

1   General measures. It is essential to spend some time with patients explaining the nature of their disability, reassuring them that they need not fear becoming crippled and that the severity of their symptoms is often caused by overuse of the joint. Consultation with an occupational therapist is advisable to outline any special problems at work or around the house. Correction of any other postural problems in the legs or back should be undertaken.
    Weight loss, if the patient is obese, is a rational form of therapy designed to take some load off the patient's hip.
2   Rest. The patient needs to avoid excessive weight-bearing and should be advised to stand and walk less on the affected hip if pain, particularly at night, is a problem. The patient should lie down in the prone position for approximately half an hour a day to inhibit a flexion deformity. Acute episodes of pain are usually best managed with a few days of rest in bed.
3   Aids and supports. A walking stick carried in the opposite hand will allow weight to be redistributed onto the normal hip and ease pain in the affected hip [38]. Crutches or a walking frame are only rarely necessary. A heel raise on a shoe may be necessary if there is any disparity in leg length.

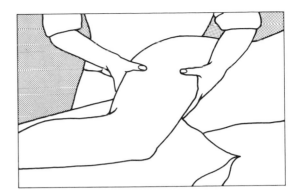

Figure 9.25 Treatment of osteoarthritis of the hip with gentle lateral movement

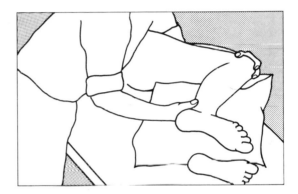

Figure 9.26 Treatment of osteoarthritis of the hip with gentle medial rotation

4   Regular simple analgesics should be given at first. Anti-inflammatory drugs are added to this regimen only if required.
5   Physical methods. Physical methods of therapy such as heat usually bring only a short-term relief of pain and have little place to play in the long-term management. Exercise therapy should be given only with well-defined objectives, is of no value when pain is the dominant feature and should not be persevered with if it causes exacerbation of pain. Exercises to increase the range of hip movement, particularly rotation, often produce exacerbation of pain. Patients with weakness and wasting in the thigh and gluteal muscles should be taught isometric exercises, especially if they have difficulty in walking or a feeling of instability in the leg. To overcome stiffness, they may be combined with assisted exercises, e.g. the use of a sling to stretch the hip in extension or abduction [39].

6 Manual therapy. When pain is the dominant problem, treatment first uses small amplitude passive movements without provoking any further pain. The patient lies with the painful hip uppermost. The therapist places the thumbs over the greater trochanter and uses posteroanterior, anteroposterior, longitudinal movements and lateral movement of the femoral head away from the acetabulum (Figure 9.25). As pain settles, treatment is progressed using rotational movements (Figure 9.26) and their amplitude is gradually progressed until a full rocking from medial to lateral rotation is attained. When pain and stiffness are major problems, the hip is first treated in flexion and adduction (Figure 9.9) and accessory movements are used at the end of the range. As the condition improves, medial rotation is the treatment method, using large-amplitude movements at the end of the range, and other movements can then be added at the limit of range.

7 Surgery. This should be considered in patients with severe degrees of pain or disability or who fail to respond to conservative measures. Total hip replacement is the treatment of choice in older patients, but in younger patients a femoral osteotomy may still have a role [40].

Septic arthritis

This is relatively uncommon and is usually caused by *Staphylococcus aureus*, but other causative organisms include streptococcal, gonococcal and pneumococcal infections. Tuberculosis of the hip has now fortunately become rare.

The patient usually presents with a sudden onset of severe hip pain that is constant, worse at night and with marked restriction of hip movement. Associated features include a raised temperature, a leucocytosis and an elevated erythrocyte sedimentation rate. Investigations include hip aspiration for cell count and culture and blood cultures. Radiography may be normal at first but usually severe destructive changes are seen later, especially if the diagnosis is delayed, as may easily happen in this joint [41]. Hence other imaging methods are necessary [44]. Treatment consists of surgical drainage, immobilization and appropriate antibiotic cover for at least 6 months.

Monoarthritis of the hip

This rare and apparently unique form of arthritis involves only one hip. The patient, usually middle-aged, presents with a rapid onset of hip pain and stiffness that gradually settle over the next 2–3 years. Radiographs reveal gross narrowing of the joint space with destructive changes in the acetabulum and femoral head but no osteophyte formation. The erythrocyte sedimentation rate is always elevated and aspirated samples of synovial fluid show inflammatory changes. Synovial biopsy shows numerous inflammatory foci in hypertrophic villi and vascular dilatation. This disease is distinct from other important causes of monoarthritis of the hip such as infections, chondrocalcinosis, rheumatoid arthritis and spondyloarthritis.

Disorders of the hip bones

Osteonecrosis of the femoral head

Osteonecrosis of the femoral head may follow trauma or occur as a rare complication of many different diseases, but in a quarter of cases no underlying cause can be found [42].

The initial change is an area of subchondral osteolysis in the femoral head; in the early stages, the articular cartilage remains normal [43,44]. The underlying subchondral bone becomes necrotic and liable to collapse and a bony sequestrum may form [45]. Beneath the subchondral bone an area of vascular granulation tissue forms in an attempt to resorb the necrotic bone and lay down new bone. As the lesion progresses, the articular cartilage may separate from the femoral head and become reattached to the collapsed subchondral bone. The femoral head becomes irregular in shape and degenerative changes may ultimately develop.

These changes are consistent with an ischaemic necrosis of bone from vascular occlusion [43] but it

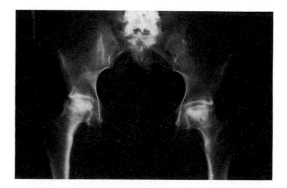

Figure 9.27 Bilateral avascular necrosis of the hip in a long-distance runner

has not been possible to demonstrate such an occlusion in all cases, including the primary form of disease. The intraosseous pressure is raised [46] and so the capillary perfusion pressure becomes insufficient in the rather tenuous microcirculation of the femoral head. Interruption of the arterial blood supply may follow trauma, e.g. a fracture of the femoral neck, slipped femoral epiphysis and dislocation of the hip, but it may follow simple trauma such as a fall on the hip. It may also occur in deep-sea divers, when bubbles of nitrogen gas are formed and cause emboli or direct compression of the vascular channels. Vasculitis, coagulation defects and haemoglobinopathy also produce vascular occlusion. Vasculitis may be the underlying cause of avascular necrosis in several of the inflammatory arthropathies, especially systemic lupus erythematosus, even if it has not been treated by corticosteroids.

Fat emboli, which may occur in many diseases associated with a disorder of lipid metabolism, such as hyperlipoproteinaemia, Gaucher's disease, gout, chronic alcoholism, prolonged corticosteroid therapy or Cushing's disease, have been suggested as a cause.

CLINICAL FEATURES
Symptoms are identical regardless of the cause. The onset may be gradual, but often there is a sudden, dramatic, onset of hip pain that usually becomes severe and incapacitating and disturbs sleep. Pain may be felt in the hip or thigh but is often felt only at the knee. At first the range of hip movement may remain normal, although pain may be exacerbated by hip movements. After a time, a marked limitation of hip movement and wasting of thigh muscles are usually found.

DIAGNOSIS
Osteonecrosis as a result of ischaemic changes, with death of osteocytes and marrow, leads to increased bone marrow pressure which then can produce more ischaemia. Patchy osteoporosis and sclerosis are usually the first radiographic signs but these changes, necessary to confirm the diagnosis, may take quite some time to develop [47,48]. During this time a radionuclide bone scan [47,49], CT scan or especially MRI [50–52] are the most useful confirmatory tests but measurement of intra-osseous pressure and/or venography may also help [42].

MANAGEMENT
Investigations are necessary to establish any underlying cause [45]. In the early stages the patient may need to be admitted to hospital for bed rest and relief from weight-bearing. Analgesics and anti-inflammatory drugs are given for pain relief. If pain settles, the patient can then be mobilized with the aid of crutches and later a walking stick [53]. If not, decompression by removing a small core of cancellous bone to reduce intra-osseous pressure may help [54,55]; subsequent replacement of the femoral head is usually necessary.

Paget's disease

Paget's disease commonly involves bones around the hip. Pain is the usual presenting symptom and is often worse at night. Pain may be due to the Paget's disease or its complications, such as pathological fracture. If juxta-articular bone is involved osteoarthritis of the hip usually develops, producing mechanical hip pain [56].

Acute osteoporosis

This condition occurs mainly in middle-aged men, usually in the absence of any recognizable cause or rarely after trauma [57]. The patient presents with severe pain and stiffness in the hip or thigh, often of sudden onset, which becomes gradually progressive over the next few months so that walking becomes increasingly difficult. The course is one of slow resolution over the next 6 months [58]. Radiographic changes are necessary for diagnosis and show rarefaction in the hip, especially the femoral head. The joint space remains well preserved, thus helping to differentiate it from arthritis or joint infection. Radiographic changes are present for some time after clinical remission.

Stress fractures

Stress fractures of the femoral neck are not uncommon [59] and tend to occur in two types of patient. The first is in young active males, such as army recruits or joggers [60]. The second is in the elderly, who may also have osteoporosis. Two types of fracture have also been described. One is a compression fracture that tends to occur at the lower border of the neck in the young and responds well to rest. The second is a transverse fracture across the upper border of the neck in the elderly that tends to become displaced and requires surgical treatment.

Diagnosis is made by radiography, bone scan and CT scans.

Entrapment neuropathy

Lateral cutaneous nerve of the thigh

The lateral cutaneous nerve of the thigh is derived mainly from the L2 and L3 nerve roots and supplies the skin over the anterolateral aspect of the thigh. The nerve usually enters the thigh by passing through a tunnel in the inguinal ligament near its attachment to the anterior superior iliac spine. The most common site for entrapment is in this tunnel, as the nerve angulates to enter the thigh, and it may be compressed or kinked by the inguinal ligament. The degree of angulation is increased by extension of the hip. Many other causes of compression here have been described including direct trauma, pregnancy, alteration in weight [61] or activity after prolonged bed rest. Less commonly, the nerve may be entrapped at other sites along its course from the spinal canal.

Symptoms occur mainly in middle-aged males. The patient describes a typical burning pain with numbness or paraesthesia in the distribution of the nerve over the anterolateral aspect of the thigh to just above the knee. An unusual sensation of itching or formication may be present which leads the patient to rub the area of skin involvement so producing a rash. Symptoms may be intermittent and tend to be brought on by periods of prolonged standing or by alterations of posture which usually involve hip extension.

MANAGEMENT
The patient needs to rest from those movements or positions of the hip that are known to cause exacerbation of symptoms. Injections of 5 ml of local anaesthetic and 1 ml corticosteroid may be infiltrated around the nerve as it passes through the inguinal ligament, approximately one fingerbreadth medial to the anterior superior iliac spine.

Mobilization of the tissues in the entrapment area may relieve the patient's symptoms. Heat, ice and other physical modalities are of no value. Microsurgery to decompress the nerve may be necessary in those patients whose symptoms continue [62].

Hip diseases in childhood

These include [62,63]:

1 Congenital dislocation of the hip and acetabular dysplasia.

2 Juvenile chronic polyarthritis.
3 Perthes' disease.
4 Transient synovitis.
5 Slipped femoral epiphysis.

Congenital

Congenital dislocation of the hip

Failure of normal hip development may result in congenital dislocation, subluxation of the hip or acetabular dysplasia, any of which may be associated in later life with osteoarthritis.

In congenital dislocation, the underdeveloped femoral head dislocates upwards onto the ilium. It is approximately six times more common in females and is predominantly a disorder of the Caucasian population, especially Scandinavians. It is bilateral in about one-third and the left hip is more commonly and more severely involved. Ideally it should be diagnosed at birth by either Barlow's test (pushing laterally to dislocate the head) or Ortolani's test (reducing it in abduction) [64,65], and the diagnosis confirmed on radiographs or ultrasound [65]. If dislocation is reduced early, the chances of subsequent osteoarthritis are considerably lessened [65].

Congenital subluxation

Subluxation is present when the femoral head moves upwards and outwards, losing contact with the underdeveloped acetabulum. Radiographs will demonstrate these changes and there is an interruption in Shenton's line (Figure 9.20).

Acetabular dysplasia

Here the acetabulum is shallow with an inadequate sloping roof, and may be associated with coxa valga and anteversion of the femoral neck. It can be measured radiologically by reduction in the vertical angle VCE to less than 20 degrees and an increase in the horizontal angle HTE to more than 10 degrees (Figure 9.28). Inadequate covering of the femoral head predisposes to osteoarthritis in later life.

Juvenile chronic polyarthritis

Hip involvement is an important cause of loss of functional capacity in children with this condition. It usually occurs comparatively early in the course of the polyarticular form of disease, and monoarticular

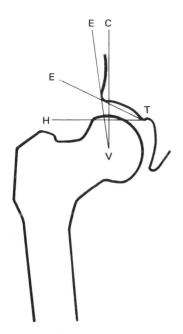

Figure 9.28 In acetabular dysplasia the vertical angle (VCE) is reduced and the horizontal angle (IITE) increased

a widening of the medial joint space owing to an effusion in the hip, which may be a causative factor in the development of ischaemia [78]. Later a line of separation in the subchondral bone develops, and the epiphysis becomes necrotic and dense. Healing occurs as vascular buds grow out into the epiphysis and produce an appearance of fragmentation of the head. This continues for several years leaving a residual oval mushroom shaped deformity of the femoral head, coxa plana, and a wide, thick femoral neck. The acetabular fossa becomes too small for the femoral head and osteoarthritis commonly develops after the age of 50 years.

MANAGEMENT
Management remains controversial [79] and early cases can be managed with rest and without surgery [74]. Later, the aim is to contain the femoral head within the acetabulum while repair takes place, using either an abduction brace [80] or surgery [81,82]. Prolonged bracing is difficult [67] and innominate or femoral osteotomy [83,84] may be preferable to minimize the residual deformity of the femoral head and acetabulum [85] and maintain femoral head mobility [74,86].

hip disease is rare. Radiographic features include growth defects in the femoral head, protrusio acetabuli and coxa valga.

Perthes' disease

Perthes' disease, one of the group of juvenile osteochondroses, occurs usually in male children aged from 3 to 10 years and may be bilateral. The child presents with a limp, associated usually with a minor degree of pain and some limitation of hip movement. The aetiology and natural course are uncertain. Loss of blood supply to the proximal epiphysis [5,66] produces episodes of infarction and necrosis, but reasons for this have not been identified [67]. Boys often have a delay in skeletal age and impaired skeletal growth [68], which may be associated with raised serum somatomedin activity [69,70]. They are often of low socioeconomic status [71] and nutritional changes [72], including low manganese levels [73], have been described. Prognosis is better for the younger ages and for boys [74].

Diagnosis is confirmed on radiography but it may take some time for typical changes to develop and bone scans [75], ultrasound [76] or MRI [77] are more helpful. The first radiographic change may be

Transient synovitis

This condition, also known as irritable hip [87], results from a benign self-limiting synovial inflammation [78,88]. The child presents with sudden onset of hip pain and limp, with painful limitation of hip movements. There may be a history of minor trauma and it may represent a form of reactive arthritis involving the hip [89].

Laboratory tests are always normal but the radiograph may show soft tissue swelling, especially bulging over the intrapelvic aspect of the acetabulum [78,90,91]. Isotope scanning [92,93] or ultrasound [94] are useful to differentiate it from other conditions such as infective arthritis or Perthes' disease. These conditions usually become evident after repeated investigations, whereas transient synovitis settles within a few days with bed rest and analgesics, without any sequelae [78].

Slipped femoral epiphysis

This disorder, of unknown aetiology, is a displacement of the upper epiphysis of the femoral head in a medial, posterior and then inferior direction. The slip must occur before this epiphysis unites, usually

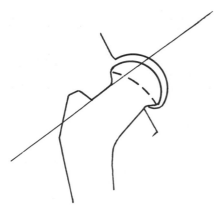

Figure 9.29 Tracing of a radiograph of the right hip. Normally, a line drawn along the superior surface of the femoral neck transects the femoral head

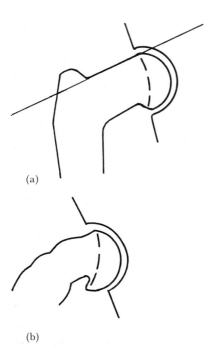

(a)

(b)

Figure 9.30 Tracings of radiographs of the hip. (a) In slipped epiphysis, this line passes above the femoral head; (b) in the lateral view, the slipped femoral head is extruded from the confines of the acetabulum

at about the age of 16 years. It is bilateral in approximately 25% of cases, and some genetic or hormonal predisposition is considered likely [95]. It occurs more commonly in males, aged usually 11–15 years, who are usually either obese [96] with poorly developed secondary sexual characteristics or tend to be lean and tall [5]. The onset may be insidious or

trauma may produce a shearing strain on the femoral head resulting in an acute slip. The child usually presents with pain, often felt in the knee rather than in the hip, and a limp with the hip maintained in a position of adduction and lateral rotation. Examination may reveal a Trendelenburg gait and restricted hip movements, particularly medial rotation [64]. As the hip is flexed, the femur characteristically goes into lateral rotation and abduction.

Routine and frog views are necessary to confirm the diagnosis (Figures 9.29 and 9.30). In the anteroposterior view the head may appear to be tilted medially so that the medial third of the metaphysis is displaced out of the acetabulum. In this view a line drawn along the superior surface of the femoral neck should transect a portion of the femoral head. If the head has slipped medially a line drawn along the superior aspect of the femoral neck will fall outside the head of the femur. Subsequently, bone is laid down on the medial side of the neck and resorbed on its lateral aspect, producing a characteristic radiological appearance of the femoral head which appears to be tilted.

MANAGEMENT

The aim of treatment is to stabilize and prevent additional slipping; stimulate early closure and prevent complications [96]. In the acute stages the patient should be admitted to hospital for bed rest and traction to the leg in medial rotation. Manipulative reduction of the displacement under anaesthesia may be successful, especially in patients with an acute slip and the epiphysis is held in place by pins. If not, an osteotomy may be necessary.

Complications of slipped epiphysis include cartilage necrosis [97], avascular necrosis of bone and osteoarthritis.

References

1   Radin, E.L. (1980) Biomechanics of the human hip. *Clinical Orthopaedics and Related Research*, **152**, 28–34

2   Frankel, V.H. (1986) Biomechanics of the hip joint. *Instructional Course Lectures*, **25**, 3–9

3   Hodges, D.L., McGuire, T.J. and Kumar, V.N. (1987) Diagnosis of hip pain, an anatomic approach. *Orthopaedic Review*, **16**, 109–113

4   Wan, A. (1988) Retro-peritoneal haemorrhage presenting as hip pain. *Archives of Emergency Medicine*, **5**, 246–247

5   McBeath, A.A. (1985) Some common causes of hip pain. Physical diagnosis is the key. *Postgraduate Medicine*, **77**, (i) 189–192; (ii) 194–195; (iii) 198

6   Friberg, O. (1983) Clinical symptoms and biomechanics of lumbar spine and hip joint in leg length inequality. *Spine*, **8**, 643–651

7   Lavyne, M.H., Voorhies, R.M. and Coll, R.II. (1982) Femoral neuropathy caused by an iliopsoas bursal cyst. Case report. *Journal of Neurosurgery*, **56**, 584–586

8   Sartoris, D.J., Danzig, L., Gilula, L. *et al.* (1985) Synovial cysts of the hip joint and iliopsoas bursitis: a spectrum of imaging abnormalities. *Skeletal Radiology*, **14**, 85–94

9   Maitland, G.D. (1991) *Peripheral manipulation* (3rd edn), Butterworth-Heinemann, Oxford, p. 223

10   Pitt, M.J., Lund, P.J. and Speer, D.P. (1990) Imaging of the pelvis and hip. *Orthopedic Clinics of North America*, **21**, 545–559

11   Haller, C.C., Coleman, P.A., Estes, N.C. *et al.* (1989) Traumatic trochanteric bursitis. *Kansas Medicine*, **90**, 17–18

12   Little, H. (1979) Trochanteric bursitis: a common cause of pelvic girdle pain. *Canadian Medical Association Journal*, **120**, 456–458

13   Roberts, W.N. and Williams, R.B. (1988) Hip pain. *Primary Care*, **15**, 783–793

14   Raman, D. and Haslock, I. (1982) Trochanteric bursitis – a frequent cause of 'hip' pain in rheumatoid arthritis. *Annals of Rheumatic Diseases*, **41**, 603

15   Schapira, D., Nahir, M. and Scharf, Y. (1986) Trochanteric bursitis: a common clinical problem. *Archives of Physical and Medical Rehabilitation*, **67**, 815–817

16   Karpinski, M.R. and Piggott, H. (1985) Greater trochanteric pain syndrome. A report of 15 cases. *Journal of Bone and Joint Surgery*, **67**, 762–763

17   Rasmussen, K.J. & Fano, N. (1985) Trochanteric bursitis. *Scandinavian Journal of Rheumatology*, **14**, 417–420

18   Underwood, P.L., McLeod, R.A. and Ginsburg, W.W. (1988) The varied clinical manifestations of iliopsoas bursitis. *Journal of Rhematology*, **15**, 1683–1685

19   Harper, M.C., Schberg, J.E. and Allen, W.C. (1987) Primary iliopsoas bursography in the diagnosis of disorders of the hip. *Clinical Orthopaedics*, **221**, 238–241

20   Pellman, E., Kumari, S. and Greenwald, R. (1986) Rheumatoid iliopsoas bursitis presenting as unilateral leg edema. *Journal of Rheumatology*, **13**, 197–200

21   Binek, R. and Levinsohn, E.M. (1987) Enlarged iliopsoas bursa. An unusual cause of thigh mass and hip pain. *Clinical Orthopaedics*, **224**, 158–163

22   Reid, D.C. (1988) Prevention of hip and knee injuries in ballet dancers. *Sports Medicine*, **6**, 295–307

23   Sammarco, G.J. (1983) The dancer's hip. *Clinics in Sports Medicine*, **2**, 485–498

24   Lyons, J.C. and Peterson, L.F.A. (1984) The snapping iliopsoas tendon. *Mayo Clinic Proceedings*, **59**, 327–329

25   Zoltan, D.J., Clancy, W.G. Jr. and Keene, J.S. (1986) A non-operative approach to snapping hip and refractory trochanteric bursitis in athletes. *Annals of Journal of Sports Medicine*, **14**, 201–204

26   Griffiths, H.J., Utz, R., Burke, J. *et al.* (1985) Adhesive capsulitis of the hip and ankle. *American Journal of Roentgenology*, **144**, 101–105

27   Gamble, J.G., Simmons, S.C. and Freedman, M. (1986) The symphysis pubis: Anatomic and pathologic considerations. *Clinical Orthopaedics and Related Research*, **203**, 261–272

28   Scott, S.T. and Watt, I. (1984) Gas at the symphysis pubis: A sign of occult pelvis trauma. *British Journal of Radiology*, **57**, 173–176

29   Walheim, G.G., Olerud, S. and Ribbe, T. (1984) Mobility of the pubic symphysis. *Acta Orthopaedica Scandinavica*, **55**, 203–208

30   Walheim, G.G. and Selvik, G. (1984) Mobility of the pubic symphysis. *Clinical Orthopaedics and Related Research*, **191**, 129–135

31   Webb, L.X., Gristina, A.G., Wilson, J.R. *et al.* (1988) Two-hole plate fixation for traumatic symphysis pubis diastasis. *Journal of Trauma*, **28**, 813–817

32   Sequeira, W. (1986) Diseases of the pubic symphysis. *Seminars in Arthritis and Rheumatism*, **16**, 11–21

33   Tauber, C., Geltner, D., Noff, M. *et al.* (1987) Disruption of the symphysis pubis and fatigue fractures of the pelvis in a patient with rheumatoid arthritis. *Clinical Orthopaedics and Related Research*, **215**, 105–108

34   Laban, M.M., Meerschaert, J.R., Taylor, R.S. *et al.* (1975) Symphyseal and sacroiliac joint pain associated with pubic symphysial instability. *Archives of Physical Medicine and Rehabilitation*, **59**, 40–42

35   Olerud, S. and Walheim, G.G. (1984) Symphysiodesis with a new compression plate. *Acta Orthopaedica Scandinavica*, **55**, 315–318

36   Lange, R.H. & Hansen, S.T. (1985) Pelvic ring disruptions with symphysis pubis diastasis. *Clinical Orthopaedics and Related Research*, **201**, 130–137

37   Harris, W.H. (1986) Etiology of osteoarthritis of the hip. *Clinical Orthopaedics*, **213**, 20–33

38   Brady, L.P. (1988) Hip pain. Don't throw away the cane. *Postgraduate Medicine*, **83**, (i) 89–90; (ii) 95–97

39   Leivseth, G., Torstensson, J. and Reiker, O. (1989) Effect of passive muscle stretching in osteoarthritis of the hip. *Clinical Science*, **76**, 113–117

40   Hackenbroch, M.H. (1989) Intertrochanteric osteotomy for the treatment of coxarthrosis. *Archives of Orthopaedic and Trauma Surgery*, **108**, 125–131

41   Shiv, V.K., Jain, A.K., Taneja, K. *et al.* (1990) Sonography of hip joint in infective arthritis. *Canadian Association of Radiology Journal*, **41**, 76–78

42   Zivic, T.M., Marcoux, C., Hungerford, D.S. *et al.* (1986) The early diagnosis of ischemic necrosis of bone. *Arthritis and Rheumatism*, **29**, 1177–1186

43   Solomon, L. (1985) Mechanisms of idiopathic osteonecrosis. *Orthopedic Clinics of North America*, **16**, 655–667

44   Spencer, J.D., Humphreys, S., Tighe, J.R. *et al.* (1986) Early avascular necrosis of the femoral head: Report of a case and review of the literature. *Journal of Bone and Joint Surgery*, **68B**, 414–417

45   Meyers, M.H. (1988) Osteonecrosis of the femoral head: Pathogenesis and long-term results of treatment. *Clinical Orthopaedics and Related Research*, **231**, 51–61

46   Pedersen, N.W., Kiaer, T., Kristensen, K.D. *et al.* (1989) Intraosseous pressure, oxygenation, and histology of arthrosis and osteonecrosis of the hip. *Acta Orthopaedica Scandinavica*, **60**, 415–417

47   Conklin, J.J., Alderson, P.O., Zizic, T.M. *et al.* (1983) Comparison of bone scan and radiograph sensitivity in detection of steroid-induced ischemic necrosis of bone. *Radiology*, **147**, 221–226

48   Kenzora, J.E. and Glimcher, M.J. (1985) Pathogenesis of idiopathic osteonecrosis: The ubiquitous crescent sign. *Orthopedic Clinics of North America*, **16**, 681–699

49 Tawn, D.J. and Watt, I. (1989) Bone marrow scintigraphy in the diagnosis of post traumatic avascular necrosis of bone. *British Journal of Radiology*, **62**, 790–795

50 Markisz, J.A., Knowles, R.J., Altcheck, D.W. *et al.* (1987) Segmental avascular necrosis of the femoral heads: early detection with MR imaging. *Radiology*, **162**, 717–720

51 Mitchell, D.G., Rao, V.M., Dalinda, M.K. *et al.* (1987) Femoral head avascular necrosis: correlation of MR imaging, radiographic staging, radionuclide imaging and clinical findings. *Radiology*, **162**, 709–715

52 Brower, A.C. and Kransdorf, M.J. (1990) Imaging of hip disorders. *Radiology Clinics of North America*, **28**, 955–974

53 Musso, E.S., Mitchell, S.N., Schink-Ascani, M. *et al.* (1986) Results of conservative management of osteonecrosis of the femoral head. *Clinical Orthopaedics and Related Research*, **207**, 209–215

54 Colwell, C.W. (1989) The controversy of core decompression of the femoral head for osteonecrosis. *Arthritis and Rheumatism*, **32**, 797–800

55 Hungerford, D.S. (1989) Response: The role of core decompression in the treatment of ischemic necrosis of the femoral head. *Arthritis and Rheumatism*, **32**, 801–805

56 Ludkowski, P. and Wilson-McDonald, J. (1990) Total arthroplasty in Paget's disease of the hip. A clinical review and review of the literature. *Clinical Orthopaedics*, **255**, 160–167

57 Lakhanpel, S., Ginsbury, W.W., Luthra, H.S. *et al.* (1987) Transient regional osteoporosis: a study of 56 cases and review of the literature. *Annals of Internal Medicine*, **106**, 444–450

58 Kaplan, S.S. and Stegman, C.J. (1985) Transient osteoporosis of the hip. *Bone and Joint Surgery*, **67A**, 490–493

59 Pavlov, H. (1987) Roentgen examination of groin and hip pain in the athlete. *Clinics in Sports Medicine*, **6**, 829–843

60 Hajek, M.R. and Noble, H.B. (1982) Stress fractures of the femoral neck in joggers. *American Journal of Sports Medicine*, **10**, 112–116

61 Baldini, M., Raimondi, P.L. and Princi, L. (1982) Meralgia paraesthetica following weight loss. Case report. *Neurosurgical Reviews*, **5**, 45–47

62 Chung, S.M. (1986) Diseases of the developing hip joint. *Pediatric Clinics of North America*, **33**, 1457–1473

63 Hodges, D.L. and McGuire, T.J. (1988) Hip pain in children: an anatomic approach. *Orthopaedic Reviews*, **17**, 251–256

64 Gross, R.H. (1984) Hip problems in children: aids to early recognition. *Postgraduate Medicine*, **76**, 97–105

65 Clarke, C.M.P. (1989) Management of neonatal hip instability. *Postgraduate Update*, October, 41–46

66 Herring, J.A. (1989) Legg–Calve–Perthes disease: a review of current knowledge. In *American Academy of Orthopaedic Surgeons: Instructional Course Lectures*, **38**, 309–315

67 Editorial (1986) Perthes' disease. *Lancet*, pp. 895–896

68 Cannon, S.R., Pozo, J.L. and Catterall, A. (1989) Elevated growth velocity in children with Perthes' disease. *Journal of Pediatric Orthopaedics*, **9**, 285–292

69 Burwell, R.G., Vernon, C.L., Dangerfield, P.H. *et al.* (1986) Raised somatomedin activity in the serum of young boys with Perthes' disease revealed by bioassay.

A disease of growth transition? *Clinical Orthopaedics*, **209**, 129–138

70 Rayner, P.H., Schwalbe, S.L. and Hall, D.J. (1986) An assessment of endocrine function in boys with Perthes' disease. *Clinical Orthopaedics*, **209**, 124–128

71 Barker, D.J. and Hall, A.J. (1986) The epidemiology of Perthes' disease. *Clinical Orthopaedics*, **209**, 89–94

72 Hall, A.J. and Barker, D.J. (1989) Perthes' disease in Yorkshire. *Journal of Bone and Joint Surgery (Br)*, **71**, 229–233

73 Hall, A.J., Margetts, B.M., Barker, D.J. *et al.* (1989) Low blood manganese levels in Liverpool children with Perthes' disease. *Paediatric and Perinatal Epidemiology*, **3**, 131–135

74 Catterall, A. (1985) Legg–Calve–Perthes disease: morbid anatomy and natural history. In *American Academy of Orthopaedic Surgeons: Instructional Course Lectures*, **38**, 297–303

75 Paterson, D. and Savage, J.P. (1986) The nuclide bone scan in the diagnosis of Perthes' disease. *Clinical Orthopaedics*, **209**, 23–29

76 Linnenbaum, F.J., Woltering, H., Karbowski, A. *et al.* (1989) Ultrasonography of the hip for Perthes' disease. *Archives of Orthopaedic and Trauma Surgery*, **108**, 166–172

77 Pinto, M.R., Peterson, H.A. and Berquist, T.H. (1989) Magnetic resonance imaging in early diagnosis of Legg–Calvert–Perthes disease. *Journal of Pediatric Orthopedics*, **9**, 19–22

78 Mukamel, M., Litmanovitch, M., Yosipovich, Z. *et al.* (1985) Legg–Calvert–Perthes' disease following transient synovitis. How often? *Clinical Pediatrics (Phila)*, **24**, 629–631

79 Saito, S., Takaoka, K., Ono, K. *et al.* (1985) Residual deformities related to arthritic change after Perthes' disease. A long-term follow-up of fifty-one cases. *Archives of Orthopaedic and Trauma Surgery*, **104**, 7–14

80 Nava, L.C. (1985) IMA II brace for deambulatory treatment of Legg–Perthes disease. *Journal of Biomedical Engineering*, **7**, 71–74

81 Harrison, M.H. (1986) A preliminary account of the management of the painful hip originative from Perthes' disease. *Clinical Orthopaedics*, **209**, 57–64

82 Karpinski, M.R. and Piggott, H. (1986) Greater trochanteric pain syndrome. A report of 15 cases. *Journal of Bone and Joint Surgery (Br)*, **67**, 762–763

83 Menelaus, M.B. (1986) Lessons learned in the management of Legg–Calve Perthes disease. *Clinical Orthopaedics and Related Research*, **209**, 41–48

84 Lack, W., Feldner-Busztin, H., Ritschl, P. *et al.* (1989) The results of surgical treatment for Perthes' disease. *Journal of Pediatric Orthopedics*, **9**, 197–204

85 Schoenecker, P.L. (1986) Legg–Calvert–Perthes disease. *Orthopaedic Reviews*, **15**, 561–574

86 MacEwen, G.D. (1985) Conservative treatment of Legg–Calvert–Perthes' condition. *Hip*, 17–23

87 Sharwood, P.F. (1981) The irritable hip syndrome in children. A long-term follow-up. *Acta Orthopaedica Scandinavica*, **52**, 633–638

88 Haveisen, D.C., Weiner, D.S. and Weiner, S.D. (1986) The characterization of transient synovitis of the hip in children. *Journal of Pediatric Orthopedics*, **6**, 11–17

89 Jones, D.A. (1989) Irritable hip and *Campylobacter* infection. *Journal of Bone and Joint Surgery*, **71B**, 227

90 Kallio, P., Ryoppy, S. and Kunnamo, I. (1986) Transient synovitis and Perthes' disease. Is there an aetiological connection? *Journal of Bone and Joint Surgery (Br)*, **68**, 808–811

91 Landin, L.A., Danielsson, L.G. and Wattsgard, C. (1987) Transient synovitis of the hip. Its incidence, epidemiology and relation to Perthes' disease. *Journal of Bone and Joint Surgery (Br)*, **69**, 238–242

92 Carty, H., Maxted, M., Fielding, J.A. *et al.* (1984) Isotope scanning in the irritable hip syndrome. *Skeletal Radiology*, **11**, 32–37

93 Hasegawa, Y., Wingstrand, H. and Gustafson, T. (1988) Scintimetry in transient synovitis of the hip in the child. *Acta Orthopaedica Scandinavica*, **59**, 520–525

94 Miralles, M., Gonzales, G., Pulpeiro, J.R. *et al.* (1989) Sonography of the painful hip in children: 500 consecutive cases. *American Journal of Roentgenology*, **152**, 579–582

95 Rappaport, E.B. and Fife, D. (1985) Slipped capital femoral epiphysis in growth hormone-deficient patients. *American Journal of Diseases of Children*, **139**, 396–399

96 Crawford, A.H. (1988) Slipped capital femoral epiphysis. *Journal of Bone and Joint Surgery*, 1422–1427

97 Domingue, R., Oh, K.S., Young, L.W. *et al.* (1987) Acute chondrolysis complicating Legg–Calvert–Perthes disease. *Skeletal Radiology*, **16**, 377–382

10 Knee

The knee joint, the largest synovial joint in the body, combines considerable mobility and strength with the stability necessary to lock the knee in the upright position. The joint is made up of three functional units, the medial and lateral tibiofemoral compartments and the patellofemoral joint, each lined by articular cartilage and all enclosed in a common capsule lined by synovial membrane.

The medial and the lateral compartments of the knee joint have a similar basic structure. Each contains an intra-articular meniscus and each compartment is enclosed by a capsular ligament that runs anteriorly from the patellar ligament to the posterior cruciate ligament. The inner aspect of each capsular ligament is attached to the intra-articular meniscus, and the outer aspect is strengthened and supported by a strong collateral ligament and the surrounding musculotendinous insertions.

The capsular ligaments supporting the two tibiofemoral compartments have similar anatomical arrangements. The medial compartment is bounded medially by the medial capsular ligament and laterally by the posterior cruciate ligament. The medial capsular ligament is divided into anterior, middle and posterior thirds (Figure 10.1). The anterior third is thin and loose. The thick middle third runs from the femur above to the medial meniscus as the meniscofemoral ligament, and then from the meniscus to the tibia below as the meniscotibial ligament (Figure 10.2). The posterior third, also known as the posterior oblique ligament, is supported by the semimembranosus muscle and its aponeurosis which is also known as the oblique popliteal ligament.

The medial capsular ligament is strengthened in its medial side by the more superficially placed medial collateral ligament, which runs from medial femoral epicondyle to the tibia.

The lateral joint compartment has a similar arrangement of its capsular ligaments. It is bounded laterally by the lateral capsular ligament, and on its medial aspect by the anterior cruciate ligament.

The lateral capsular ligament can also be divided into anterior, middle and posterior thirds. The anterior third is supported laterally by the iliotibial band. The middle third is divided into a meniscofemoral and a meniscotibial ligament, and is supported by the lateral collateral ligament which runs from the lateral epicondyle of the femur to the head of the fibula. The posterior third has also been called the arcuate ligament, because of its shape as

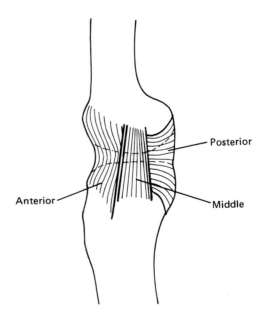

Figure 10.1 Medial aspect of the knee. The medial capsular ligament is made up of three ligaments

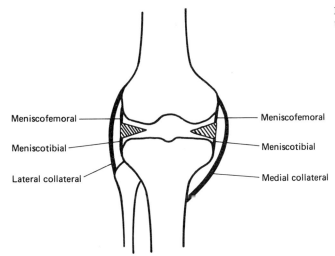

Figure 10.2 Ligaments shown on section through the knee joint

Meniscofemoral — — Meniscofemoral

Meniscotibial — — Meniscotibial

Lateral collateral — — Medial collateral

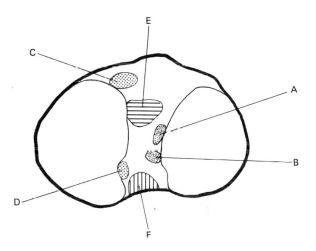

Figure 10.3 Upper surface of right tibia showing tibial condyles and the intercondylar area with its attachments. (A) Anterior horn of lateral meniscus; (B), posterior horn of lateral meniscus; (C), anterior horn of medial meniscus; (D), posterior horn of medial meniscus; (E), anterior cruciate ligament; (F), posterior cruciate ligament

it arches up across the popliteus muscle. It is supported by the biceps and popliteus muscles.

The cruciate ligaments, so named because they cross each other, occupy the central intercondylar area of the knee. They are named according to their tibial attachments, so that the anterior cruciate is inserted more anteriorly on the tibia than the posterior cruciate (Figure 10.3).

The anterior cruciate ligament arises from the medial aspect of the lateral condyle of the femur and passes downwards to be inserted on the anterior aspect of the intercondylar area of the tibia between the anterior horns of the two semi-lunar cartilages. The ligament is composed of three bundles, each of different length and each taut in different degrees of flexion: a long anteromedial band, a short posterolateral band and an intermediate band.

It has five major functions [1,2]:

1 It controls and resists medial rotation of the tibia on the femur.
2 It resists anterior tibial displacement on the femur.
3 It prevents hyperextension of the knee.
4 It guides the knee-locking mechanism.
5 It acts as a secondary restraint against valgus and varus strains in knee flexion.

The posterior cruciate ligament arises by a fanlike attachment from the lateral aspect of the medial condyle of the femur and is inserted into the posterior aspect of the intercondylar fossa of the tibia, posterior to the posterior horns of the two semilunar cartilages. It receives more ligamentous support than the anterior cruciate by virtue of attachments to the posterior capsular ligaments and the accessory ligaments. It is situated in the centre of the knee, is taut in all degrees of flexion and extension, provides 95% of the total restraint to posterior displacement of the tibia [3] and appears to be the axis around which the knee moves [3,4].

Knee joint movements

Two active movements take place in the knee joint: (1) flexion–extension, and (2) axial rotation.

Flexion–extension

These take place around a transverse axis running through the femoral condyles, but also involve a spiral action and are not simple hinge movements. Movement involves a complex set of actions in all of the surrounding structures.

Tibiofemoral joints

Each tibial plateau on bony specimens is nearly flat. The presence of articular cartilage alters this shape and the lateral plateau becomes curved. The menisci attached to their tibial plateau further modify these shapes. The curved medial meniscus deepens the medial compartment so that its ball and socket arrangement also allows axial rotation to take place. With the knee fully flexed, the extreme posterior portions of the two femoral condyles lie on the posterior portion of the corresponding articular surface of the tibial condyles. Knee extension from this flexed position involves a rolling and sliding action of the femoral condyles on the tibia. The two femoral condyles are of unequal sizes, with the medial condyle being longer, narrower and more curved than the lateral condyle. Accordingly, during extension, the movement in the lateral condyle is completed first leaving approximately 1.5 cm of movement available in the medial femoral condyle. Thus, during the last 20 degrees of knee extension the femur can passively medially rotate on the tibia, producing the 'screw-home' locking mechanism. Similarly, on flexion of the knee from the fully extended position the femur must first laterally rotate on the tibia. The centre for this condylar motion, the so-called 'instant centre', varies during movements and between individuals.

Patellofemoral joint

During flexion and extension of the knee, the patella moves in its femoral groove. During flexion it moves downwards and backwards on the femoral trochlear surface, which extends down on to the articular surface of the medial and lateral femoral condyles. The patella moves in the deep groove formed by the femoral condyles and comes to lie within the intercondylar notch. The range of patellar excursion is about twice its length, so that on full knee flexion the patella comes to lie under the femoral condyles and faces upwards. Its excursion and stability are controlled by the quadriceps muscle (see p. 164).

Muscles

The fine muscular control of this movement is supplied by knee muscles, the vastus medialis and medial hamstrings, which rotate the tibia medially while flexing the knee, and the popliteus, which stabilizes the former while flexing the knee.

Cruciate ligaments

The cruciate ligaments form a functional unit [5] that helps to control flexion and extension, acting as a guide rope to maintain the femur and tibia on their spiral movement and guide the femoral condyle as it slides into the 'screw-home' position. In this position the knee is locked and all ligaments are taut.

Menisci

The menisci have firm attachments to tibia, joint capsule and cruciate ligaments. These attachments form a functional unit to control meniscal movements. The menisci play only a passive role in flexion and extension. During extension the menisci move forwards and on flexion they move backwards so that on full flexion they are compressed between the posterior aspects of the femur and tibia. The lateral meniscus is not as firmly attached to its collateral ligament and has greater mobility. The tendon of the popliteus muscle, interposed between the lateral meniscus and the capsule, produces an increased excursion of the meniscus.

Infrapatellar fat pad

The fat pad lies deep to the patellar ligament in the space between the tibial condyles and femur. It lies within the joint capsule but outside the synovial membrane, which is reflected over the lateral margins of the fat pad as the alar ligaments. This mobile cushion is important in aiding knee movements, by changing its shape as it is moved by its alar ligaments.

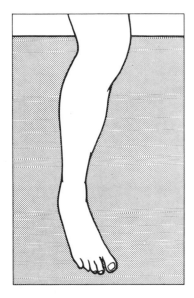

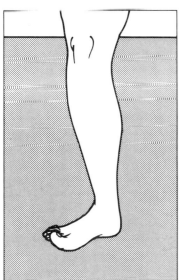

Figure 10.4 Axial rotation in the flexed knee

Axial rotation

Axial rotation of the knee about the long axis of the leg occurs only when the knee is flexed and is normally impossible with the knee extended. This movement can best be observed on sitting with the knee flexed over the edge of a couch. The active range of medial rotation is normally about 30 degrees and lateral range about 40 degrees (Figure 10.4). On rotation, the menisci move with the femur as rotation takes place in the lower compartment of the joint. On lateral rotation, the lateral meniscus moves anteriorly in its compartment and the medial meniscus moves posteriorly in its compartment. These movements are reversed during medial rotation. They can be easily felt to move by palpating the joint line while the flexed knee is laterally and medially rotated.

Symptoms

Perhaps in no other joint is a detailed history as important as in the knee, and it should provide an appreciation of the underlying type and degree of abnormality. Important points in the history include:

1   Whether the onset of pain is sudden or gradual.
2   The relationship of pain to any trauma and the mechanism of such trauma.
3   The presence of any swelling and how rapidly or gradually it develops.
4   A feeling of instability or 'giving way' of the knee during use.
5   Any locking of the knee.
6   Clicking or catching, especially if it reproduces pain.
7   Whether the knee problem is stable, progressive, recurrent or intermittent, or brought on only by certain activities.
8   The presence of any stiffness.
9   Whether any other joints are involved.
10 Any other illnesses that may have been present.
11 The effects of any previous treatments.

Knee pain

The knee is the largest synovial joint in the body and is a common site for traumatic, degenerative and inflammatory disorders. Pain may also be felt in the knee as the result of disease in more proximal structures. Pain from hip disease may be referred as a dull aching pain in the knee or suprapatellar region. Patients with an L3 or L4 intervertebral disc prolapse may first complain of pain in the knee.

Disorders of the knee joint usually produce pain within the knee itself. Pain arising from the tibiofemoral joint is often worse when the patient first stands up and starts to walk or after walking for some distance, is often worse with weight-bearing on the affected leg and is worse going up or down stairs. Pain may also be associated with stiffness, especially after sitting for a time. In medial meniscal tears, pain may be felt at night especially when the knees touch in bed. Disorders of the patellofemoral joint usually produce pain in the retropatellar area, made worse either by activities that involve this joint such as walking, running, riding a bike or going up stairs; or after a prolonged period of sitting, for example in a car or theatre.

Locking

A history of locking of the knee, if present, is of considerable diagnostic significance but a careful evaluation of this symptom is essential. Locking means a sudden complete block to full extension of the knee, which is nevertheless able to flex fully. The knee usually lacks about 30 degrees of extension, but this can range from 10 to 45 degrees, and the screw-home mechanism is lost. The end-feel of extension in a locked knee provides a characteristic rubbery sensation with an associated protective muscle spasm. Locking may be acute, recurrent or chronic. It is not an appropriate term as it implies that no movement at all should be possible and also because the patient may use the word to describe an inability to move the knee owing to stiffness or pain. A history of unlocking of the joint is of considerable value in establishing whether locking has occurred. Unlocking may occur either spontaneously or after manipulation of the knee and the patient reports a sensation of something slipping or snapping back into place. Locking may result from a torn meniscus, a loose bony fragment, e.g. from an osteochondritis dissecans, a torn cruciate ligament or avulsed anterior tibial spine, chondromalacia patellae, a dislocated patella or a medial plica.

Catching

This is a sensation which indicates that something is getting in the way of joint movement, and it may be painful. Its mechanism of production is similar to locking.

Instability

Stability is provided by ligaments (static stability) and surrounding muscles (dynamic stability) with the quadriceps muscle being the major stabilizer. A feeling of instability, giving way or 'buckling' of the knee on use, is a common symptom. It may be produced by chondromalacia patellae, a torn meniscus, (usually a tear of the posterior horn of the medial meniscus), a loose bony foreign body or arthritis. A feeling of instability may also arise after cruciate ligament tear with true rotatory instability. The knee usually gives way suddenly without any warning or pain but often with a feeling that one bone has moved or slipped on the other. This tends to occur on walking down stairs or over uneven ground when the leg supports the body-weight. It is particularly common when a runner changes direction or steps off the involved leg. Instability may also occur with weakness or inhibition of the quadriceps mechanism, particularly of the vastus medialis, and after injuries to the capsular ligaments of the knee with subsequent loss of normal proprioceptive feedback from knee ligaments.

Synovial swelling

Swelling as a result of synovial effusion should always be asked about as it usually indicates the presence of some intra-articular damage. Haemarthrosis comes on more rapidly after an injury than does synovitis so that its onset is measured in minutes rather than hours. The knee is usually extremely painful, warm, tender and held in some degree of flexion. The most common cause of a haemarthrosis is a ruptured anterior cruciate ligament. So much so, that a traumatic haemarthrosis should be regarded as arising from a ruptured anterior cruciate ligament until proved otherwise. Less common causes are tears in the capsular ligament, a torn meniscus, an osteochondral fracture, or a dislocated patella. Non-traumatic causes are rare and include blood dyscrasias, anticoagulant therapy, pigmented villonodular synovitis or neoplasms. Haemarthrosis may need to be differentiated from crystal deposition diseases, inflammatory arthritis and septic arthritis. Diagnosis is then made after aspirating the knee joint and examining the synovial fluid.

Examination

Before the knee joint is tested, the lower limb and lumbar spine should first be examined. The knee forms a part of a link system in which the femur acts as a supporting pedestal that transmits forces into the lower leg and foot. As the knee is the midjoint in the link, alterations in other lower limb structures can produce alterations in the biomechanical load on the knee and result in pathological changes. Movement in the spine and hip is tested for any limitation in their range and for any reproduction of the knee pain. The strength and extensibility of the thigh muscles, the flexors and abductors of the hip and the hamstrings for any tightness, should be tested routinely. Any deficiency in their structures may be associated with knee pain and especially retropatellar pain. Gait and the presence of any structural deformities in both lower limbs are observed. The whole length of both lower limbs is inspected first with the patient standing, walking, sitting with knees over the edge of the couch and finally, with the patient supine for any deformities, swelling or muscle wasting.

Examination of the knee joint

1 Inspection.
  (a) Deformities.
  (b) Swelling.
  (c) Muscle wasting.
2 Movements.
  (a) Active.
  (b) Passive.
  (c) Accessory.
  (d) Isometric tests.
3 Palpation.
4 Special tests.
  (a) Ligamentous instability.
  (b) Meniscus tears.
  (c) Patellofemoral joint.

Inspection

Knee deformities

The knee is inspected for the presence of any deformities, such as genu valgum, genu varum (Figure 10.5), genu recurvatum or flexion deformity. The patella is best inspected with the patient seated and the knees flexed to a right angle over the edge of the couch. The size and shape of the patella, its relationship to the tibiofemoral joint and the direction in which it points are noted. The Q angle (see p. 165) is measured.

Swellings

Swellings around the knee are usually evident in certain characteristic sites. A synovial effusion in the knee bulges into the suprapatellar pouch where the synovium is reflected along the femoral shaft. It obliterates the normal suprapatellar depression and appears as a moon-shaped swelling extending up to 6 cm above the border of the patella (Figure 10.6). This swelling is easily seen on inspection especially in

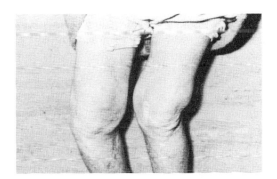

Figure 10.5 Genu varum of right leg and genu valgum of left leg

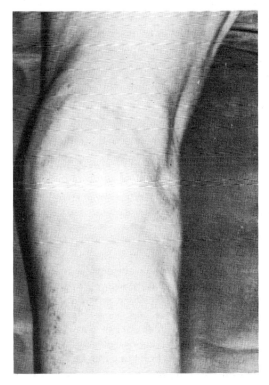

Figure 10.6 Synovial effusion in the knee seen bulging in the suprapatellar area

the presence of quadriceps wasting and by comparing the swollen knee with the opposite one.

Swellings in other areas of the knee include: a Pellegrini–Stieda lesion associated with a swelling at the upper attachment of the medial collateral ligament; a prepatellar bursitis, which points forward over the anterior aspect of the patella; cysts of the menisci, which are often best appreciated with the patient sitting with the knees flexed over the edge of the couch and the swelling becomes most apparent over the joint line, with the knees flexed to 45 degrees; Osgood–Schlatter's disease, which is associated with a swelling of the tibial tubercle below the knee; a popliteal cyst, which with the patient standing may be seen bulging into the popliteal space; a calf cyst, which can be easily appreciated, usually as a swelling in the medial aspect of the calf.

Muscle wasting

The size and tone of the quadriceps muscle in each leg are compared and the presence of any muscle wasting is usually detected on inspection.

Movements

These should be first assessed by functional movements such as gait and squatting. The examiner should ask the patient to walk towards him and then away from him assessing any abnormality or asymmetry of gait. This test may also be repeated by having the patient walk backwards, at first away from and then towards the examiner. Loss of knee extension is often more readily visible on walking backwards on the heels.

Active movements

The ranges of flexion, extension and axial rotation are tested. The knee should normally extend to a straight line, referred to as zero degrees of extension, and some degree of active hyperextension may at times be possible. The active range of flexion, approximately 140 degrees, may be assessed with the patient lying either supine or prone and then actively flexing the knee. The distance of the heel from the buttock may also be used as a measure of knee flexion. The degree of axial rotation of the knee is measured with the patient seated with the knee flexed over the edge of the couch. The normal active range is approximately 40 degrees of external rotation of the tibia and 30 degrees of internal rotation.

Quadriceps lag

This is tested with the patient supine, heel supported on a small block and the knee sags into full extension without touching the couch. The patient is then asked to lift his heel off the block without lifting his knee. It should be possible to do this before the knee starts to lift. With quadriceps lag, the knee will be observed to lift first. Inability to extend the knee fully in this manner is often due to pain inhibition and is usually associated with loss of knee accessory movements. They often respond well to manual therapy techniques, with a return of pain-free knee movements, and the lag disappears.

Passive movements

More information may be derived from testing the passive ranges of extension, flexion, and axial rotation. First, the range of hyperextension is tested with the patient lying supine and the examiner holds the patient's knee with one hand and lifts the lower

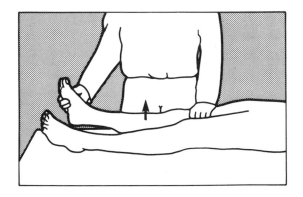

Figure 10.7 Passive hyperextension of the knee

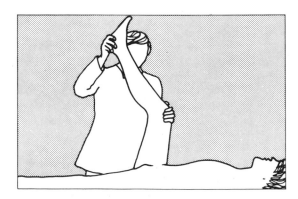

Figure 10.8 Test for the degree of hamstring tightness

leg upwards with his other hand. The range of this movement is compared in both legs, and normally up to 15 degrees of passive hyperextension is possible (Figure 10.7). This test should then be repeated with overpressure. Unilateral hyperextension may indicate a tear of the cruciate ligament and posterior capsule.

Second, the passive range of flexion is tested. The patient lies prone and the examiner grasps the lower limb above the ankle and moves the heel towards the buttock. Normally the heel should approximate the buttocks, as the passive range of this movement is approximately 20 degrees greater than the active range. A decrease in this passive range may be associated either with intrinsic knee disorders or a lesion in the quadriceps muscle causing a loss of extensibility or a contracture of the muscle.

Third, the degree of hamstring tightness should be tested with the patient lying supine and the hip flexed to 90 degrees. The examiner than passively extends the knee (Figure 10.8). The normal range of this movement varies with age, physical activity and the normal extensibility of the hamstrings, but may also be reduced in disorders of the knee joint.

Fourth, the passive range of axial rotation is tested, with the knee firstly in extension and then flexed to 90 degrees. Loss of this range occurs in many intrinsic knee disorders and an increased range with the knee flexed may be associated with a rotary instability of the knee.

Accessory movement

There are ten accessory movements in the tibiofemoral joint:

1 Abduction. The patient lies supine and the examiner produces a valgus movement of the tibia on the femur.
2 Adduction. A varus movement of the tibia is produced (see Figure 10.9).
3 Anteroposterior. The tibia is moved backwards on the femur (Figure 10.10).
4 Posteroanterior. The tibia is moved forwards on the femur.
5 Lateral movement of the tibia on the femur, produced by counter-pressure between the examiner's two hands (Figure 10.11).
6 Medial movement of the tibia on the femur, produced by counter-pressure in the opposite direction (Figure 10.12).
7 Longitudinal caudad is produced by distraction of the tibia from the femur (Figure 10.13).
8 Longitudinal cephalad is produced by compression of the tibia.

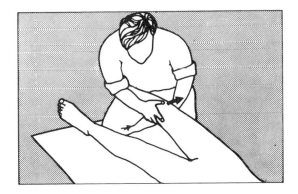

Figure 10.9 Adduction accessory movement

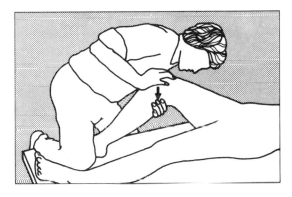

Figure 10.10 Anteroposterior accessory movement

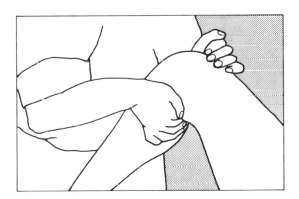

Figure 10.11 Lateral accessory movement

9 Medial rotation of the tibia on the femur is produced by the examiner with the patient supine and the knee flexed to 90 degrees (Figure 10.14).
10 Lateral rotation is produced by reversing the hands.

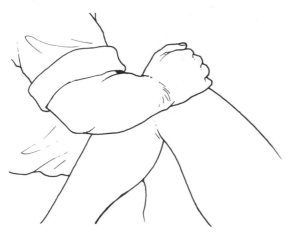

Figure 10.12 Medial accessory movement

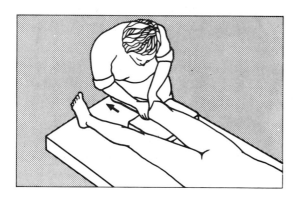

Figure 10.13 Longitudinal caudad accessory movement

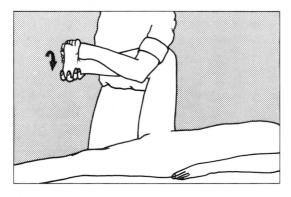

Figure 10.14 Medial rotation accessory movement

Isometric tests

Isometric tests assess the strength of the quadriceps and hamstring muscles. Normal quadriceps development, essential for knee function, is best detected by having the patient sit with the knees flexed over the edge of the couch. The examiner places one hand above the ankle and resists attempted extension. The bulk of the quadriceps muscle can be appreciated on inspection and its tone may be evaluated by palpation. Special attention is given to the size and tone of the vastus medialis muscle, as it plays an important role in knee stability. Hamstring strength is tested with the patient lying prone and the examiner resists the patient's attempt to flex the knee. Finally, as part of normal knee examination, the strength of the hip flexors and hip abductors should be tested.

Palpation

The knee joint is palpated for the presence of any fluid; synovial thickening; warmth, swellings; end-feel; crepitus, clicking; and tenderness.

Fluid

The knee joint is palpated to confirm the presence of any synovial fluid bulging into the suprapatellar pouch and having a characteristic fluctuant sensation. A large effusion is best appreciated by placing the index finger and thumb of the right hand on either side of the patella and the left hand placed over the suprapatellar pouch squeezes the fluid distally. The finger and the thumb of the right hand are separated, producing a fluctuant feeling. A small effusion is not so readily appreciated on inspection and is best demonstrated by the bulge sign (Figure 10.15).

Bulge sign

The examiner first empties the normal gutter over the medial compartment of the knee joint just under the medial border of the patella by stroking out any fluid upwards into the suprapatellar pouch. The left hand is then used to compress the suprapatellar pouch, which forces any fluid present distally where it can be seen to bulge this gutter outwards in a wave-like motion. This test should then be repeated but this time with the thumb and index finger of the right hand placed on either side of the patella so that the index finger can confirm the presence of fluid.

Patellar tap

Patellar tap (Figure 10.16) is of no great clinical value because it requires only a certain amount of

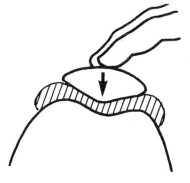

Figure 10.16 Patellar tap

fluid within the joint and if insufficient or excessive fluid is present the patella cannot be suitably tapped.

Chronic synovial thickening

Chronic synovial thickening may be palpated about the synovial reflection along the superior margins of the suprapatellar pouch where it presents a characteristic doughy sensation as it is rolled under the fingers. The synovial membrane may also be palpated over the medial joint compartment in the gutter that lies on the medial side of the patella just above the medial tibiofemoral joint line. To palpate the synovium in this area, the examiner uses both thumbs, placing one hand below the patella and the other hand above the patella over the suprapatellar pouch.

Warmth

The synovial membrane is palpated for any increased warmth, easier to detect by comparison with the opposite knee. It may be caused by an effusion, haemarthrosis, infections or malignancy. Routine palpation of the inguinal lymph nodes should also be made at this time.

Swellings

Many swellings are best appreciated on inspection, but palpation is necessary to confirm their presence and to differentiate them from synovitis or other swellings around the knee. Types of swellings are:

1 A tender swelling of the tibial tubercle is present in Osgood–Schlatter's disease (see p. 171).

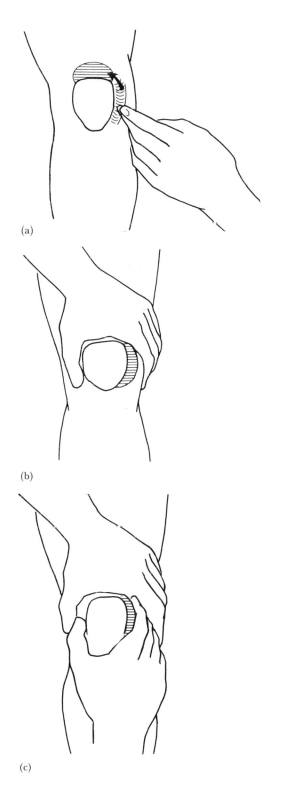

Figure 10.15 The bulge sign. (a) Fluid is stroked out of the medial gutter; (b), the suprapatellar pouch is compressed; (c), fluid bulges out into the medial gutter

2   Cysts of the menisci usually involving the lateral meniscus with a tender swelling over the joint line (see p. 160).

3   A Pellegrini–Stieda lesion produces a tender swelling over the upper attachment of the medial collateral ligament to the femoral condyle (see p. 153).

4   Bursitis may be present as a soft tissue swelling anterior to the patella, known as prepatellar bursitis or housemaid's knee; or bulging on either side of the patellar ligament (infrapatellar bursitis); or as a semi-membranous bursitis with a soft tissue swelling bulging posteriorly into the popliteal fossa where it may need to be differentiated from an aneurysm of the popliteal artery.

5   Osteochondromatosis can usually be palpated as bony swellings within the synovial cavity and needs to be differentiated from other loose bony bodies.

6   Soft tissue swellings in the synovial cavity, which may be caused by pigmented villonodular synovitis and pedunculated swellings as a result of rheumatoid nodules, a ganglion or a benign tumour, e.g. fibroma or a giant cell tumour, are often palpable as they protrude through the joint line.

End-feel

End-feel is tested with the patient lying supine with the knee fully extended and relaxed. The knee is passively flexed approximately 20 degrees and then allowed to drop back into full extension. The normal knee can fall into full extension with a typical painless bony end-feel. In patients with osteoarthritis a similar bony end-feel may be found but the joint lacks full extension. The end-feel of the movement produced on adduction and abduction of the knee is also characteristic as the collateral ligaments allow a small range of normal joint movement. If a collateral ligament is ruptured this is replaced by a 'mushy' end-feel and an excessive range of movement.

Crepitus

Crepitus is best appreciated by palpating over the patellofemoral joint while flexing and extending the knee. In the young it occurs in chondromalacia patellae; in the elderly a fine crepitus is common, whereas a coarse crepitus may indicate osteoarthritis. In osteoarthritis of the tibiofemoral joint, a coarse crepitus may be palpable over the joint line. If osteoarthritis results in instability of the knee a coarse creaking or crunching sensation may be felt.

Clicking

An audible and palpable click, which may also be painful, can be produced by many of the soft tissue structures around the knee. The extensor retinaculum may be seen to click over the front of the lateral femoral condyle; the biceps tendon over the head of the fibula; the popliteus tendon in and out of its groove on the lateral femoral condyle; the iliotibial band over the lateral epicondyle of the femur; a normal vacuum joint click associated with the patellofemoral joint; and a torn or discoid meniscus.

Tenderness

Palpation of the knee for tenderness is best achieved with the patient supine with the hip and knee flexed. The joint line and the upper and lower attachments of the ligaments are easily accessible to the palpating fingers. Injuries of the meniscus may produce tenderness over the anterior, middle or posterior thirds of the joint line. Ligament sprains are usually tender over the upper or lower attachments but tenderness is sometimes found over the middle third of the joint line, and tenderness in this area does not help in differentiating between a ligamentous or meniscus injury. The articular margins of the tibiofemoral joint can also be palpated for tenderness and the presence of osteoarthritic bony lipping.

The retropatellar area is next palpated with the quadriceps relaxed, best achieved by having the patient lie supine while the examiner sits on the couch to support the slightly flexed knee over his

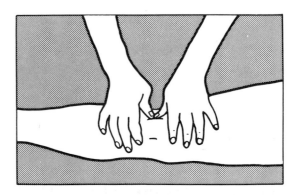

Figure 10.17 Palpation of the retropatellar surface

thigh. The patella can be readily moved laterally or medially while tenderness is sought in the retropatellar articular surfaces (Figure 10.17).

The popliteal space is examined for cystic swellings by having the patient stand with the knee extended.

Classification of knee lesions

1   Soft tissues injuries.
  (a) Ligament injuries.
      (i)   Collateral ligaments.
      (ii) Anterior cruciate.
      (iii) Posterior cruciate.
      Ligament instability.
      Pellegrini–Stieda lesion.
      Breast-stroke swimmer's knee.
  (b) Musculotendinous lesions.
      Quadriceps weakness.
      Quadriceps tendon tear.
      Gastrocnemius tendinitis.
      Bicipital tendinitis.
      Popliteal tendinitis.
      Iliotibial tract.
  (c) Bursitis.
      Prepatellar.
      Infrapatellar.
      Anserine.
      Semimembranosus.
      Bicipital.
2   Lesions of the tibiofemoral joint.
  (a) Menisci.
      Tears.
      Cysts.
      Discoid meniscus.
  (b) Chondral injuries.
  (c) Osteochondral injuries.
      Osteochondral fractures.
      Osteochondritis dissecans.
  (d) Osteonecrosis.
  (e) Loose bodies.
  (f) Osteoarthritis.
3   Patellofemoral joint.

Soft tissue injuries

Ligament injuries

Collateral ligament injuries

Collateral ligament sprains of the knee are common soft tissue injuries. These ligaments are important as static stabilizers of the knee which is normally stable in extension. The flexed knee is less stable and some degree of axial rotation is possible, so abnormal stresses then are most liable to cause ligament injury.

A history of the mechanism of injury should be obtained. There are two common mechanisms which may, of course, be combined. The medial ligament is usually injured in body-contact sports by a direct valgus force applied to the outside of the knee as in collision or a football tackle. The second mechanism involves a twisting injury with the foot stuck in the ground and the leg in lateral tibial rotation, as in skiing. In lateral rotation injuries the medial capsular ligament tends to tear before the anterior cruciate [6].

FIRST DEGREE SPRAINS
Only a few ligament fibres are torn and diagnosis and assessment usually present no great difficulty. Pain and tenderness are localized over the site of the injury, either over the joint line or at its upper or lower attachments. Pain is reproduced by stressing the ligament. For sprains of the medial ligament a valgus strain is applied to the joint; for sprains of the lateral ligament, a varus strain. The knee joint is stable and there is no synovial effusion, although some swelling over the site of the injury may be present.

Management   The sprained ligament needs to be protected from further damage by resting the knee for 24–36 h after the injury and ice is applied to minimize haemorrhage and swelling. Isometric quadriceps and hip exercises are commenced during this time. Subsequently, complete rest is neither justified nor necessary and the patient should continue isometric exercises. Gentle slow painless movements are used in the direction of the ligament fibres to encourage healing and lessen fibrous tissue with adhesion formation. Active exercises can be commenced as pain and discomfort settles, and the patient should be encouraged first to walk and then jog. Heat or ice may be applied before the exercise regimen. Full activity can be resumed when there is a full painless range of movement, usually within 3 weeks.

SECOND DEGREE SPRAINS
These may be more difficult to assess as there is often a synovial effusion which may be blood stained and it is necessary to determine whether any other intra-articular structure is damaged. Pain, tenderness and disability are greater than in first-degree

sprains and a mild degree of instability with a definite end point may be present. An isolated ligament tear generally produces less instability than a combined lesion.

Management The early treatment of this injury is similar to that outlined above and a compression bandage should be applied to control swelling. A large effusion, if present, may be drained to ease discomfort. The patient should rest and avoid weight-bearing on the injured leg for 24–48 h and the degree of injury then be reassessed. The knee is tested by applying a valgus stress with the knee in extension and then at 30 degrees of flexion (see p. 151).

If there is no damage to any other knee ligaments and instability resulting from a collateral tear is limited, surgery is not indicated [7,8], and an active exercise and rehabilitation programme with special attention to the quadriceps is instituted. If pain is severe or the knee feels unstable a derotational brace should be worn [8].

This degree of injury takes approximately 6 weeks to heal even after the original symptoms subside. If return to full activity is too early, pain and effusion may result and the ligament may be further injured. In most patients a gradual return to weight-bearing activity is possible.

THIRD DEGREE SPRAINS
These result from complete rupture of the capsular ligament. The medial ligament is usually torn from its upper femoral attachment; the lateral ligament is usually torn from its lower fibular attachment. Immediate pain and disability are usually severe and the diagnosis can be readily made if the patient is seen immediately. Subsequently, the diagnosis can be easily missed as pain may not then be marked and the patient may be able to walk into the surgery. Moreover, a synovial effusion may be absent as fluid and blood can escape from the synovial cavity through the capsular tear. Clinical tests to stress the ligament (see below) demonstrate instability and subluxation of the tibiofemoral joint with a mushy end-feel. Radiographs are necessary and may demonstrate an avulsion of bone and stress films may be helpful. Arthroscopy is needed for assessment and to show if other joint structures are injured.

Management Management of acute rupture may be conservative or surgical [10]. Prolonged conservative treatment in a cast has been advocated [11] but surgical repair in athletes is the treatment of choice. Surgery also permits other damaged knee structures such as the cruciate ligaments and meniscus to be inspected. The medial ligament is reconstructed and surrounding capsular structures, especially in the posteromedial corner, tightened.

Anterior cruciate ligament injuries

Partial midsubstance tears of this ligament may occur [12,13] usually associated with gross haemarthrosis. If the knee remains clinically stable, an active muscle rehabilitation programme is instituted, a knee brace is used for 6 weeks and then a graduated weight-bearing programme is commenced before a return to sport.

An isolated rupture of the anterior cruciate ligament may also occur [14], but it is much more common for this ligament to be damaged with other knee ligaments and/or the posterior horns of the meniscus. A tear of the anterior cruciate places additional stress on its other soft tissue supports, which may then give way, leading to an anterolateral rotational instability.

The mechanism of injury involves [15]:

1 Landing from a jump or when running, suddenly side-stepping or changing direction by decelerating, flexing and internally rotating the knee.
2 Hyperextension of the knee occurs in gymnasts or in basketballers when landing awkwardly on coming down from a height.
3 A twisting injury in contact sports with a valgus force applied to the outer knee in lateral rotation. In these injuries the medial ligament tends to tear before the anterior cruciate [6].
4 Acute hyperflexion of the knee is uncommon.

CLINICAL FEATURES
The player usually feels a sudden audible 'pop' or 'snap' or that the knee is 'coming apart' and is unable to continue running. He usually needs to be assisted from the field but at that stage the knee may feel stable to him and he can stand without difficulty. Within a few hours the knee has become painfully swollen with a tense haemarthrosis (see p. 140) owing to damage to its surrounding vascular supply. A knee radiograph may reveal avulsion fracture from the lateral tibial condyle. If the diagnosis remains in doubt or damage to other structures is suspected arthroscopy, CT [16] or MRI [17] should be performed.

In acute injuries examination of the knee should reveal evidence of haemarthrosis. The Lachman test [18] tests for anterior translation of the tibia on the femur at 20 degrees of flexion and is by far the most reliable and least painful test of instability.

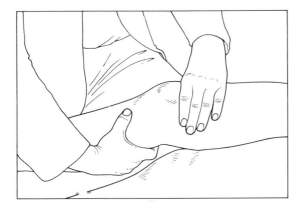

Figure 10.18 Testing for ruptured anterior cruciate ligament, modified Lachman test

METHOD

The patient lies supine with the knee flexed to 20 degrees supported over the end of the couch (Figure 10.18). The distal femur is held down with one hand and the upper tibia held with the other to pull the tibia directly forward. A test is positive if the tibia can be subluxed forward on the femur with a soft 'mushy' end-feel. The test may be limited by pain or hamstring spasm.

Other tests include an anterior drawer test (see p. 152) [19] and a pivot shift test.

PIVOT SHIFT TEST

This is a specific test which reproduces the patient's sensation of instability, but is more difficult to perform. The patient lies supine with hip flexed to 45 degrees and knee to 90 degrees. The foot is grasped and fully medially rotated. A valgus stress is applied to the proximal end of the tibia and the knee is then gradually straightened. At about 30 degrees of flexion the lateral tibiofemoral compartment may be seen to sublux or 'jerk' suddenly forward. As the knee is further extended the tibia returns to its former position.

MANAGEMENT

Despite the huge volume of literature over the past decade, management as to surgical or non-surgical treatment remains controversial [2,20–24]. It may be summarized as follows:

1 An avulsed bony fragment should be repositioned surgically.
2 In active sportsmen an acute rupture, seen within 2 weeks, should be considered for repair [6,24,25]. Only rarely can a primary suture of the ligament be successfully undertaken and an arthroscopic augmentation using a bone–tendon–bone preparation from the central third of the patellar tendon is performed [6,14,24,26–29].
3 An extra-articular procedure may also need to be considered [28,30].
4 If the patient is not so active or more elderly, or if the knee remains clinically stable and asymptomatic, management may consist of a derotational brace [20,31–34] with an active rehabilitation programme [35] with emphasis particularly on hamstring strengthening [36].
5 Chronic insufficiency of the ligament with instability in a young and active sportsman with a positive pivot test should be treated by arthroscopic repair and an extra-articular reconstruction [14].

Late complications Overstretching of other capsular ligaments, rotational instability and meniscus tears can lead finally to osteoarthritis [37].

Posterior cruciate ligament rupture

Posterior cruciate rupture may occur as an isolated event [38,39] but more commonly is associated with injury to other knee structures [3,38,40]. It is a common sporting injury especially following falls or collisions in contact sports [41]. It most commonly results from a direct blow to the anterior tibia with the knee flexed [42], e.g. a motor vehicle dashboard injury, but it can also arise as a hyperextension injury [3] or a twisting injury with a valgus or varus force.

The posterior capsule is also commonly torn so that no effusion may be evident on initial examination. Pain often presents late with retropatellar pain as the tibia falls backwards on the femur [14] or pain and difficulty on running downhill. Pain can also be felt through the knee, especially posteriorly.

MAJOR SIGNS

1 Posterior sag. The patient is supine with both knees flexed to 90 degrees. The lateral contours of the knees are observed for any posterior sag backwards of the involved tibia.
2 Posterior drawer sign. With the knee flexed to 90 degrees the tibia is passively subluxed posteriorly on the femur. Care must be taken as this may easily be mistaken for an anteroposterior movement.
3 A reverse pivot has been described [43] for this injury.
4 In patients with a combined rupture of the medial ligament the abduction test (see p. 147) is positive with the knee in full extension.

MANAGEMENT

This remains controversial, although most agree that acute ruptures diagnosed within 2 weeks should be surgically repaired [38,44]. If the diagnosis is delayed numerous surgical reconstructions have been described [38] but are not generally satisfactory [14]. Conservative treatment with immobilization and active rehabilitation may be sufficient, at least in the short term [40,44].

Knee ligament instability

Ligament instability of the knee is a common, often underdiagnosed, condition associated with a considerable loss of function [45]. There is usually previous trauma to the knee but, in late cases, a history of such trauma cannot always be obtained as the patient may have forgotten the incident. The terminology used can be confusing. For example, medial instability refers to the injury sustained by the medial ligament structures that become disrupted. This then allows the tibia to sublux in a valgus, or lateral, direction from the femur. Thus the direction of the resultant subluxation, which is the important clinical finding, differs from the commonly used descriptive title. Similarly, an anteromedial instability results from an injury to the medial capsular ligament. The test for it depends, however, on demonstrating a subluxation of the anteromedial tibial condyle in an anterior and a lateral direction.

Instability of the knee may be classified as either: (1) straight, non-rotary, or (2) rotary [4].

1   Straight, non-rotary instability is classified into four groups (Figures 10.19–10.21).
    (a) Medial.

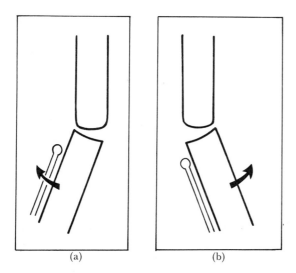

Figure 10.19 (a), Medial instability; (b), lateral instability

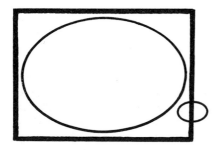

Figure 10.20 Diagrammatic representation of the normal relationship of the femoral condyles (square) to the tibial condyles (large oval) and fibula (small oval), viewed from above

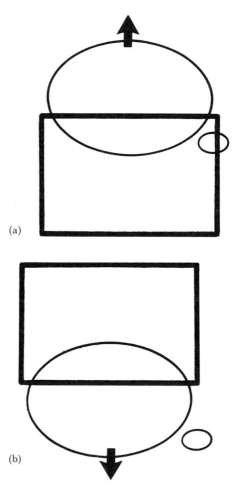

Figure 10.21 (a), Anterior instability; (b), posterior instability. Key as in Figure 10.20

(b) Lateral.
(c) Anterior.
(d) Posterior.
2 Rotary instability is classified into four groups (Figures 10.22–10.24).
   (a) Anteromedial.
   (b) Anterolateral.

(c) Posterolateral.
(d) Combined instabilities.

Testing for instability requires the patient and his muscles to be relaxed and examination needs to be gentle. The normal leg is always examined first to assess the degree of laxity present. A gross effusion, if present, should be aspirated. The degree of laxity should be assessed either in millimetres or as a scale. Thus laxity may be measured as up to 5 mm or 1+, or 5–10 mm or 2+. Third degree rupture will be more than 10 mm separation or 3+.

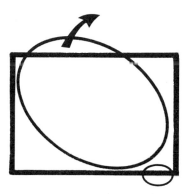

Figure 10.22 Anteromedial rotary instability. Key as in Figure 10.20

STRAIGHT INSTABILITY

Medial instability Disruption of the ligaments of the medial compartment results in a valgus subluxation of the tibia on the femur (Figure 10.19a). It is diagnosed by a positive abduction stress test. This is performed in two positions, first with the knee in 30 degrees of flexion and then fully extended.

Initial position. The patient lies supine with the hip slightly abducted. The knee is flexed to 30 degrees over the side of the couch. The examiner hugs the patient's lower leg under his right arm and the right hand steadies the lower leg. The left hand is placed over the lateral aspect of the patient's knee (Figure 10.25a).

Method. The knee is gently moved in abduction until pain is produced over the medial compartment or subluxation and gapping of the medial joint line are shown. This test is then repeated with the knee straight (Figure 10.25b).

Interpretation. With the knee fully extended in the screw-home position, ligament supports should be taut. Significant laxity here demonstrates that the cruciate and capsule ligaments are torn. Flexion relaxes the posterior capsule so allowing a true test of collateral ligament stability. If this test is positive with the knee flexed to 30 degrees but negative with the knee fully extended it implies that the medial collateral ligament has been damaged. If the test is positive with the knee both at 30 degrees of flexion and in full extension it implies damage to the cruciate and the medial capsular ligaments.

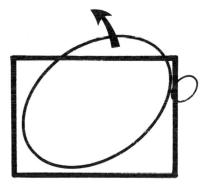

Figure 10.23 Anterolateral rotary instability. Key as in Figure 10.20

Lateral instability Disruption of the lateral compartment ligaments with varus subluxation of the tibia on the femur (Figure 10.19b) is not as common as medial instability. It is diagnosed by a positive adduction stress test with the hands changed around to apply an adduction stress to the knee.

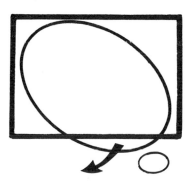

Figure 10.24 Posterolateral rotary instability. Key as in Figure 10.20

Interpretation. If the test is positive with the knee flexed to 30 degrees, but negative with the knee fully extended, it implies that the lateral collateral

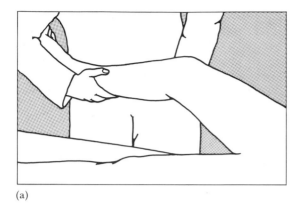

(a)

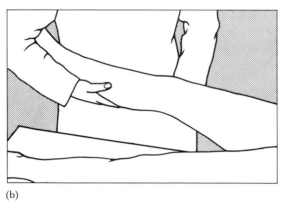

(b)

Figure 10.25 Abduction stress test. (a), Knee flexed; (b), knee extended

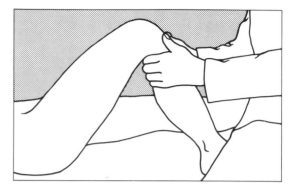

Figure 10.26 Test for anteroposterior instability

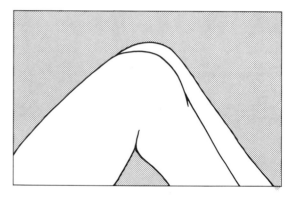

Figure 10.27 Ruptured posterior cruciate ligament of the right knee

ligament has been damaged. If it is positive also in extension it implies damage both to the cruciate and lateral capsular ligaments.

Anterior instability This is diagnosed if both tibial plateaux can be displaced anteriorly in relation to the femur while the tibia is maintained in the neutral position. It is diagnosed by the presence of a positive anterior drawer test.

Starting position. The patient lies supine with the hip flexed to 45 degrees and the knee to 90 degrees; the examiner sits on the dorsum of the foot to stabilize it, the upper tibia is grasped and hamstring tendons palpated to ensure that they are relaxed (Figure 10.26).

Method. The tibia is gently pulled and pushed to and fro to determine the degree of anterior movement. The knee must be kept in neutral position during this test.

Interpretation. A positive anterior drawer test is traditionally held to be synonymous with rupture of the anterior cruciate ligament. This is no longer tenable, as patients with a negative test may be found at operation to have a ruptured cruciate ligament. A positive anterior drawer test with the knee in flexion may suggest anterior cruciate ligament injury but a negative test does not rule it out [46].

A positive test should be regarded as detecting a torn anterior cruciate in which its secondary restraints, especially the lateral ligaments, are also torn [46]. A markedly positive test may be from a tear of the medial and lateral capsular ligaments that produces a combined anteromedial and antero-lateral rotational instability.

Variations. The anterior drawer test is performed at three separate angles of rotation: first in neutral rotation, then with the foot medially rotated by approximately 30 degrees; and finally with the foot laterally rotated approximately 15 degrees.

Lateral rotation of the tibia tightens the medial capsular ligament and medial rotation of the tibia tightens the lateral capsular ligament. Excessive movement in either of these two positions indicates a rotary instability, discussed below. This degree of movement is accentuated in the presence of a torn anterior cruciate.

Posterior instability This implies that the tibia can be displaced posteriorly on the femur while maintained in the neutral position (Figure 10.21b). It is diagnosed by a positive posterior drawer test. The tibia is now pulled to and fro to disclose any backwards movements of the tibia on the femur.

Interpretation. This test is positive after disruption of the posterior cruciate ligament together with a tear of the posterior capsular ligaments. This test can, at times, be difficult to differentiate from the anterior drawer test, as the tibia is originally subluxed posteriorly (Figure 10.27) and the test movements will then draw the tibial plateau forwards.

ROTARY INSTABILITY

Rotary instability of the knee from ligament injury results in an excessive degree of rotation of the tibia on the femur. This may either be an inwards rotation or, more commonly, an outwards rotation. The patient usually presents with a history of sudden giving way of the knee, usually without any warning or pain but often with a feeling that one bone in the knee has moved or slipped on the other. This tends to occur on walking down stairs or over uneven ground when the leg is supporting body-weight. It is particularly common when a runner suddenly changes direction or steps off the involved leg. There may be a history of pain and swelling of the knee after trauma, when the patient may have been conscious of a sudden snapping sensation in the knee.

Anteromedial rotary instability This is an anterior subluxation of the medial tibial condyle which also moves into lateral rotation on the femur (Figure 10.22). It follows a tear of the capsular ligament of the medial joint compartment, which is then unable to limit the degree of lateral rotation of the tibia on the femur. This may occur as an isolated lesion but the degree of instability is accentuated if the medial collateral or cruciate ligaments are also ruptured.

Anteromedial instability is diagnosed in the presence of a positive anterior drawer test, which is performed while the tibia is held in lateral rotation.

Anterolateral rotary instability This is an anterior subluxation of the lateral tibial condyle, which moves into internal rotation on the femur (Figure 10.23). It is caused by insufficiency of the anterior cruciate ligament and the degree of instability is increased if the lateral capsular ligament is also torn.

Posterolateral rotary instability This is a posterior subluxation of the lateral tibial condyle that also rotates medially (Figure 10.24). It follows a tear of the arcuate complex and is diagnosed by a lateral rotation–hyperextension test.

Starting position. The patient lies supine with the knees straight and the leg is lifted by the toes to produce hyperextension.

Method. The tibia may then be seen to rotate laterally so that the knee develops a varus deformity. This test requires considerable experience to evaluate.

Complications of rotary instability A tear in the posterior horn of the meniscus occurs as it is repeatedly caught by the abnormal movement now possible between the femur and tibia. The blocking of knee movements by the torn meniscus may mask the presence of a rotary instability produced by the torn ligament. After meniscectomy the rotary instability becomes obvious and the patient complains of his knee letting him down. As a further complication osteochondral injuries and osteoarthritis may develop in the tibiofemoral or patellofemoral joint [21].

Pellegrini–Stieda lesion

This relatively common condition with ossification in the upper attachment of the tibial collateral ligament usually follows a direct injury with haematoma formation but may occasionally follow a first or second degree sprain. The patient, often involved in body-contact sports, presents with pain on the medial side of the knee or, stiffness or may be conscious of a tender lump. Examination reveals a tender swelling at the upper end of the attachment of the tibial collateral ligament and pain is reproduced by applying an abduction stress to the knee. Radiographs confirm the ossification related to the medial femoral condyle.

MANAGEMENT

Treatment is with ultrasound and isometric quadriceps exercises at first, followed with mobilizing exercises. The painful area in the upper attachment responds well to an injection of local anaesthetic and corticosteroid which may be repeated a few times at intervals of 1 month. The pain usually settles but a slightly tender lump may persist for some months and the patient needs to be reassured about its benign nature. Surgery is not indicated.

Breast-stroke swimmer's knee

This overuse syndrome involves the medial collateral ligament of the knee. In breast-stroke swimming the

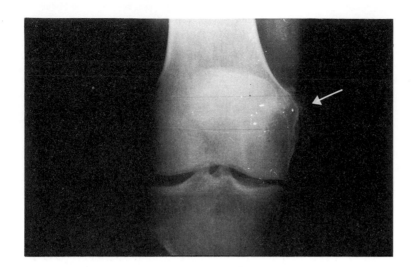

Figure 10.28 Pellegrini–Stieda

hips are first abducted with the knees medially rotated. The hips are then actively laterally rotated, so placing considerable strain on the medial compartment of the knee resulting in inflammation of the upper attachment of the ligament. Pain is well localized over the medial knee compartment and made worse by continuing activity.

MANAGEMENT
The patient needs to rest from breast-stroke swimming and other swimming strokes may be substituted. Ultrasound applied over the painful ligament helps to ease pain and localize the area of tenderness, which should then be injected with 1 ml corticosteroid. The patient usually returns to full activity in 2–3 weeks.

Musculotendinous lesions of the knee

Quadriceps weakness

In any injury to the quadriceps mechanism or after any knee joint disorder, the quadriceps rapidly loses bulk and strength, especially the vastus medialis which is necessary to maintain balance in the quadriceps group. This, in turn, may lead to a self-perpetuating painful knee problem which may then be confused with an intrinsic knee disorder or lead to retropatellar pain. Treatment to strengthen the quadriceps by a full passive and active exercise programme is essential.

Quadriceps tendon

Partial or complete rupture of the quadriceps tendon at its insertion into the upper border of the patella [47] is a major injury as the quadriceps is unable to maintain stability of the knee. The tendon may tear if the knee is actively flexed while maintaining a maximum quadriceps contraction, as may happen during an unexpected fall. It occurs more commonly in elderly males and may be bilateral [48,49]. The tear usually extends into the quadriceps expansion on either side of the patella. If untreated there may be some degree of repair, but the patient will be unable to climb stairs or walk up hills without the knee giving way.

MAJOR SIGN
The patient sits over the edge of the couch with the knee fully extended and is unable to sustain an isometric contraction of the quadriceps muscle. A gap may be palpable in the tendon above the patella.

MANAGEMENT
Partial tears may be treated conservatively but treatment of a complete tear requires urgent surgery.

Gastrocnemius tendinitis

This little known lesion involves the musculotendinous origin of the gastrocnemius, more commonly its medial head. It is an overuse injury, e.g. in distance runners. Pain is usually well localized but when severe may radiate down the leg. The underlying bursa may also be inflamed.

MAJOR SIGN

The patient lies prone and pain is reproduced by fully resisting knee flexion. Tenderness is well localized over the gastrocnemius head, best felt by placing one finger over the gastrocnemius origin and then fully flexing the knee. It needs to be differentiated from semimembranosus tendinitis [50].

Bicipital tendinitis

The biceps tendon is inserted into the fibular head. Tendinitis follows an overuse injury usually from running and may be associated with a bursitis

MAJOR SIGN

Pain is reproduced by resisting flexion of the knee. Tenderness is well localized on palpation over the tendon insertion.

Popliteal tendinitis

The popliteus muscle runs from the posterior surface of the tibia and is attached by its tendon into the lateral surface of the lower femur. Pain is felt at the posterolateral corner of the knee joint and may be extreme for the first 24 h after running but then usually improves. At times, the tendon may slip in and out of its groove on the femoral condyle, which produces a painful click.

MAJOR SIGN

Pain may be reproduced on contraction of the muscle. The patient lies supine, the hip flexed, abducted and laterally rotated and the knee at right angles. Active flexion of the knee is fully resisted with one hand while palpating the tendon just posterior to the lateral collateral ligament with the other (Figure 10.29). Tenderness may be felt just above the joint line in the posterolateral corner of the knee joint.

Iliotibial tract

The iliotibial tract is a thickened strip of fascia lata that passes down the lateral aspect of the thigh to a tubercle on the lateral tibial condyle. Overuse of the iliotibial tract is relatively common, especially in distance runners [51]. As the knee is flexed and extended, the iliotibial tract rubs over the lateral femoral condyle. Pain is felt over the lateral compartment of the knee where the iliotibial band passes over the lateral femoral epicondyle. Pain is characteristically brought on after running a few miles along a flat surface or on running downhill but may also occur after the completion of a run and then becomes worse [52]. Pain may radiate either distally or proximally and the patient may complain of a clicking hip (see p. 124).

Major signs Compression over the iliotibial band while flexing and extending the knee should reproduce the patient's pain. The patient's knee is first flexed to 90 degrees and the examiner places his thumb over the iliotibial band just proximal to the lateral epicondyle [53]. The knee is then gradually extended and at approximately 30 degrees of flexion pain is reproduced. This is increased by additional medial rotation of the tibia. Associated leg deformities include especially hyperpronation of the feet and tibia vara.

Confirmatory signs The diagnosis may be confirmed on palpation; there will be a localized area of tenderness over the lateral femoral epicondyle approximately 3 cm proximal to the joint line. This may also be associated with a sensation of crepitus, creaking or clicking.

MANAGEMENT

1 Rest. The patient usually needs to rest from distance running, especially if it involves hills, but other activities are usually possible, including swimming and cycling.
2 Anti-inflammatory drugs and analgesics are prescribed.
3 Physical methods including heat or ice are usually of benefit. Stretching the iliotibial band is also necessary using windmill techniques (see Figure 10.30); quadriceps and hamstring exercises are begun.
4 Injections of local anaesthetic and corticosteroid into the tender area usually produce marked relief and may be repeated at intervals.

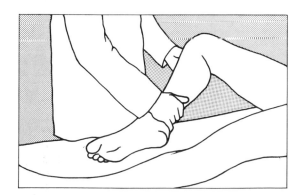

Figure 10.29 Test for popliteal tendinitis

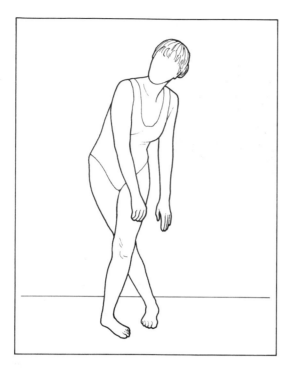

Figure 10.30 Stretching of the iliotibial tract

5   Correction of foot biomechanical disorders with appropriate orthotics. Overstriding is common and training errors need to be corrected.
6   Correction of training errors or running mechanics such as running on cambered roads is usually necessary.
7   Surgery. If the conservative methods fail, or if it is recurrent, surgery to free the posterior fibres of iliotibial tract over the lateral epicondyle may be very successful [54].

Bursitis

Prepatellar bursitis

This bursa lies between the anterior surface of the patella and the skin. It is commonly involved by direct trauma, often of a chronic repetitive nature producing the 'housemaid's knee'. Examination shows a distinctive prominent swelling in front of the patella, which can grow to a large size. Acute bursitis may also be caused by infections or gout.

Infrapatellar bursitis

This bursa lies between the patellar tendon and the infrapatellar fat pad. Bursitis is produced by the same mechanism as patellar tendinitis. Pain may be reproduced on full extension or full passive flexion of the knee. The distended bursa is best seen with the knee fully extended bulging on either side of the patellar tendon and cross-fluctuation between the two sides may be demonstrated.

Superficial infrapatellar bursitis

The superficial infrapatellar bursa lies between the tibial tubercle and the skin. Bursitis is not common and is produced by overuse of the patellar tendon. In young people it needs to be differentiated from Osgood–Schlatter's disease and board-rider's knee.

Anserine bursitis

This bursa lies between the tibial collateral ligament and its attachment to the tibia, and the overlying insertion of sartorius, gracilis and semitendinosis, the pes anserinus tendon insertion. Bursitis may be produced by direct trauma but is more common after an overuse injury or as a complication of knee arthritis [55]. Pain tends to be well localized and may be made worse by resisting knee flexion.

Semimembranosus bursitis (popliteal cyst)

This bursa is found on the medial side of the popliteal fossa between the medial head of the gastrocnemius and the semimembranosus tendon. It usually communicates with the knee joint. Swelling from the bursitis is best seen and felt while standing with the knee in extension (Figure 10.31). This popliteal cyst results from any condition that produces synovitis in the knee. Fluid then tracks into the bursa and a ball-valve arrangement prevents its return. It may track into the calf (see p. 179). Children differ in that the larger cystic popliteal swelling is often bilateral and most often resolves spontaneously.

Bicipital bursitis

The bicipital bursa lies between the insertion of the biceps tendon and fibular collateral ligament into the head of the fibula. Bursitis may complicate an overuse injury of the biceps tendon or a sprain of the ligament. The small swelling can be made more obvious by resisted flexion of the knee. It needs to be differentiated from a cyst of the lateral meniscus which lies over the joint line.

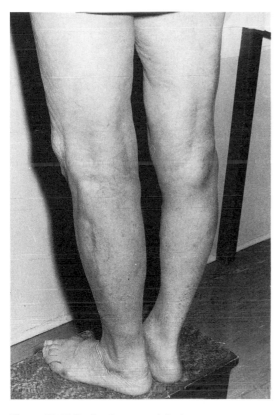

Figure 10.31 Popliteal cyst on right leg

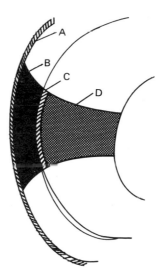

Figure 10.32 Peripheral attachments of the medial meniscus. (A), joint capsule; (B), vascular parameniscal zone; (C), a fibrous zone; (D), avascular fibrocartilage

Lesions of the tibiofemoral joint

Menisci

The medial and lateral compartments of the knee each contain a fibrocartilaginous meniscus (Figure 10.32) that help to absorb the compressive forces that develop as body-weight is transmitted. During compression of the knee joint the menisci may carry a substantial proportion of the applied load. They increase the load-bearing surface by making the joint surfaces more congruent and thus reduce the load per unit area on the articular cartilage.

The menisci also act as an intra-articular fibro-cartilaginous washer. The convex femoral condyles cause a lack of bony symmetry between the femur and the tibia. The space is filled by the menisci. They play an important role in stabilizing the knee throughout its range of motion and also aid in the control of rotary stability. This may be confirmed clinically in patients with a previous cruciate injury who then develop a rotary instability after menisc-ectomy.

The menisci form a functional unit with the surrounding ligaments and move with movement of the knee joint. They are commonly considered to aid joint lubrication and the symmetrical distribution of pressure within the joint.

Meniscal tears: aetiological factors

AGE
The peak age for a torn meniscus is 20–30 years, and a tear in a normally developed meniscus is rare under the age of 16 years.

SITE
The medial meniscus is much more commonly torn than the lateral meniscus.

OCCUPATION
This is a common sporting injury; it may occur in any type of sport but contact sports are the most common and skiing a relatively uncommon cause. People whose occupation involves prolonged squatting or kneeling, such as miners or floor carpeters, are particularly liable to develop cartilage degeneration. Degenerative changes occur with age and play a role in cartilage tears in the more elderly age group.

HISTORY OF TRAUMA
There may be a history of a previous knee ligament sprain or of a fracture of the tibial plateau.

MECHANISM OF INJURY

The usual combination is to have the knee in some degree of flexion while weight-bearing, so that the tibia is held fixed and usually in a position of external rotation. The medial meniscus can then be drawn into the centre of the joint space, where it is firmly held between the condyles of the femur and the tibia. As the patient then straightens up by extending the knee, the femur is forced into medial rotation, the meniscus is caught in the centre of the joint and torn. Injuries of the lateral meniscus are less common because injuries of the lateral compartment are less common and the lateral meniscus is more mobile because it is not attached to its collateral ligament.

Associated injuries

1 The forces that produce a tear of the meniscus with flexion, rotation and abduction are also the same forces that produce knee ligament sprains. The same type of injury may damage the ligaments or meniscus or both, and meniscal tears may be associated with a sprain of the middle capsular ligaments.
2 Instability of the knee may ultimately result in a meniscal tear.
3 Chondral lesions. The articular cartilage lining the surface of the femoral condyle may also be damaged. This relatively common complication is found usually on the femoral surface opposite the site of the meniscal tear.
4 Patellofemoral pain may be associated with a torn meniscus, as normal patellofemoral rhythm is disturbed.
5 Osteoarthritis may develop as a late complication, especially with any chondral injury.

Types of tear

The cartilage may tear in either a longitudinal or a horizontal direction. Longitudinal tears are the more common and may involve either the anterior or the posterior horn or the cartilage substance. The longitudinal tear may involve only a small area of the meniscus and can then become displaced. If sufficiently long to pass from the anterior to the posterior horn it produces a 'bucket-handle tear' and the detached inner fragment can become displaced into the centre of the joint, where it may produce locking. At times the meniscus may be detached from its peripheral attachments.

Transverse horizontal tears occur more commonly in the lateral meniscus, usually at the junction of the anterior and middle thirds. The tear commences on the concave edge and extends backwards and laterally into the midzone. This parrot-beak tear may be associated with a cyst of the meniscus. Only rarely does a transverse tear become complete.

Horizontal cleavage tears occur over the age of 40 years as a degenerative lesion usually in the posterior half. They may remain asymptomatic but are associated later with osteoarthritis in that compartment.

A history to disclose the exact mechanism of injury and subsequent knee disability is of paramount importance. Diagnosis can usually be made clinically but arthroscopy is indicated for accurate assessment.

Pain is usually sudden in onset, severe and located over the involved joint compartment or felt 'somewhere in the knee'. It may be associated with a tearing sensation or an audible click, and the patient is unable to continue his activities. It may be difficult to differentiate clinically from a ligament sprain.

Different symptoms develop in the elderly in whom a tear is associated with degeneration in the meniscus. The history is usually one of pain in the knee that increases over a period of time, tends to be worse with activity and is often present at night, especially if the affected knee is twisted or if one knee rests on the other. Walking up stairs may be painful. A knee effusion usually develops, especially after activity, and may gradually resolve only to return later after another period of prolonged use.

SWELLING

An effusion is nearly always present.

LOCKING

A history of locking and unlocking of the knee is of considerable importance (see p. 140) indicating that a fragment of the meniscus is trapped between the femoral and tibial condyles, so preventing full extension. A history of locking is more likely if the tear involves the anterior two-thirds of the meniscus. If the displaced fragment lies within the intercondylar space no locking may occur.

CLICKING

There may be a history of recurrent, painful, often audible clicks or a snapping sensation in the knee.

INSTABILITY

The patient may be conscious of a sudden giving way and instability of the knee, or that something slips in the joint.

EXAMINATION

Examination usually reveals a synovial effusion and quadriceps atrophy. Normal knee movement is usually lost, either as a loss of hyperextension or of the last few degrees of full extension, or loss of the last 10 degrees of full knee flexion. Pain may be reproduced with these movements. A meniscal tear also results in a loss of the range of passive axial rotation. Lesions of the anterior half of either meniscus produce a block to lateral rotation, and lesions of the posterior half of the meniscus produce a block to full passive medial rotation.

SPECIAL TESTS

Various manoeuvres have been described to reproduce symptoms by manipulating the meniscus between the bony condyles. However, they may be negative in the presence of a torn meniscus and so do not necessarily exclude the diagnosis.

1 Rotation. The patient lies supine with the hip and knee flexed. The lower leg is rapidly medially and laterally rotated while the examiner palpates over the joint line for pain and tenderness. The test is repeated with the knee in varying degrees of flexion.
2 McMurray's test. This test is most useful for tears in the posterior or middle third of the meniscus. The patient lies supine with the hip and knee flexed. In a suspected tear of the medial meniscus, the lower leg is laterally rotated and abducted (Figure 10.33) and the knee is then slowly extended. As it extends from 90 degrees of flexion, a painful click, which may be palpable or audible, indicates a positive test. In suspected lateral meniscus tears the knee is medially rotated and then slowly extended while the examiner palpates over the lateral joint line.
3 Apley's test. The patient lies prone with the hip extended and the knee flexed to 90 degrees. The lower leg is rotated medially and laterally while at the same time applying first a downwards compression (Figure 10.34) and then upwards traction. If rotation of the knee with downwards compression produces pain a tear of the meniscus is indicated. Pain reproduced on rotation with upwards traction indicates a ligament sprain.
4 Shearing strain. The patient lies supine with the knee flexed to a right angle. The heel of one hand is placed over the lower femur and the heel of the other over the upper tibia (Figure 10.35). The hands are forced together, producing a shearing strain across the joint. The hands are then reversed and the shearing strain imposed from the opposite direction.

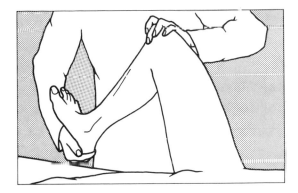

Figure 10.33 McMurray's test

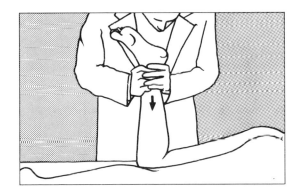

Figure 10.34 Apley's test: downwards compression

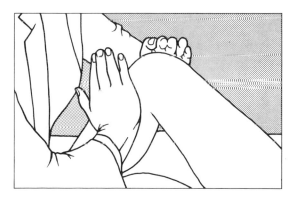

Figure 10.35 Shearing strain being produced across the knee joint

Confirmatory tests

The patient lies supine with the hip and knee flexed while the joint line is palpated. Tenderness over the anterior or posterior thirds of the joint line tends to confirm a meniscus tear, but tenderness over the middle third may indicate a meniscus or ligament injury. Routine radiographs are taken to exclude bony injury or the presence of a loose body. Arthroscopy is used to inspect the menisci and other joint structures and has revolutionized the operative approach.

Management

Meniscectomy is not a benign procedure and should never be undertaken without very careful assessment [56]. Loss of its normal weight-bearing and stabilizing functions can lead to rotary instability and osteoarthritis in later life, especially in children, the elderly, with lateral meniscectomies and in total rather than in partial meniscectomy. Many menisci that would previously have been resected are now spared [57]. The aim is to correct symptoms, return patients to their former activity and prevent future problems. Assessment and treatment by arthroscopy have many advantages over open arthrotomy [14,56]. Not all meniscal tears need to be removed; some can be repaired with arthroscopic suturing and peripheral tears can be reattached. The success of meniscus repair will depend on a lack of degenerative changes and an adequate blood supply [56]. Otherwise, partial meniscectomy may suffice; meniscal repair decreases the incidence of articular cartilage degeneration [58]. The majority of reparable meniscal tears occur in unstable knees [14] and with ACL-deficient knees the cartilage retear rate is high and so it may need to be reconstructed also.

A locked knee caused by a meniscus tear should be treated by arthroscopic surgery as soon as practicable. If not, manipulative reduction should be undertaken.

STARTING POSITION
The patient lies supine and relaxed. The knee is flexed with the hip at a right angle, the left hand is placed over the knee to stabilize it and the heel grasped with the right hand. The medial compartment of the knee is opened up by fully abducting and laterally rotating the lower leg (Figure 10.36a).

METHOD
The knee is suddenly extended with a snap as it is turned into medial rotation (Figure 10.36b). The torn meniscus can usually be felt or heard to click, and after the knee is unlocked the patient can extend the knee without pain. Occasionally, the displaced fragment can be felt to reduce while the knee is either flexing or rotating.

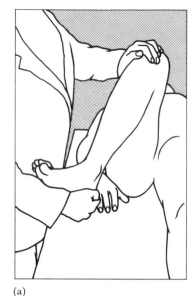

(a)

(b)

Figure 10.36 Reduction of a locked knee. (a), Starting position; (b), final position

Cysts of the meniscus

A cyst of the meniscus involves the lateral much more commonly than the medial meniscus in a ratio of approximately 9 : 1. They are usually traumatic in origin and a parrot-beak tear can usually be demonstrated in the outer zone of the meniscus. Synovial fluid can then enter the tear, producing a ganglion-like swelling filled with hyaluronic acid and thick gelatinous fluid.

Symptoms are usually highly characteristic. The patient is often a young sportsman who presents with localized knee pain and may be conscious of a swelling. However, it can present at any age. Pain may be intermittent and occurs especially during running or climbing stairs, with a sudden severe painful 'catch' in the knee so that it may give way. Pain is usually dull and aching, made worse by activity and is often present at night, when it will disturb sleep. A tender lump is usually present in the middle third of the joint line and it may vary in size over a period of time. This swelling is most obvious over the joint line when the patient sits with the legs over a couch and the knee held at about a 45 degree angle of flexion. It is generally absent at full flexion and extension. Synovial effusion is usually absent.

These cysts need to be differentiated from pseudo-cysts of the lateral meniscus owing to displacement of an extensive horizontal cleavage tear or a bucket-handle tear which can also occur [18,59].

Management requires arthroscopy for accurate diagnosis, assessment and treatment to exclude other pathology. Surgical management to remove the cyst and repair the meniscus brings good results.

Discoid meniscus

In this the meniscus is discoid in shape rather than semilunar. It may be a congenital variation showing persistence of the foetal state. It usually involves the lateral meniscus which is more liable to damage and minor trauma may result in a tear, most commonly of the parrot-beak variety. The patient, usually in his late teens, complains of a painful snapping or clicking on knee movement, usually in a few degrees of flexion. This snapping can be easily palpated over the joint line. Surgical removal or sauccrization is usually necessary.

Chondral injuries

Injuries to the articular cartilage in adults can involve joint surfaces of the femur, tibia or patella. They can follow a torsion injury, sudden severe compression, repetitive scarring or direct trauma and may be associated with meniscal or ligament injuries. They are, of course, translucent on radiographs and require arthroscopy or MRI for definitive diagnosis.

Osteochondral injuries

These involve both the articular cartilage and subchondral bone of the femoral condyle or less commonly the patella [60].

Osteochondral fractures

Acute fractures usually involve the lateral femoral condyle in adolescents usually following a twisting injury, although the degree of trauma may at times seem minor. There is immediate detachment of the articular surface and haemarthrosis. Diagnosis is made on radiographs. This condition needs to be differentiated from osteochondritis dissecans which involves a gradual separation of the fragment with the line of separation extending through ischaemic bone rather than the normal bone of osteochondral fractures.

Osteochondritis dissecans

Despite its name, this disorder, in which a fragment of cartilage and bone separates partially or completely, is not an inflammatory lesion. Osteochondritis dissecans tends to occur on the convex surfaces of joints and in the knee most cases involve the lateral side of the medial femoral condyle. Less commonly the lateral femoral condyle is involved, usually on its weight-bearing surface. There is considerable speculation as to its aetiology and it may have more than one cause, although the most likely single cause is trauma, and the site of this lesion is consistent with such an origin. Hereditary factors, ischaemia, anomalies of ossification and repetitive microtrauma have been incriminated. It most commonly follows a twisting injury while playing sport. Osteochondritis dissecans tends to occur in better class athletes and its incidence mirrors the degree of sport participation. It may be produced by the medial tibial spine impinging against the lateral surface of the medial femoral condyle, especially when the lower leg is in a position of abduction and lateral rotation with the knee held slightly flexed, e.g. when pivoting on one leg. Whatever the original mechanism, ischaemia and avascular necrosis are a final common pathway. It occurs more often in young males and symptoms are determined according to whether the osteochondral fragment becomes separated. If the fragment remains attached pain tends to be of insidious onset, dull and aching, poorly localized within the knee, made worse by activity and may be present at night. The knee may be swollen especially after activity. Symptoms may be those of a loose body with intermittent pain and swelling in the knee. Pain may be present only on exertion and is difficult to differentiate from other intra-articular lesions.

A loose fragment may also produce locking or giving way of the knee, usually with a synovial effusion and may be difficult to distinguish clinically from a torn meniscus. Radiographs, including intercondylar views, are necessary to confirm the diagnosis and the presence or absence of a loose bony fragment. Arthroscopy or MRI may be necessary to confirm the diagnosis and its extent.

MANAGEMENT

If the diagnosis is made early, and the osteochondral fragment is still in position, treatment consists of rest to the knee with avoidance of weight-bearing. Extra rest by use of a plaster cast with the knee flexed is rarely indicated. If symptoms persist or if the fragment appears to be separating, arthroscopy is necessary. It may be possible to drill the lesion with wires. If a fragment is small and loose it may be possible to remove it through the arthroscope. The crater that is left is smoothed out and its base drilled to promote healing with fibrocartilage. Pinning of the fragment has been advocated if a large segment of bone is involved.

Osteonecrosis

Spontaneous osteonecrosis of the femoral condyle involves the weight-bearing surface of the medial femoral condyle in elderly, usually female, patients (Figure 10.37) [61]. The aetiology is unknown but the original lesion may be an occlusion of the arterial supply to this area in a previously normal knee. The onset of pain is usually sudden and severe, so that the patient can often remember the exact time it started. Pain usually becomes persistent, is often worse at night and is accompanied by swelling and stiffness of the knee. The diagnosis may be suspected with the typical history and the finding of marked bony tenderness localized over the medial femoral condyle. Diagnosis needs to be confirmed by radiographs which may be normal at first, typical changes possibly taking several months to become evident. Flattening of the condyle is followed later by a radiolucent defect in the condyle, subsequently surrounded by a sclerotic margin. Additional information may be obtained from a CT or MRI scan, or a radionuclide bone scan, which is positive before radiological changes become evident. Synovial fluid examination shows non-inflammatory fluid. The subsequent history may depend on the amount of rest from weight-bearing that the patient can take, but degenerative changes develop in the medial joint compartment and result in a genu varum.

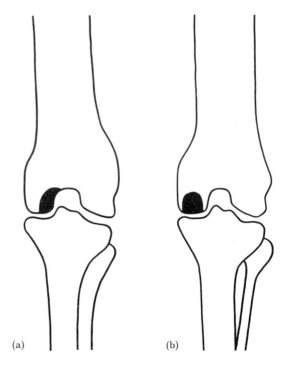

(a)　　　　　　　　(b)

Figure 10.37 Usual site of involvement in (a) osteochondritis dissecans and (b) in osteonecrosis

MANAGEMENT

Management in the initial stages depends on the patient not bearing weight on the affected knee, and in some cases pain may settle at this stage. Degenerative changes in the medial compartment often develop rapidly and surgery is then necessary.

Loose body formation

Intra-articular loose bodies in the knee may be formed from cartilage, bone or osteochondral fragments (Figure 10.38). They occur in osteochondritis dissecans, osteochondral fractures, chondromalacia patellae, osteoarthritis or synovial osteochondromatosis. In general, small loose bodies cause more trouble than larger ones and in osteoarthritic joints may be responsible for attacks of synovitis. They present as recurrent attacks of knee pain with locking and swelling. Diagnosis can be made by radiographs, if the fragment contains bone, or on arthroscopy.

Osteochondromatosis is a benign tumour in which the synovium proliferates and becomes hyperplastic. Cartilage forms in the synovial fronds which are

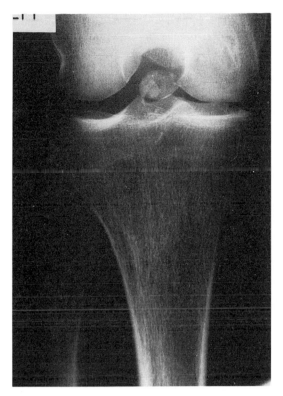

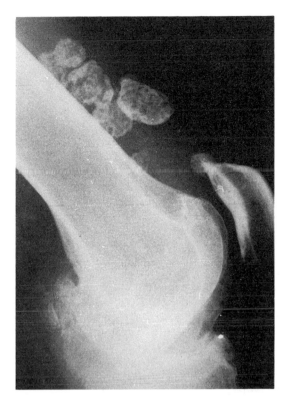

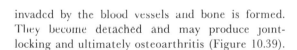

Figure 10.38 Loose body formation

Figure 10.39 Osteochondromatosis of the knee

invaded by the blood vessels and bone is formed. They become detached and may produce joint-locking and ultimately osteoarthritis (Figure 10.39).

Osteoarthritis of the knee

The knee is a very common site of osteoarthritis in sportspeople, possibly because it is so often subjected to varus or valgus deformities and trauma. Previous tears of the meniscus, injuries of the joint surfaces or ligament instability may all be complicated by subsequent degenerative changes. These may involve either the medial or lateral tibiofemoral compartment, the patellofemoral joint or any combination of these. Osteoarthritis usually commences in one compartment and in the tibiofemoral compartment may follow meniscal tears. Lateral compartment degeneration produces a valgus deformity, whereas medial compartment disease produces a varus deformity. As the disease progresses the degenerative changes in either compartment tend to increase the degree of any existing deformity. If there is any disparity in leg lengths the knee on the longer side is usually involved.

In the tibiofemoral compartment the menisci may be involved in the degenerative process; as the joint space narrows increased pressure is carried by the weight-bearing surface of the meniscus, which develops increased degenerative changes and a horizontal cleavage type of tear may occur. The meniscus is slowly ground away and its anterior part may disappear.

MANAGEMENT
The general management of patients with osteoarthritis of the knee is similar to that previously outlined for osteoarthritis of the hip (see p. 127) and includes rest, weight loss, aids, supports, anti-inflammatory drugs and physical therapy, especially passive mobilization and quadriceps exercises.

Mobilization techniques using large-amplitude painless techniques aid in easing knee pain and stiffness. Small-amplitude stretching movements used at the limit of range are of most value. For example, if knee flexion is most limited, treatment is commenced using anteroposterior pressures into extension. As the range of flexion improves, so usually does the range of extension.

Surgery is indicated in patients in whom pain and stiffness are severe with loss of function. The choice of operation lies between a total knee replacement or an osteotomy in patients with unicompartmental disease and a marked deformity.

Patellofemoral joint

Patellofemoral function

The patella has several functions. It is a sesamoid bone linking the quadriceps tendon to the patella tendon, increasing the quadriceps lever arm and its mechanical advantage. To function efficiently, the patella must remain aligned in the trochlear notch of the femur during movement and remain under muscle control. The retropatellar articular surface is divided into small medial and larger lateral facets by a vertical ridge. The medial patellar facet is further divided by a ridge into two facets, the smaller and more medial facet called the odd facet because of peculiarities of its articulation with the femur (Figure 10.40). The lateral facet of the patella articulates with the femur throughout the range of flexion movement, but the odd facet articulates only at 135 degrees of flexion.

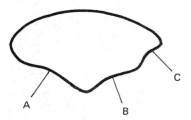

Figure 10.40 Retropatellar surface. (A), lateral patellar facet; (B), medial patellar facet with its 'odd facet' (C)

While standing with the knee extended, the patella normally lies above the articular margins on the femoral condyle. As the patella descends during knee flexion, different areas of its particular surface come into contact with the femur. At 20 degrees of flexion the medial and lateral facets on its lower pole become opposed and at 90 degrees of flexion the medial and lateral facets of the upper pole of the patella do so. As the knee is flexed past 90 degrees the patella comes to lie under the femoral condyles, rotates and moves laterally. At 135 degrees of flexion the areas of contact are its lateral facet and medially the odd facet articulates with the medial femoral condyle.

Dynamic and static factors are involved in patellofemoral stability and tracking. The dynamic factors result from the pull of the surrounding muscles and their patellar attachments. The quadriceps and its tendon exert the main pull. The vastus lateralis exerts a dynamic pull on the lateral side, aided by the iliotibial tract. The vastus medialis, but especially the vastus medialis oblique (VMO) whose fibres insert more distally and horizontally on the patella than do those of the lateralis, are the primary medial stabilizers.

Static factors are: (1) extra-articular – the patella ligament, joint capsule and surrounding medial and thicker lateral retinacula which connect the patella to femur, tibia and collateral ligaments; and (2) intra-articular – the patella facets and the femoral trochlea.

Patellar pain

Anterior knee pain arising from the patellofemoral joint is a very common symptom [62,63]. In older ages the most likely cause is osteoarthritis [64,65]. In young patients, usually runners [66], it occurs mainly from abnormalities of tracking or an increase in retropatellar pressure. It has been commonly termed chondromalacia patellae, but this is but one cause of dysfunction and should only be applied to the pathological articular cartilage changes which in turn can only be recognized on arthroscopy or at surgery. Chondromalacia is a pathological diagnosis then, that has been converted to and confused with a clinical diagnosis [63].

Moreover, patients with typical retropatellar pain may have normal arthroscopic findings [67]. Alternatively, articular changes may be present but the patient may be asymptomatic [65,67–71]. Chondromalacia patellae should be diagnosed only in patients with typical clinical findings and typical changes on arthroscopy [69] or MRI. Hence other causes of retropatellar dysfunction, especially malalignment and maltracking, must be searched for, but may be difficult to determine [69]. If articular cartilage is not the source of pain [64], other changes such as increased pressure, changes in the lateral retinaculum or synovitis should be considered.

Examination

The patellofemoral joint is to be regarded as part of the link system of joints in the lower limb that may be subjected to great pressure. Pressures may be increased by knee flexion (Figure 10.41) and also by many structural abnormalities or rotational deformities in the leg that lead to increased loading on the patellofemoral joint. A flexion deformity of the hip or tight hamstrings alter components in the link system. Special attention is pain to the subtalar joints. Any of these conditions may lead to patellar pain, and all patients with retropatellar pain must undergo a full examination of the whole of the lower limb.

Inspection

DEFORMITIES

Varus or valgus deformities of the knee should first be looked for with the patient standing. The quadriceps or Q angle is measured with the patient lying down (Figure 10.42). The combination of an increased Q angle with femoral anteversion and pronated feet is known as the malignant malalignment syndrome (Figure 10.43). With the patient

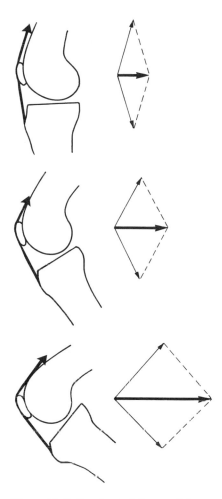

Figure 10.41 Resultant of the parallelogram of forces on the patellofemoral joint is increased as the knee is progressively flexed

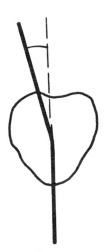

Figure 10.42 Q angle

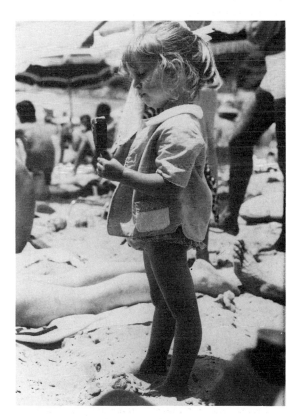

Figure 10.43 Genu recurvatum

sitting and knees flexed to 90 degrees over the edge of the couch, the patella is viewed: with patellar subluxation, it may be medially rotated ('squinting') or laterally rotated ('grasshoppers' eyes'). The height of the patella, patella alta or baja, is assessed. Patellar tracking on flexion and extension of the knees is observed.

SWELLING

Swellings around the patella include synovial effusions (see p. 144) and bursitis (see p. 156).

WASTING

Particular note is taken of any quadriceps wasting, especially involving the VMO.

Movements

These are active, passive and accessory.

ACTIVE MOVEMENT

Active movements in sitting or squatting may be performed while observing patellar movements.

PASSIVE MOVEMENT

Tightness in the hamstrings and iliotibial tract should be tested for. With the patient lying supine with the knee in extension and the muscles around the patella relaxed, test: (1) side to side movements of the patella. These may be increased or decreased, (2) a cephalad and caudal movement of the patella, and (3) these tests are then repeated using compression.

Pain may be reproduced by moving the undersurface of the patella against the femur by one of three manoeuvres:

1 Direct manual compression of the patella against the femoral groove with actively resisted extension of the knee.
2 Passive hyperextension of the knee (Figure 10.7).
3 McConnell's test is most useful [72,73]. The patient lies with the knees flexed to 20 degrees and the quadriceps are isometrically contracted to reproduce pain. This can be repeated with the patient squatting or going up or down stairs. Pressure is then applied to the lateral surface of the patella gliding it medially. This pressure should relieve pain for the test to be considered positive.

ACCESSORY MOVEMENT

Six accessory movements of the patella are lateral rotation, medial rotation, axial rotation, sagittal rotation, translation and compression.

Palpation

Retropatellar tenderness may be elicited (Figure 10.17) under the lateral or medial surface and retropatellar crepitus may be felt or heard. Wasting of the quadriceps and VMO is assessed.

Lesions of the patellofemoral joints

1 Chondromalacia patellae.
2 Patellofemoral dysfunction.
3 Instability of the patellofemoral joint.
4 Synovial plicae.
5 Osteochondritis dissecans.
6 Bipartite patella.
7 Stress fractures.
8 Reflex sympathetic dystrophy.

Extensor mechanism

Lesions of this mechanism may include:

1 Quadriceps tendon.
2 Patellar tendinitis.
3 Jumper's knee.
4 Rupture of the patellar tendon, partial or complete.
5 Osgood–Schlatter's disease.
6 Infrapatellar bursitis.
7 Osteochondritis of the patella.
8 Infrapatellar fat pad injuries.

Chondromalacia patellae

This disorder of the patellar articular cartilage is no longer regarded as a common cause of patellar pain (see p. 167). The cartilage lesion is a degeneration with softening and fibrillation, somewhat similar pathological changes to those in osteoarthritis although there are important differences [67,71]. Whether these are the result of excess or too little pressure is still not resolved [70]. Chondromalacia usually involves the medial patellar surface, is somewhat more common in females usually in the late teens, and often occurs in certain occupations or sports such as ballet dancing, distance running and bicycle riding.

Pain is usually described as a deep-seated ache, localized around the retropatellar area. It may be felt on going up or down stairs, on prolonged activity or after sitting for a prolonged time with the knees flexed, e.g. as in a car, at the theatre or on squatting. Some complain that they need an aisle seat in a theatre to keep their knee extended or else they have to get up and walk around during the show. In distance runners pain may come on only after running a certain distance. Pain is normally not present in the morning or after rest. Associated symptoms include stiffness, catching, locking, swelling or a sensation of insecurity or giving way of the knee. Synovitis may be caused by synovial irritation produced by flakes of cartilage.

Retropatellar dysfunction

Retropatellar dysfunction is a worthwhile term to describe any condition that interferes with normal patellofemoral movements and produces a retropatellar pain syndrome. These may result from anatomical alterations in: (1) the patella, (2) surrounding soft tissues, and (3) outside the joint.

Patella changes may be the result of:

1 Direct trauma to the patella that may result in chondral damage.
2 Misalignment and maltracking. While standing with the knee extended, the patella is at its most proximal point above the articular margins of the femoral condyle. It does not sit into the trochlea until approximately 20 degrees of flexion. On full flexion the patella glides 7–8 cm on the femur and only the most medial and lateral aspects of the proximal patella contact the femur [71]. The patella is potentially unstable during its first 20 degrees of flexion [74] and in some may become progressively tilted during further flexion [74].

The patella may be malaligned with the intercondylar sulcus of the femur [75]. Diagnosis is made on radiographs or MRI [76,77]. Several different radiographic angles have been described but they lack precision [78–80].

Maltracking laterally of the patella may occur with an excessive Q angle (see below) and/or a tight lateral retinaculum plus a weak VMO or may be a result of structural abnormalities of the trochlear groove [81].

Maltracking and misalignment may produce patellar pain, especially in athletes. Abnormal movement may be observed clinically as a sudden abrupt movement, especially during the first 30 degrees of flexion as the patella enters or leaves the femoral trochlea.

Surrounding soft tissues include muscles and retinaculae. Tightness occurs in:
1 The iliotibial band (see p. 155) which pulls the patella laterally during flexion.

2 The hamstrings which cause increased knee flexion during running, increasing patellofemoral joint reaction force.
3 The lateral retinaculum [82].
4 Gastrocnemius.

These may cause disturbed patellofemoral rhythm.

Alternatively, the VMO is the only dynamic medial stabilizer of the patella [83]. Any insufficiency of this muscle will increase the lateral drift of the patella.

Changes outside the patella may result from:

1 Altered Q angle. The Q angle is formed by the intersection of the line of the pull of the quadriceps at the centre of the patella and the patellar tendon. Normally about 10 degrees, it should never exceed 20 degrees. An increase may be associated with femoral anteversion, coxa vara, genu valgus, lateral displacement of the tibial tubercle or external tibial torsion. An increase in the Q angle from any cause will increase the lateral pull on the patella and so predispose to increased lateral pressure and subluxation.
2 Subtalar joint. Excessive or prolonged pronation of the subtalar joint [84] will result in prolonged medial rotation of the tibia and femur, but the tibia rotates faster than the femur and results in abnormal patellar movement which is pulled laterally in its groove by the quadriceps, also producing an increase in the Q angle.
3 Overuse. In some cases no definite underlying cause is demonstrable [69] and overuse alone may be responsible. Most sports involve knee movements with a full range of normal patellofemoral movement, often under load. Huge surface contact forces, up to eight times body-weight, may be generated during activity [72,85] and repetitive compressive and shearing stresses may initiate articular damage [67].

Investigations

Plain radiographs are taken to assess the site and size of the patella, the Q angle and the relative height of the patella: patella alta or baja. Retropatellar views can be taken using several different views in varying degrees of flexion [67,77,86,87], CT scan [74,86], or MRI [77]. Arthroscopy remains the definitive method of diagnosis and assessment.

Management

Most aspects of management remain controversial, more so as the cause of pain also remains undetermined. Conservative treatment is always undertaken first, and needs to be continued for a prolonged time. Surgery is only rarely indicated. General measures include:

1 Mobilization techniques may be useful to reduce pain and allow the exercise programme to be instituted. The first treatment session must be performed gently without pain, so assessing the irritability. If it is very painful or irritable, gentle passive movements are performed with distraction of the patella from the femur (Figure 10.44). As pain improves, passive movements are increased with movements of the patella in more than one direction, with varying degrees of compression of the patella, and by varying degrees of knee flexion while performing the movements against different surfaces of the femur.

2 Pain-free exercises to strengthen the quadriceps, especially the VMO, are essential and form the basis of conservative management [62,66,67, 69,72,77,78,83,88,89]. Isometric quadriceps exercises may need to be given first, supervised by a physiotherapist, as they involve only minimal movement of the patella, should not exacerbate pain and do strengthen the VMO. Exercises that include knee flexion using progressive resisted exercises or squats place an increased loading on the patellofemoral joint and exacerbate pain. Eccentric pain-free exercises [90] to strengthen the VMO are performed according to the McConnell technique [72,88] to change the timing of the quadriceps contraction [73]. A cybex evaluation of knee strength should be obtained as a baseline. Exercises are not progressed in the presence of pain or a knee effusion. General fitness is maintained, especially with a swimming programme.

3 Stretching exercises are given to tight structures in the leg and around the knee, especially the iliotibial band or hamstring muscles to reduce the forces at the patellofemoral joint during active quadriceps contraction.

4 Use of shoe orthotics if foot deformities, such as excessive or prolonged pronation, are present is helpful in most cases.

5 Avoidance of activities known to provoke pain, such as running on hills or stairs, and exercises involving flexion, such as bicycling or deep knee bends.

6 Non-steroidal anti-inflammatory drugs are given for pain relief, especially if an effusion is present.

7 Aftercare. Conservative management usually produces satisfactory results and the patient can then be gradually remobilized but should continue to perform at a progressively increasing pace on a good surface. He should also continue to perform the isometric quadriceps exercises and may wear a knee support with a patellar hole [64,89,91].

8 Surgery may be necessary [63] if symptoms are recurrent but careful patient selection after arthroscopy is necessary. Arthroscopy may include lavage with shaving of the articular cartilage to remove loose material and leave an even surface [60]. Why this relieves pain is uncertain. Many other operations have been devised and include either proximal or distal realignment:

(a) Lateral retinacular fibre release [82,92–95] may be combined with reefing of the medial capsule or advancement of the vastus medialis. The exact indications for this procedure are still not settled and careful selection of cases is necessary [85,96]. It may be done as an open or a closed procedure [97].

(b) Operations to relocate the insertion of the patellar tendon into the tibial tubercle include anterior advancement of the tibial tubercle or transfer of its insertion medially [94,98,99]. This may produce subsequent problems from abnormal tibial rotation.

(c) Total excision of the affected area of articular cartilage or facet [100].

(d) Patellectomy seriously weakens the knee and should very rarely be contemplated [101].

Patellofemoral instability

This may be caused by (1) acute dislocation, (2) recurrent subluxation or dislocation, or (3) chronic subluxation or dislocation.

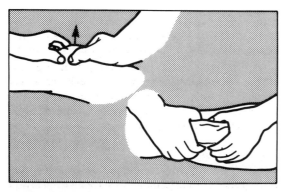

Figure 10.44 Patellofemoral distraction

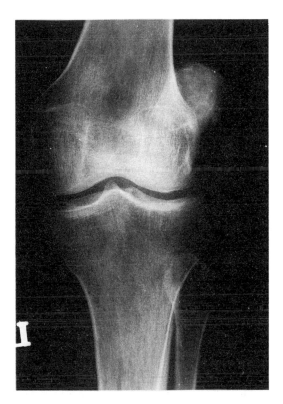

Figure 10.45 Recurrent dislocation of the patella

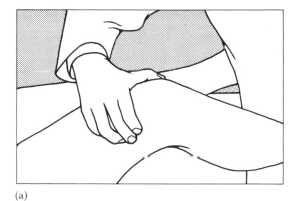

(a)

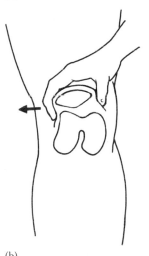

(b)

Figure 10.46 The apprehension test. (a), As the knee is flexed the patella is pushed laterally; (b), as the knee is flexed the patella is pushed laterally

Acute dislocation occurs mainly in knees with pre-existing anatomical dysplastic abnormalities. It is rare in normal knees and requires a violent action in sportspeople to produce it. The patella can be palpated on the lateral side of the knee, which is locked in flexion. Treatment is by reduction and immobilization.

RECURRENT SUBLUXATION OR DISLOCATION OF THE PATELLA

Recurrent subluxation of the patella (Figure 10.45) is common and tends to occur either in knock-kneed teenage girls or more commonly in athletes [79,102]. Pain, locking and a sensation of instability in the knee can be most difficult to distinguish from a torn meniscus.

Examination Postural abnormalities such as genu valgum or wasting of the vastus medialis muscle may be seen. With the knees over the edge of the couch, the patella may be shown to be abnormally seated, e.g. either high or directed laterally (Figure 10.45). The patella is excessively mobile, best tested with the knee flexed to 30 degrees and lying across the examiner's thigh to relax the quadriceps muscle. It is then easier to apply pressure to the medial aspect of the patella to assess the degree of hypermobility and apprehension.

MAJOR SIGN: THE APPREHENSION TEST

The examiner pushes outwards against the medial border of the patella while flexing the knee with his other hand (Figure 10.46). As the patella begins to subluxate laterally, the patient feels pain and becomes acutely aware that the patella is about to dislocate. Any further attempts to move the patella are actively resisted by contracting the quadriceps.

Confirmatory signs The patella is examined for painful crepitus, retropatellar tenderness. Retropatellar radiographic views should reveal a subluxed or abnormally seated patella as a result of dysplastic changes such as a shallow sulcus angle [79,103]. An avulsion injury of the patella may be present.

Management   Conservative treatment consists at first of making movements pain free and then an isometric exercise regimen to strengthen the quadriceps, the hip flexors and abductors is given with the use of a knee brace. This is followed by an active exercise programme of concentric and eccentric exercises [91].

If symptoms are recurrent surgery is indicated, the type of operation depending on the underlying pathology. The capsule and lateral retinaculum usually needs to be released and the medial structures tightened. Other procedures include realignment of the patellar tendon insertion.

Synovial plicae

A plica is a reduplicated fold of synovium within the knee joint, a remnant of a normal embryological septum [60,104,105]. There are three distinct folds: infra-, supra- and medial patellar. The suprapatellar plica may separate the suprapatellar bursa from the joint cavity and may then become a source of loose bodies. The infrapatellar plica runs across the infrapatellar fat pad. The medial plica (or shelf) [105] runs as a band from the anteromedial side of the knee obliquely down to the synovium over the fat pad. This band may become inflamed, thickened and fibrotic [104], especially after trauma and haemorrhage, and project into the joint over the medial femoral condyle. Here it can impede normal patellar movements as the knee moves from full flexion towards extension, and causes pain and snapping. Impingement on the patella produces patellar pain. Diagnosis may be made by palpation when the band can be felt as a thickened cord one fingerbreadth medial to the medial border of the patella or on arthroscopy. Treatment, if indicated, is by arthroscopic division.

Osteochondritis dissecans of the patella

This is rare, occurs mainly in active young boys and may be bilateral. It presents with an aching anterior knee pain, made worse by activity and crepitus. X-rays show fragmentation of the patellar surface [106]. Osteochondritis dissecans may also rarely involve the femoral trochlea.

Bipartite patella

This is usually a chance finding on radiographs but may be a cause of retropatellar pain (Figure 10.47).

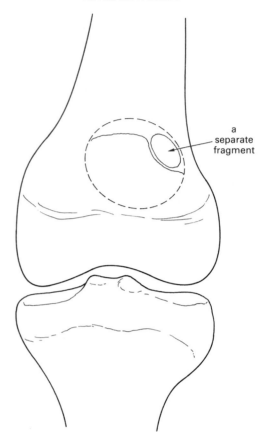

"BIPARTITE PATELLA"

a separate fragment

Figure 10.47 Bipartite patella

It should not cause any confusion with a stress fracture of the patella which occurs usually after exercise or following a knee replacement [107].

Reflex sympathetic dystrophy

This involves the patella after trauma or especially surgery. Pain is severe and patellar movements severely restricted. Diagnosis is made on radiographs or scan.

Lesions of the extensor mechanism

Patellar tendinitis

Tendinitis occurs in active sportsmen after the apophysis of the tibial tubercle has fused as an overuse injury, particularly in runners, fast bowlers and ballet dancers. Degenerative changes may occur in the patellar tendon, which will show an area of focal degeneration similar to that seen in the Achilles tendon (see p. 182).

Jumper's knee

This occurs commonly in sports such as jumping, basketball, volleyball or weight-lifting whose action requires repeated jumping off one leg [108]. It is associated with a small area of degeneration at the tendon attachment at the lower pole of the patella, characterized by pain and extreme local tenderness. Pain may be present at first only after activity, but in severe degrees it begins during activity and severely limits athletic performance and may be associated with a weakness or 'giving way' of the knee.

Clinical signs Pain is reproduced on resisting active knee extension. Crepitus may be present on passive movement of the patellar tendon. Tenderness, usually marked, is found localized at the lower pole of the patella, especially if the patella is pushed distally. Radiographs are normal but are necessary to exclude any patellar abnormality, stress fracture or an elongated lower pole of the patella.

MANAGEMENT

1 Rest. Symptoms are usually brought on by activity, e.g. running, jumping or kicking, and these may need to be curtailed. In younger patients other activities can be substituted but in professional sportsmen this is extremely difficult.
2 Anti-inflammatory drugs are given.
3 Physical measures such as heat or ice may help to relieve symptoms.
4 The patella should be mobilized using the techniques described above.
5 Exercises are essential. Isometric quadriceps exercises may be used first, followed by eccentric knee exercises [109].
6 Injections of corticosteroid may be given around the tender area in the tendon but never into the tendon substance. Extra rest is advised after the injection, which should be given as infrequently as possible and with at least 1 month between each injection. The injections are stopped if symptoms do not improve significantly.
7 Surgery is indicated if conservative measures fail or if tendinitis is recurrent and prevents full participation in sport [110]. Surgical treatment consists of decompression of the tendon and removal of any area of focal degeneration, adhesions around the tendon or an area of chondromalacia. Operation is followed by an intensive programme of rehabilitation and the patient can usually return to full activity.

COMPLICATIONS OF TENDINITIS
The patellar tendon may undergo partial or complete rupture. Complete rupture is quite rare and occurs mainly in patients who have had tendinitis for a considerable period of time. An incomplete tear also occurs but is difficult to distinguish from tendinitis alone.

Osgood–Schlatter's disease

This is associated with repetitive stress leading to tears and partial avulsion of the patellar tendon at its insertion into the tibial tubercle before the apophysis unites [111,112]. It occurs mainly in young active boys aged 9–14 years with a gradual onset of pain and a tender lump over the tibial tubercle. Pain is made worse by running, kneeling and stairs, and is relieved by rest [113]. It tends to run a protracted course over several years before gradually settling as the tuberosity is ossified.

MAJOR SIGNS
A tender swelling is present over the tibial tubercle and pain is reproduced on resisting active quadriceps extension. Stretching the quadriceps by fully flexing the knee with the hip in full extension reproduces pain and may demonstrate a shortening of the quadriceps. Radiographic changes, produced by separation of the tendon from the tibial tubercle with fragmentation of the apophysis and occasional loose bodies, take some time to develop.

MANAGEMENT
This is often difficult as the patient is young and active, and symptoms may not fully resolve until the apophysis is fully united. Pain usually prevents participation in activities requiring running or jumping but complete immobilization of the knee is neither necessary nor practical. Isometric quadriceps exercises with the knee straight are essential. Gentle, carefully controlled stretching and passive movement techniques to the knee may reduce pain and hamstrings are strengthened and stretched. Non-steroidal anti-inflammatory drugs and corticosteroid injections are contraindicated.

This condition usually settles after a prolonged time without any additional active therapy, but is apt to recur on return to activity and then requires a careful balance between rest and activity. Surgery remains controversial but removal of loose bony bodies which fail to unite may be necessary. Rarely the patellar tendon may be avulsed [114].

Osteochondritis dissecans of the patella

This relatively uncommon condition in teenagers is also known as Sindig–Larsen–Johansson disease. The usual mechanism of production is a traction injury to the lower pole of the patella. It occurs mainly in active boys aged 10–14 years, may at times be bilateral, and a similar condition occurs rarely at the upper pole of the patella. The patient presents with an aching pain, made worse by activity and localized to one pole of the patella, usually the lower. Radiographs show fragmentation of the pole of the patella.

Injury to the infrapatellar fat pad

The infrapatellar fat pad plays an important role in facilitating knee movements. It may be injured by direct injuries with haemorrhage and oedema. As the fat pad becomes enlarged it can rarely be more readily traumatized and its synovial folds can also become entrapped within the knee. Ultimately, fibrotic changes with loss of elasticity develop which limit its movements and the knee may feel unstable [115]. Knee pain is usually dull and aching, related to activity and relieved by rest. Swelling is evident on inspection as it bulges on either side of the patellar ligament, and is usually accentuated in genu recurvatum or by forced passive extension of the knee.

References

1 Dye, S.F. and Cannon, W.D. Jr. (1988) Anatomy and biomechanics of the anterior cruciate ligament. *Clinics in Sports Medicine*, **7**, 715–725
2 King, J.B. and Aitken, M. (1988) Treatment of the torn anterior cruciate ligament. *Sports Medicine*, **5**, 203–208
3 Van Dommelen, B.A. and Fowler, P.J. (1989) Anatomy of the posterior cruciate ligament: a review. *American Journal of Sports Medicine*, **17**, 24–29
4 Hughston, J.C., Andrews, J.R., Cross, M.J. *et al.* (1976) Classification of knee ligament instabilities. *Journal of Bone and Joint Surgery*, **58A**, 159–172
5 Solomonow, M., Baratta, R. Zhou, B.H. *et al.* (1987) The synergistic action of the anterior cruciate ligament and thigh muscles in maintaining joint stability. *American Journal of Sports Medicine*, **15**, 207–213
6 Cross, M.J., Pinczewski, L.A. and Bokor, D.J. (1989) Acute knee injury in a rock musician. *Physician and Sports Medicine*, **17**, 79–82
7 Hastings, D.E. (1980) The non-operative management of collateral ligament injuries of the knee joint. *Clinical Orthopaedics and Related Research*, **147**, 22–28
8 Hastings, D.E. (1986) Knee ligament instability – a rational anatomical classification. *Clinical Orthopaedics and Related Research*, **208**, 104–107
9 Wojtys, E.M., Goldstein, S.A., Redfern, M. *et al.* A biomechanical evaluation of the Lenox Hill knee brace. *Clinical Orthopaedics*, **220**, 179–184
10 Ritter, M.A., McCarroll, J., Wilson, F.D. *et al.* (1983) Ambulatory care of medial collateral ligament tears. *Physician and Sports Medicine*, **11**, 47–51
11 Kannus, P. (1989) Non-operative treatment of grade II and III sprains of the lateral ligament compartment of the knee. *American Journal of Sports Medicine*, **17**, 83–88
12 Farquharson-Roberts, M.A. and Osborne, A.H. (1983) Partial rupture of the anterior cruciate ligament of the knee. *Journal of Bone and Joint Surgery*, **69**, 32–34
13 Buckley, S.L., Barrack, R.L. and Alexander, A.H. (1989) The natural history of conservatively treated partial anterior cruciate ligament tears. *American Journal of Sports Medicine*, **17**, 221–225
14 Zarins, B. and Adams, M. (1988) Knee injuries in sports. *New England Journal of Medicine*, **318**, 950–961
15 Gersoff, W.K. and Clancy, W.G. Jr. (1988) Diagnosis of acute and chronic anterior cruciate ligament tears. *Clinics in Sports Medicine*, **7**, 727–738
16 Buttner-Janz, K., Schellnack, K. and Rieder, T. (1989) Non invasive diagnosis of cruciate ligament damage with particular reference to computer tomography with arthrography. *American Journal of Sports Medicine*, **17**, 501–504
17 Lee, J.K., Yao, L. and Wirth, C.R. (1990) Magnetic resonance imaging of major ligamentous knee injuries. *Physician and Sports Medicine*, **18**, 97–100
18 Cross, M.J. and Crichton, K.J. (1987) *Clinical Examination of the Injured Knee*, Gower Medical Publishing, London
19 Jonsson, T., Althoff, B., Peterson, L. *et al.* (1982) Clinical diagnosis of ruptures of the anterior cruciate ligament. *American Journal of Sports Medicine*, **10**, 100–102
20 Coughlin, L., Oliver, J. and Berretta, G. (1987) Knee bracing and anterolateral rotatory instability. *American Journal of Sports Medicine*, **15**, 161–163
21 Kannus, P. and Jarvinen, M. (1987) Conservatively treated tears of the anterior cruciate ligament. *Journal of Bone and Joint Surgery*, **69A**, 1007–1012
22 Pattee, G.A., Fox, J.M., del Pizzo, W. *et al.* (1989) Four to ten year follow-up of unreconstructed anterior cruciate ligament tears. *American Journal of Sports Medicine*, **17**, 430–435
23 Lorentzon, R., Elmqvist, L., Sjostrom, M. *et al.* (1989) Thigh musculature in relation to chronic anterior cruciate ligament tear: Muscle size, morphology and mechanical output before reconstruction. *American Journal of Sports Medicine*, **17**, 423–429
24 Andersson, C., Odensten, M., Goods, L. *et al.* (1989) Surgical or non-surgical treatment of acute rupture of the anterior cruciate ligament. *Journal of Bone and Joint Surgery*, **71A**, 965–974
25 Bilko, T.E., Paulos, L.E., Feagin, J.A. *et al.* (1986) Current trends in repair and rehabilitation of complete (acute) anterior cruciate ligament injuries. *American Journal of Sports Medicine*, **14**, 143–147

26 Gollehon, D.L., Warren, R.F. and Wickiewicz, T.L. (1985) Acute repairs of the anterior cruciate ligament – past and present. *Orthopedic Clinics of North America*, **16**, 111–125

27 Higgins, R.W. and Steadman, J.R. (1987) Anterior cruciate ligament repairs in world class skiers. *American Journal of Sports Medicine*, **15**, 439–447

28 Sherman, M.F. and Bonamo, J.R. (1988) Primary repair of the anterior cruciate ligament. *Clinics in Sports Medicine*, **7**, 739–750

29 Wilcox, P.G. and Jackson, D.W. (1987) Arthroscopic anterior cruciate ligament reconstruction. *Clinics in Sports Medicine*, **6**, 513–524

30 Carson, W.G. (1988) The role of lateral extra-articular procedures for anterolateral rotatory instability. *Clinics in Sports Medicine*, **7**, 751–772

31 Mishra, D.K., Daniel, D.M. and Stone, M.L. (1987) The use of functional knee braces in the control of pathologic anterior knee laxity. *Clinical Orthopaedics*, **241**, 213–220

32 Miller, C.W. and Drez, D.J. (1988) Principles of bracing for the anterior cruciate ligament-deficient knee. *Clinics in Sports Medicine*, **7**, 827–833

33 Maltry, J.A., Noble, P.C., Woods, G.W. *et al.* (1989) External stabilization of the anterior cruciate ligament deficient knee during rehabilitation. *American Journal of Sports Medicine*, **17**, 550–554

34 Stuller, J. (1985) Bracing the unstable knee. *Physician and Sports Medicine*, **2**, 142–156

35 Steadman, J.R., Forster, R.S. and Silferskiold, J.P. (1989) Rehabilitation of the knee. *Clinics in Sports Medicine*, **8**, 605–627

36 Solomonow, M., Baratta, R. and D'Ambrosia, R. (1989) The role of the hamstrings in the rehabilitation of the anterior cruciate ligament-deficient knee in athletes. *Sports Medicine*, **7**, 42–48

37 Kannus, P. and Jarvinen, M. (1989) Posttraumatic anterior cruciate ligament insufficiency as a cause of osteoarthritis in a knee joint. *Clinical Rheumatology*, **8**, 251–260

38 Barton, T.M., Torg, J.S. and Das, M. (1984) Posterior cruciate ligament insufficiency. A review of the literature. *Sports Medicine*, **1**, 419–430

39 Frank, C. and Strother, R. (1989) Isolated posterior cruciate ligament injury in a child: literature review and a case report. *Canadian Journal of Surgery*, **32**, 373–374

40 Torg, J.S., Barton, T.M., Pavlov, H. *et al.* (1989) Natural history of the posterior cruciate ligament-deficient knee. *Clinical Orthopaedics and Related Research*, **246**, 208–216

41 Keene, J.S. (1985) Diagnosis of undetected knee injuries. *Postgraduate Medicine*, **85**, 153–163

42 McCarroll, J.R., Ritter, M.A., Schrader, J. *et al.* (1983) The 'isolated' posterior cruciate. *Physician and Sports Medicine*, **11**, 146–151

43 Feagin, J.A. (1989) The office diagnosis and documentation of common knee problems. *Clinics in Sports Medicine*, **8**, 453–459

44 Fowler, P.J. and Messieh, S.S. (1987) Isolated posterior cruciate ligament injuries in athletes. *American Journal of Sports Medicine*, **15**, 553–557

45 Simonet, W.T. (1984) Current concepts in the treatment of ligamentous instability of the knee. *Mayo Clinic Proceedings*, **59**, 67–76

46 Rong, G. and Wang, Y. (1987) The role of cruciate ligaments in maintaining knee joint stability. *Clinical Orthopaedics*, **215**, 65–71

47 Kaye, J.J. and Nance, E.P. Jr. (1987) Pain in the athlete's knee. *Clinics in Sports Medicine*, **6**, 873–883

48 Keogh, P., Shanker, S.J., Burke, T. *et al.* (1988) Bilateral simultaneous rupture of the quadriceps tendons. A report of four cases and review of the literature. *Clinical Orthopaedics*, **234**, 139–141

49 Pillemer, R.H. (1984) Rupture of the quadriceps tendon. *Medical Journal of Australia*, **141**, 398–399

50 Ray, J.M., Clancy, W.G. and Lemon, R.A. (1988) Semimembranosus tendinitis: An overlooked cause of medial knee pain. *American Journal of Sports Medicine*, **16**, 347–351

51 Sutker, A.N., Jackson, D.W. and Pagliano, J.W. (1981) Iliotibial band syndrome in distance runners. *Physician and Sports Medicine*, **9**, 69–73

52 Lindenberg, G., Pinshaw, R. and Noakes, T.D. (1984) Illiotibial band friction syndrome in runners. *Physician and Sports Medicine*, **12**, 118–130

53 Noble, H.B., Najek, M.R. and Porter, M. (1982) Diagnosis and treatment of iliotibial band tightness in runners. *Physician and Sports Medicine*, **10**, 67–74

54 Noble, H.B., Hajek, M.R. and Porter, M. (1982) Diagnosis and treatment of iliotibial band tightness in runners. *Physician and Sports Medicine*, **10**, 67–74

55 Voorneveld, C., Arenson, A.M. and Fam, A.G. (1989) Anserine bursal distention: Diagnosis by ultrasonography and computed tomography. *Arthritis and Rheumatology*, **32**, 1335–1338

56 Muckle, D.S. (1988) Meniscal repair in athletes. *Sports Medicine* **5**, 1–5

57 Andrish, J.T. (1985) Knee injuries in gymnastics. *Clinics in Sports Medicine*, **4**, 111–121

58 Graf, B., Docter, T. and Clancy, W. Jr. (1987) Arthroscopic meniscal repair. *Clinics in Sports Medicine*, **6**, 525

59 Cross, M.J. and Crichton, K.J. (1987) *Clinical Examination of the Injured Knee*, Gower Medical Publishing, London

60 Dandy, D.J. (1986) Arthroscopy in the treatment of young patients with anterior knee pain. *Orthopedic Clinics of North America*, **17**, 221–229

61 Cleland, L.G., Bowey, R.R., Henderson, D.R.F. *et al.* (1976) Spontaneous osteonecrosis in the medial femoral condyle. *Medical Journal of Australia*, **2**, 92–94

62 Bloom, M.H. (1989) Differentiating between meniscal and patellar pain. *Physician and Sports Medicine*, **17**, 95–108

63 Youmans, W.T. (1989) Surgical complications of the patellofemoral articulation. *Clinics in Sports Medicine*, **8**, 331–342

64 Chrisman, O.D. (1986) The role of articular cartilage in patellofemoral pain. *Orthopedic Clinics of North America*, **17**, 231–234

65 Jacobson, K.E. and Flandry, F.E. (1989) Diagnosis of anterior knee pain. *Clinics in Sports Medicine*, **8**, 179–195

66 Cox, J.S. (1985) Patellofemoral problems in runners. *Clinics in Sports Medicine*, **4**, 699–715

67 Bentley, G. and Dowd, G. (1983) Current concepts of etiology and treatment of chrondromalacia patellae. *Clinical Orthopaedics and Related Research*, **189**, 209–228

68 Fulkerson, J.P. (1989) Evaluation of the peripatellar soft tissues and retinaculum in patients with patellofemoral pain. *Clinics in Sports Medicine*, **8**, 197–202

69 Bourne, M.H., Hazel, W.A., Scott, S.G. *et al.* (1988) Anterior knee pain. *Mayo Clinical Proceedings*, **63**, 482–491

70 MacDonald, D.A., Hutton, J.F. and Kelly, I.G. (1989) Maximal isometric patellofemoral contact force in patient with anterior knee pain. *Journal of Bone and Joint Surgery*, **71B**, 296–299

71 Ohno, O., Naitor, J., Iguchi, T. *et al.* (1988) An electron microscopic study of early pathology in chondromalacia of the patella. *Journal of Bone and Joint Surgery*, **70A**, 883–899

72 McConnell, J. (1986) The management of chondromalacia patellae: a long-term solution. *Australian Journal of Physiotherapy*, **32**, 215–223

73 Gerrard, B. (1989) The patello-femoral pain syndrome: a clinical trial of the McConnell programme. *Australian Journal of Physiotherapy*, **35**, 71–80

74 Schutzer, S.F., Ramsby, G.R. and Fulkerson, J.P. (1986) Computed tomographic classification of patellofemoral pain patients. *Orthopedic Clinics of North America*, **17**, 235–248

75 McIntyre, D. and Wessel, J. (1988) Knee muscle torques in the patellofemoral pain syndrome. *Physiotherapy Canada*, **40**, 20–23

76 Shellock, F.G., Mink, J.H., Deutsch, A. *et al.* (1989) Kinematic magnetic resonance imaging for evaluation of patellar tracking. *Physician and Sports Medicine*, **17**, 99–108

77 Yulish, B.S., Montanez, J., Goodfellow, D.B. *et al.* (1987) Chondromalacia patellae: assessment with MR imaging. *Radiology*, **164**, 763–766

78 Moller, B.N., Krebs, B. and Jurik, A.G. (1987) Patellofemoral incongruence in chondromalacia and instability of the patella. *Acta Orthopaedica Scandinavica*, **57**, 232–234

79 Merchant, A.C. (1988) Classification of patellofemoral disorders. *Arthroscopy*, **4**, 235–240

80 Minikoff, J. and Fein, L. (1989) The role of radiography in the evaluation and treatment of common anarthrotic disorders of the patellofemoral joint. *Clinics in Sports Medicine*, **8**, 203–260

81 Yates, C. and Grana, W.A. (1986) Patellofemoral pain: A prospective study. *Orthopaedics*, **9**, 663–667

82 Fulkerson, J.P. (1989) Evaluation of the peripatellar soft tissues and retinaculum in patients with patellofemoral pain. *Clinics in Sports Medicine*, **8**, 197–202

83 Brunet, M.E. and Stewart, G.W. (1989) Patellofemoral rehabilitation. *Clinics in Sports Medicine*, **8**, 319–329

84 Carson, W.G. (1985) Diagnosis of extensor mechanism disorders. *Clinics in Sports Medicine*, **4**, 231–246

85 Busch, M.T. and DeHaven, K.E. (1989) Pitfalls of the lateral retinacular release. *Clinics in Sports Medicine*, **8**, 279–290

86 Steiner, M.E. and Grana, W.A. (1988) The young athlete's knee: recent advances. *Clinics in Sports Medicine*, **7**, 527–546

87 Dowd, G.S.E. and Bentley, G. (1986) Radiographic assessment in patellar instability and chondromalacia patellae. *Journal of Bone and Joint Surgery*, **68B**, 297–300

88 McConnell, J. (1987) Training the vastus medialis oblique in the management of patellofemoral pain. Paper read at *Tenth Congress of the World Confederation for Physical Therapy*, Sydney

89 Fisher, R.L. (1986) Conservative treatment of patellofemoral pain. *Orthopedic Clinics of North America*, **17**, 269–272

90 Bennett, J.G. and Stauber, W.T. (1986) Evaluation and treatment of anterior knee pain using eccentric exercise. *Medicine and Science in Sports and Exercise*, **18**, 526–530

91 Crocker, B. and Stauber, W.T. (1989) Objective analysis of quadriceps force during bracing of the patellae: a preliminary study. *Australian Journal of Science and Medicine in Sport*, **21**, 25–27

92 Christensen, F., Soballe, K. and Snerum, L. (1988) Treatment of chondromalacia patellae by lateral retinacular release of the patella. *Clinical Orthopaedics and Related Research*, **234**, 145–147

93 Fulkerson, J.P., Schutzer, S.F., Ramsby, G.R. *et al.* (1987) Computerised tomography of the patellofemoral joint before and after lateral release or realignment. *Arthroscopy*, **3**, 19–24

94 Fulkerson, J.P. and Schutzer, S.F. (1986) After failure of conservative treatment for painful patellofemoral malalignment: lateral release or realignment? *Orthopedic Clinics of North America*, **17**, 283–288

95 Scuderi, G., Cuomo, F. and Scott, N. (1988) Lateral release and proximal realignment for patellar subluxation and dislocation. *Journal of Bone and Joint Surgery*, **70A**, 856–861

96 Hughston, J.C. and Deese, M. (1988) Medial subluxation of the patella as a complication of lateral retinacular release. *American Journal of Sports Medicine*, **16**, 383–388

97 Schreiber, S.N. (1988) Arthroscopic lateral retinacular release using a modified superomedial portal electrosurgery, and postoperative positioning in flexion. *Orthopaedic Review*, **XVII**, 375–380

98 Engebretsen, L., Svenningsen, S. and Benum, P. (1989) Advancement of the tibial tuberosity for patellar pain: a 5-year follow-up. *Acta Orthopaedica Scandinavica*, **60**, 20–22

99 Radin, E.L. (1986) Anterior tibial tubercle elevation in the young adult. *Orthopedic Clinics of North America*, **17**, 297–302

100 Worrell, R.V. (1986) Resurfacing of the patella in young patients. *Orthopedic Clinics of North America*, **17**, 303–309

101 Kelly, M.A. and Insall, J.N. (1986) Patellectomy. *Orthopedic Clinics of North America*, **17**, 289–295

102 Hughston, J.C. (1989) Patellar subluxation: a recent history. *Clinics in Sports Medicine*, **8**, 153–162

103 Moller, B.N., Jurik, A.G., Tidemand-Dal, C. *et al.* (1987) The quadriceps function in patellofemoral disorders. *Archives of Orthopaedic and Trauma Surgery*, **106**, 195–198

104 Broom, M.J. and Fulkerson, J.P. (1986) The plica syndrome: a new perspective. *Orthopedic Clinics of North America*, **17**, 279–281

105 Patel, D. (1986) Plica as a cause of anterior knee pain. *Orthopedic Clinics of North America*, **17**, 273–278

106 Schwarz, C., Blazina, M.E., Sisto, D.J. *et al.* (1988) The results of operative treatment of osteochondritis dissecans of the patella. *American Journal of Sports Medicine*, **16**, 522–529

107 Jerosch, J.G., Castro, W.H.M. and Jantea, C. (1989) Stress fracture of the patella. *American Journal of Sports Medicine*, **17**, 579–580

108 Ferretti, A., Puddu, G., Mariani, P.P. *et al.* (1984) Jumper's knee: an epidemiological study of volleyball players. *Physician and Sports Medicine*, **12**, 97–103

109 Jensen, K. and Di Fabio, R.P. (1989) Evaluation of eccentric exercise in treatment of patellar tendinitis. *Physical Therapy*, **69**, 211–216

110 Orava, S., Osterback, L. and Hurme, M. (1986) Surgical treatment of patellar tendon pain in athletes. *British Journal of Sports Medicine*, **20**, 167–169

111 Kujala, U.M., Kvist, M. and Heinonen, O. (1985) Osgood–Schlatter's disease in adolescent athletes. *American Journal of Sports Medicine*, **13**, 236–241

112 Michelli, L.J. (1987) The traction apophysitises. *Clinics in Sports Medicine*, **6**, 389–404

113 Antich, T.J. and Lombardo, S.J. (1985) Clinical presentation of Osgood–Schlatter disease in the adolescent population. *Journal of Orthopaedic and Sports Physical Therapy*, **7**, 1–4

114 Bowers, K.D. (1981) Patellar tendon avulsion as a complication of Osgood–Schlatter's disease. *American Journal of Sports Medicine*, **9**, 356–359

115 Finsterbush, A., Frankl, U. and Mann, G. (1989) Fat pad adhesion to partially torn anterior cruciate ligament: a cause of knee locking. *American Journal of Sports Medicine*, **17**, 92–95

11 Lower leg

Superior tibiofibular joint

The two bones of the lower leg, the tibia and fibula, are joined proximally at the superior tibiofibular joint and distally at the inferior tibiofibular joint. These two joints form a functional unit involved in movements of the ankle joint.

On plantar flexion of the foot, the narrower posterior part of the trochlear surface of the talus moves forwards in the ankle mortise. To maintain stability, the lateral malleolus of the fibula needs to move inwards and downwards. On dorsiflexion of the foot, the broader anterior part of the trochlear surface of the talus presents in the ankle mortise and to accommodate it the lateral malleolus of the fibula must move outwards and upwards.

These movements are reflected in the superior tibiofibular joint, so that on dorsiflexion of the foot the superior tibiofibular joint moves upwards and inwards and on plantar flexion the superior tibiofibular joint moves downwards and outwards. Their range of movement is only small but can be readily felt by palpating over the head of the fibula with the knee flexed and then plantar and dorsiflexing the ankle.

Two other movements producing movement in the superior tibiofibular joint are inversion and eversion of the foot, and rotation of the talus in the ankle mortise (see p. 187).

Accessory movements

There are five accessory movements:

1 Anteroposterior movement, produced by pressure from the thumbs over the anterior surface of the fibular head (Figure 11.1).

2 Posteroanterior produced by pressure over the anterior surface of the fibular head (Figure 11.2).
3 Longitudinal cephalad produced by eversion of the heel.
4 Longitudinal caudad movement produced by strong inversion of the patient's heel.

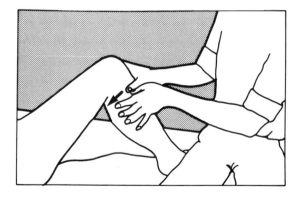

Figure 11.1 Anteroposterior accessory movement

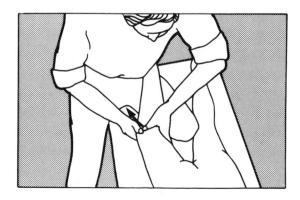

Figure 11.2 Posteroanterior accessory movement

b Compression. These movements are repeated with the fibular head compressed against the tibia with the heel of the hand.

Lesions of the superior tibiofibular joint

Direct trauma

This results in haematoma formation and may lead to calcification of the joint capsule. Joint movements are then restricted and painful especially on ankle movements. Radiographs reveal the calcified haematoma, usually on the inferior joint surface.

Subluxation

Subluxation or dislocation after a fall with an inversion strain to the ankle while the knee is held flexed and in varus occurs in parachute jumpers and footballers. Force is transmitted through the fibular shaft to the posterior tibiofibular ligament, which is ruptured and allows the fibular head to sublux forwards. Diagnosis is confirmed on radiographs, which shows undue prominence of the fibular head [1].

Instability

This uncommon condition occurs as a result of injury or rheumatoid arthritis with pain over the lateral compartment of the knee radiating down the leg. The superior tibiofibular joint clicks out of place on walking and is often mistaken for a tear of the lateral meniscus.

Compartment syndromes

The lower leg is invested with a layer of deep fascia, from which three extensions pass to the tibia and fibula (Figure 11.3) whose opposed interosseous surfaces are joined together by the interosseous membrane [2]. In this way, the muscles of the lower leg are enclosed within four fascial compartments: anterior, medial, lateral and posterior.

Compartment syndromes result from an increase in intracompartmental pressure within a closed fascial space [3]. This results in decreased capillary perfusion with decreased tissue perfusion, muscle oedema and ischaemia. This leads to further

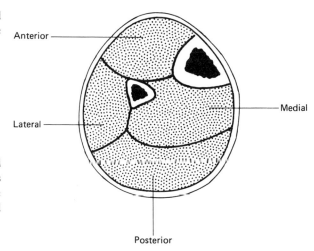

Figure 11.3 Fascial compartments of the lower leg

prolonged pressure increase with irreversible muscle and nerve damage. An acute or chronic syndrome may occur, determined mainly by the degree of swelling and distensibility of the fascial walls.

The increased compartmental pressure may be caused by: (1) increased compartmental volume with oedema or haemorrhage which may follow trauma [4] or excessive muscular exertion, or (2) external compression with decreased compartmental size.

Diagnosis of a compartmental syndrome can usually be made on clinical grounds [5,6] but should be confirmed either by MRI [7] or by measuring intracompartmental pressures at rest or exercise [8–11] with a wick or slit catheter connected to transducers.

Anterior compartment

This lies anterolaterally between the tibia and fibula, bounded deeply by the interosseous membrane and superficially by the deep fascia of the leg. It contains the tibialis anterior muscle, the toe extensors, the deep peroneal nerve and the anterior tibial artery. The deep peroneal nerve supplies the muscles in this compartment and its sensory nerve supplies the dorsal surface of adjacent sides of the first and second toes.

Acute anterior tibial syndrome

This is rare but is a medical emergency. It usually follows sudden, severe or unusual running activity often in people who have only recently commenced training [12,13]. Pain in the anterior compartment of the leg rapidly becomes severe and is made worse either by passive plantar flexion of the ankle or by isometric contraction of the dorsiflexors of the ankle. The overlying skin may be warm and oedematous. If compression is unrelieved, necrosis of muscle and a compression neuropathy of the deep peroneal nerve, with foot drop and sensory change in the first inter-digital cleft, may be produced.

MANAGEMENT

The patient is admitted immediately to hospital for an emergency fasciotomy to decompress the compartment. Wide splitting of the entire fascial sheath permits the muscles within the compartment to bulge outwards.

Chronic anterior tibial syndrome

In this syndrome pain comes on with exercise [14], usually becoming so severe that the patient is unable to continue activity. It is relieved by rest and at rest signs are usually absent. Some swelling and diffuse tenderness over the anterior tibial compartment may be evident after exercise and pain is reproduced on passive dorsiflexion of the toes or ankle.

MANAGEMENT

Activities need to be modified so that symptoms abate, otherwise an acute syndrome can be produced. If symptoms persist, fasciotomy usually produces excellent results [9,15].

Tendinitis of tibialis anterior muscle

This overuse condition involves the musculotendi-nous junction of the tibialis anterior muscle in the lower third of the leg. When running, the anterior tibial muscle is the principal decelerator of the foot at heel strike. Overuse occurs if the runner is unaccustomed to a forceful heel strike during the early stage of training, or after changing to running on a hard surface. Pain is made worse by ankle movements, and marked crepitus is palpable or audible over the involved area.

It usually responds well to rest, ultrasound or ice, anti-inflammatory drugs and injection of cortico-steroid around the anterior aspect of the lower third of the tibialis anterior muscle, stretching the anterior and posterior muscles and strengthening the tibialis anterior.

Medial compartment

The medial compartment is enclosed between the deep fascia of the medial side of the leg, the interosseous membrane and a deep transverse inter-muscular septum which separates it from the poste-rior compartment. It contains the tibialis posterior, the flexor hallucis longus and flexor digitorum longus muscles, together with the posterior tibial artery and nerve.

Medial tibial compartment syndrome

This common overuse syndrome with pain and tenderness over the medial tibial border is also termed the tibial stress syndrome, shin splints and shin soreness [16,17]. It consists of a continuum of changes starting with traction on the tibialis poste-rior origin, thickening of the overlying fascia, stress reaction in the bone through to a stress fracture of the tibia. The muscle is subjected to biomechanical stresses and stretching during dorsiflexion of the ankle and with excess pronation of the foot, which is associated with medial rotation of the lower leg. Pain often occurs in the early part of a training session, especially after running on hard surfaces or follow-ing a change of technique or running shoes.

Pain over the lower third of the medial border of the tibia, dull and aching at first, comes on with running and is relieved by rest. It gradually increases so the running stride may have to be altered by running flat footed. The pain usually becomes so intense that ultimately walking becomes difficult, and the pain is present at night.

Pain may be reproduced either by passive plantar flexion of the ankle, active dorsiflexion of the ankle or isometric contraction of the tibialis posterior muscle. Marked tenderness, sometimes with a mild degree of warmth or localized thickening is found along the posteromedial border of the tibia over its middle and lower thirds. Excessive pronation of the foot and loss of shock-absorbing capacity (see Chapter 13) is commonly found, as are varus deformities of the leg or foot.

Early radiographs are not often helpful but radionuclide bone scan is then often positive, showing the bone stress reaction, which needs to be differentiated from a stress fracture.

MANAGEMENT OF TIBIAL STRESS SYNDROME

This condition is often difficult to treat. It includes:

1   Rest from all activities that involve running. Strapping may be applied from the lower third of the leg to pass under the heel to restrict the

range of plantar flexion and produce some inversion of the foot.

2 Exercises to develop and maintain strength, flexibility and endurance of the lower leg muscles are commenced. Non-weight-bearing exercises such as swimming or bike riding are also started.

3 Anti-inflammatory drugs are usually prescribed but rarely produce any substantial benefit. Analgesics are often necessary, especially to allow sleep.

4 Physical methods. Ultrasound given over the painful, tender area is of some value, especially to help localize the painful area. Short-wave diathermy or ice are rarely of value.

5 Stretching of the medial compartment muscles, even if it provokes some degree of discomfort, is essential and is combined with stretching of the posterior calf muscles. Mobilization of the locally tender area with the therapist's thumbs may also be useful.

6 Injections. The tender area around the tenoperiosteal origin of the tibialis posterior may be injected with corticosteroid. At first the involved area is usually diffuse but after treatment the tender area becomes more localized and can then be injected using a 25-gauge needle.

7 Postural faults in the leg, especially varus deformities of the lower leg and excessive pronation of the foot, require orthotic foot devices [18].

8 As the condition improves attention must be given to running style, and hard running surfaces should be avoided.

9 Surgery. In patients with a tight fascial compartment, the thickened fascia over the medial compartment should be adequately decompressed.

Lateral compartment

This compartment contains the peroneus longus and brevis muscles and the lateral popliteal nerve. An acute peroneal compartment swelling is rare but may occur several hours after strenuous exercise. Pain is made worse by active movements and passive inversion of the foot. Swelling may compress the lateral popliteal nerve with sensory changes followed by a foot drop with inversion of the foot. This surgical emergency requires urgent decompression of the fascial compartment.

Posterior compartment

This contains the gastrocnemius, soleus and plantaris muscles, which form the Achilles tendon.

Acute posterior compartment syndrome

This is rare. Exercise produces an acute ischaemia of the soleus in the tight fascial confines of this compartment. Treatment is to split the deep fascia over the medial side of the soleus muscle.

Chronic posterior compartment syndrome

The posterior compartment syndrome may follow overuse or a previous fracture of tibia and fibula. Pain in the calf on activity may be associated with altered sensation on the plantar surface of the foot and weakness of ankle flexion.

Calf cysts

Calf cysts (Figure 11.4) are common and result from an extension of a popliteal cyst, formed (see p. 156) from a synovial swelling which tracks into the semimembranous bursa. The synovial effusion can result from any knee disorder including inflammatory, degenerative or traumatic arthritis. The synovial effusion usually accumulates rapidly and the

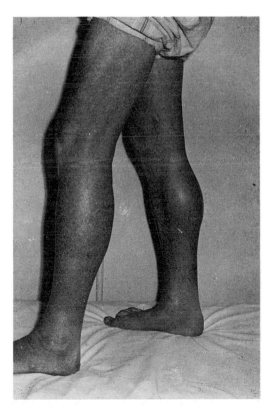

Figure 11.4 Calf cyst in right leg follows a knee effusion

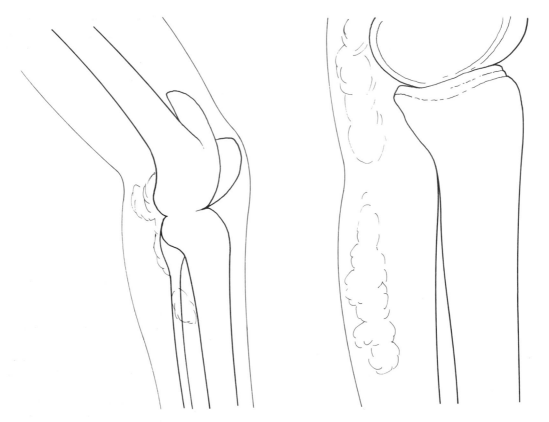

Figure 11.5 Arthrogram to show an effusion into the knee with rupture into the calf

fluid is prevented from returning to the knee because of a ball-valve arrangement. As pressure increases the cyst will extend into the posterior compartment always under the medial gastrocnemius and may grow to large proportions (Figure 11.5). It presents then as calf pain usually with ankle oedema. It is then most often confused with a deep vein thrombosis, especially with calf tenderness and a positive Homan's sign, that is, calf pain on forceful dorsiflexion of the ankle.

Complications include rupture of the knee or the cyst into the calf with a marked inflammatory reaction (pseudothrombophlebitis).

Investigations include aspiration of the knee effusion or calf cyst, arthrography, ultrasound or CT scan. Treatment is to drain the knee effusion and inject it with 3 ml of corticosteroid. The dye for arthrography can be injected at the same time, thus confirming the diagnosis and treating the underlying condition with one injection.

Tear of the gastrocnemius

A tear of the gastrocnemius is common especially in middle-aged men, usually while jogging or playing tennis ('tennis leg'). Minor degrees can also occur in the elderly while walking, especially on an uneven surface. Sudden severe calf pain is experienced during activity and the patient looks around to see if someone has hit him in the leg with a stone or other object. The degree of damage can vary from a slight tear with little resultant disability, to a moderate degree in which the patient can walk only by limping painfully on his toes, or to a severe degree of damage so that the patient is unable to walk. It usually occurs with the ankle in full dorsiflexion and with knee in extension; this stretches the gastrocnemius so that it is liable to tear as it contracts. The patient may report slight aching or stiffness in the calf a day or two beforehand, which may have been associated with some loss of muscle extensibility and probably explains why this injury is common in middle-aged patients. This injury, formerly attributed to a ruptured plantaris muscle, is now recognized as a tear of the gastrocnemius, almost always in the medial belly or at the medial musculotendinous junction.

MAJOR SIGNS

Calf pain is reproduced on stretching the gastrocnemius by passively dorsiflexing the ankle. The range of this movement is usually restricted because of spasm in the gastrocnemius. Pain can also be reproduced on active contraction by having the patient attempt to stand up on the toes, or by testing resisted plantar flexion of the ankle.

Other signs These vary according to the site of involvement and degree of the tear. In the calf, the muscle belly may be swollen, bruising may appear over the site of the tear and the lower leg may be oedematous. A gap may be palpable in a severe degree of tear. In minor degrees or in the latter stages of a severe tear, an area of tender thickening is palpable in the muscle. Swelling is uncommon in tears at the musculotendinous junction but localized pain and tenderness are often severe and prolonged. Blood may extravasate beneath the deep fascia, and appear as bruising around the ankle. It may occasionally be complicated by pressure on the calf veins resulting in a deep venous thrombosis. If suspected, because of the degree of ankle oedema, venography must be performed.

INITIAL MANAGEMENT

The patient needs to rest, ice is applied to the painful area and the leg elevated to prevent swelling. An elastic stocking is used to control ankle oedema.

SUBSEQUENT MANAGEMENT

This depends on the degree of injury. With severe degrees the patient is unable to walk freely and may need to use crutches for a few days. With moderate or minor degrees the patient can walk around. A 2.5 cm raise in the shoe reduces the strain on the muscle, which lacks extensibility, to facilitate walking. The leg should be used as normally as pain will allow. Crutches or a stick can usually be discarded within a few days and the heel raise after approximately 2 weeks. Physical methods include ultrasound or ice, and active and passive stretching exercises with passive dorsiflexion taken to the point of discomfort.

As the tear heals, exercises are progressed with increased walking or jogging with a rubber heel

inserted in the running shoe. The tear may heal with a small area of fibrosis that prevents full muscle extensibility and is apt to cause recurrent tears. This area can be readily felt on palpation as a tender thickening, best treated with an injection of local anaesthetic and corticosteroid, deep pressure massage and stretching.

AFTERCARE

The patient must not return to active sport until all pain and tenderness has subsided and the muscle has regained full painless strength and extensibility. A gradual return to full activity is advisable and a heel raise is worn in the running shoe for a few weeks.

Lesions of the Achilles tendon

The Achilles tendon is formed from an aponeurosis at the musculotendinous junction of the gastrocnemius which is joined more distally by the soleus muscle and the plantaris tendon, an unimportant vestigial remnant. The Achilles tendon curves around the concave posterior surface of the calcaneus, from which it is separated by a bursa, to be inserted into the lower part of the posterior surface of the calcaneus. The tendon does not have a surrounding tenosynovial layer but is invested by fibrous tissue that forms a paratenon which contains thin-walled blood vessels that supply part of the blood supply to the tendon.

The Achilles tendon plantar flexes the ankle and foot. This action is most efficient with the knee extended, as in the push-off phase of walking. With the foot dorsiflexed, the first point of contact of the tendon lies proximally on the posterior surface of the calcaneus, but with the foot plantar flexed the tendon uncoils from around the curved posterior surface of the calcaneus so that its efficiency is increased. As the Achilles tendon plantar flexes the ankle joint it also acts on the subtalar joint to produce supination and adduction of the foot.

The Achilles tendon is the strongest tendon in the body and can withstand forces of up to 5–10 kg mm^{-2}, or approximately 1000 kg in the average adult [19]. In the push-off phase of running the foot and ankle function as a second-class lever with body-weight distributed between the fulcrum of the Achilles tendon and force applied at the end of the foot. The effect of this lever arrangement is such that a 100 kg man may require a force of 300 kg to push off from the ground.

Classification

1 Acute tendinitis and peritendinitis.
2 Chronic paratenon thickening.
3 Focal degeneration.
4 Partial rupture.
5 Complete rupture.
6 Rare tendon lesions.
   (a) Calcification.
   (b) Ossification.
   (c) Complete avulsion.
7 Pathological conditions.
   (a) Nodule formation.
       (i)   Rheumatoid.
       (ii) Xanthomata.
       (iii) Tophi.
       (iv) Neurofibroma.
   (b) Spondyloarthritis.
8 Related conditions.
   (a) Achilles bursitis.
   (b) Tear of musculotendinous junction.
   (c) Osteochondritis of the calcaneus.

Aetiology

Achilles tendinitis [20,21] has three major groups of causes:

1 In the leg and foot. Changes may be due to varus deformities of the leg; rear foot deformities, nearly always in varus, only occasionally in valgus; pes cavus or forefoot varus. These are often associated with prolonged pronation of the foot, or subtalar or ankle joint stiffness. Calf muscle changes include weakness but more commonly tightness which also causes prolonged pronation of the foot [22,23]. Pronation results in a whipping type of action on the tendon, especially on its medial aspect, which is the usual site of pain and tenderness.
2 Localized areas of degeneration commonly develop in the tendon. These may result from age or a lack of vascular supply. A separate condition is the development of a focal area of granulomatous intratendinous degeneration (see below).
3 Training errors may arise from a sudden increase in training sessions or in their intensity or one sudden severe running session. Running on hard surfaces, changing from soft to hard surfaces, or from cross-country to track, or uneven terrain may all contribute. Shoes or their heels may be inadequate.

INVESTIGATIONS
Ultrasonography [24–26] or MRI [27] are useful in demonstrating the underlying pathology.

Acute Achilles tendinitis

Acute inflammatory changes may occur in the tendon itself, nearly always associated with similar changes in the surrounding paratenon. The patient is usually an active young or middle-aged male who presents with pain in the tendon made worse by activity. If he continues to run pain usually becomes severe and may then be worse on walking. The tendon feels stiff, especially on first getting out of bed. It appears thickened, oedematous and tender, and pain and crepitus may be produced on tendon movements.

MANAGEMENT
1 Rest. This condition usually resolves with conservative treatment. If tendinitis is only mild, it may be sufficient to curtail the amount of running but it is usually of such a degree that rest from sporting activities is essential.
2 Orthotic devices for any rear foot abnormality should be supplied [22,28]. Heel raises are not often helpful.
3 Anti-inflammatory drugs are prescribed.
4 Physical methods. Ultrasound over the inflamed tendon is an important part of treatment. It may be used in conjunction with ice or short-wave diathermy. Deep-pressure massage may be incorporated once severe pain has subsided.
5 Mobilization of the subtalar and ankle joints is combined with stretching of the gastrocnemius and soleus complex.
6 Injections. In most patients, acute tendinitis gradually settles over a few weeks. Injections of corticosteroid are never indicated in the early stages when the lesion is diffuse, and never into the tendon substance itself. A small residual area of tenderness around the medial border of the tendon usually settles well with one or two injections of corticosteroid using a 25-gauge needle.
7 Aftercare. In all patients return to activity must be gradual, so that a sudden application of the normal training load is avoided. The patient is advised to walk at first and then jog so that the distance and the pace of running are gradually progressed. In patients who do not fully respond to treatment or suffer repeated attacks of tendinitis, chronic paratenon thickening, focal degeneration or partial rupture of the tendon should be considered.

Chronic thickening of the paratenon

This condition [23,30] with chronic inflammatory changes in the paratenon may occur as a complication of acute peritendinitis or follow continued overuse. The paratenon becomes thickened and adherent to its tendon, restricting tendon movement and producing recurrent attacks of tendinitis. It may also be found in association with an area of degeneration of the tendon plus a partial tear.

MANAGEMENT
If mobilization techniques, ultrasound and local steroid injection do not produce any improvement, chronic thickening of the paratenon is best treated by operation to strip the thickened paratenon from around the tendon. The results of this operation are usually excellent [23,31].

Focal degeneration

Focal degeneration is an area of degenerated, damaged fibres which vary in size from a pin-head to a large cystic area, and is found within an area of normal tendon. It is usually peripheral and not as a central core as originally described [19]. Its cause is unknown. The athlete complains of pain on exercise, which may be severe. Surgical decompression of the tendon and removal of the focal area [30] is the treatment of choice. At operation the overlying tendon appears dull and lustreless and after incision an area of granulation tissue is found, often with cystic softening.

Rupture of the tendon

This may be: (1) complete, or (2) partial [23,32].

Complete rupture of the tendon

This is uncommon in younger patients and occurs more commonly with increasing age. The site of rupture occurs 2–5 cm from the tendon insertion (Figure 11.6), and underlying degenerative changes, evident at operation, are considered to be the predisposing cause [19]. The role of previously injected corticosteroids in the aetiology of rupture remains controversial. In theory, injections into the tendon itself could lead to a weakening of the tendon collagen or produce compression of blood vessels in the paratenon with loss of blood supply to the tendon. In practice, local corticosteroid injections do not appear

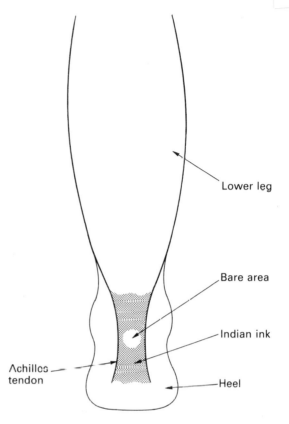

Figure 11.6 Indian ink, injected into the Achilles tendon to demonstrate its circulation, shows a bare area at its critical zone

to be commonly associated with such a rupture, which often occurs in tendons that have never received injections. Nevertheless, injections must always be given around, and not into, the tendon.

Rupture may occur during running, jumping and hurrying up stairs, when the tendon is suddenly stretched, or in a skiing accident, when the skier suddenly falls forward as the ankle is dorsiflexed with the foot anchored in the ski. Most cases occur during sporting activities, or in middle-aged joggers. As the tendon ruptures, suddenly and dramatically, the patient experiences severe pain and usually falls over. Walking becomes difficult at first because of weakness of ankle plantar flexion, but subsequently the patient may be able to walk with some limp.

CLINICAL FINDINGS
The proximal part of the ruptured tendon rolls upwards, leaving a visible and palpable gap between the ends of the torn tendon. Subsequently the gap is filled with blood clot and may not be so readily

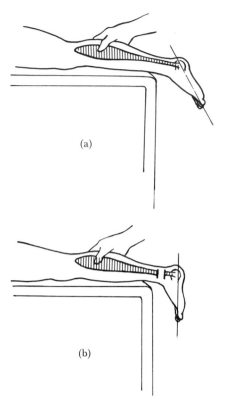

Figure 11.7 Test for ruptured Achilles tendon. (a), Normal foot movement if the tendon is intact; (b), with a ruptured tendon the foot remains stationary

appreciated. The correct diagnosis is then often not made for a considerable time and the injury is mistaken, for example as a sprain of the ankle. On inspection, the tendon is seen to be grossly swollen and the normal gutters on either side of the tendon are obliterated. After a few days, bruising appears around the ankle.

MAJOR SIGN

The patient lies prone with both feet over the edge of the couch. The calf muscles on the normal leg are squeezed by the examiner's hand and the patient's foot can be observed to plantarflex. In the affected leg, squeezing the calf fails to flex the foot as the motor power unit is disrupted (Figure 11.7).

CONFIRMATORY SIGNS

The range of passive dorsiflexion of the affected ankle is increased and there is weakness of plantar flexion, best appreciated by asking the patient to stand on tiptoe, which is virtually impossible on the affected side. A tender gap in the tendon may be palpable in the middle of the tendon, often better appreciated with the patient supine with the knee flexed rather than prone.

MANAGEMENT

This remains controversial [23] but surgery with suturing of the divided tendon ends is the treatment of choice in active people. If the patient is non-active or elderly or if the diagnosis is delayed, consideration should be made to plaster immobilization with the foot in plantar flexion. Approximately 2% of ruptures treated surgically rerupture compared with 10–35% of those treated conservatively [33].

Partial rupture of the Achilles tendon

This is becoming increasingly recognized [23,30]. The patient suffers a sudden sharp pain in the tendon, usually while running, and pain is then experienced, especially when stepping off the affected leg. Subsequently the patient usually complains of chronic tendon pain. The site of rupture usually occurs a few centimetres above the tendon insertion and a small tender thickening is felt within the tendon itself. At times, a small gap within the tendon and immediately above this a small, tender, rolled-up segment of the tendon may be palpated.

Clinical differentiation between chronic thickening of the paratenon, central core degeneration and partial rupture of the tendon may be extremely difficult, especially as they may occur together. Surgical exploration is then necessary to distinguish between them and provide definitive treatment.

MANAGEMENT

Conservative treatment is similar to that outlined for Achilles tendinitis above. However, results are not generally satisfactory and the patient often suffers recurrent pain and disability. Surgical exploration is then indicated and the tendon is debrided and repaired [30,34].

Bursitis

Two bursae, one deep and one superficial, are found in relation to the Achilles tendon. The superficial posterior calcaneal bursa lies between the skin and the tendon; bursitis is usually produced by friction from shoes, especially high-heeled ones. The deep retrocalcaneal bursa lies between the tendon and the calcaneus, sitting like a cap over the posterosuperior angle of the bone. Retrocalcaneal bursitis, which may be

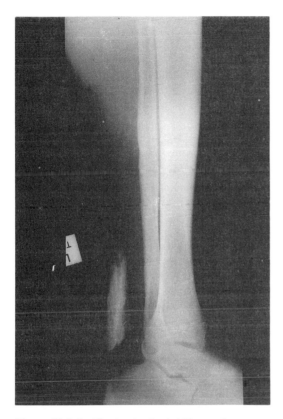

Figure 11.8 Ossification in the Achilles tendon

associated with an Achilles tendinitis, produces swelling that may be seen bulging on either side of the tendon. Tenderness may be elicited by squeezing in front of the tendon with the thumb and index finger.

MANAGEMENT

The bursa may be aspirated and injected with corticosteroid [26,35] producing rapid relief of symptoms. Surgical removal is successful [30].

Rare tendon lesions

These include calcification in degenerated tendon [26], ossification (Figure 11.8), which may also fracture [36] or complete avulsion of the tendon from the calcaneus in the elderly.

Pathological conditions

The Achilles tendon and bursa may be involved in a number of generalized conditions. Spondyloarthritis may produce, or present with, tendinitis or bursitis. Rheumatoid bursitis may produce erosive changes in the calcaneus. The tendon may rarely be thickened owing to the presence of a rheumatoid nodule, tophaceous deposits, xanthomas or, rarely, a neurofibroma.

References

1 Keene, J.S. (1985) Diagnosis of undetected knee injuries. *Postgraduate Medicine*, **85**, 153–163

2 Bourne, R.B. and Rorabeck, C.H. (1989) Compartment syndromes of the lower leg. *Clinical Orthopaedics*, **240**, 97–104

3 Aschoff, A., Steiner-Milz, H. and Steiner, H.H. (1990) Lower limb compartment syndrome following lumbar discectomy in the knee-chest position. *Neurosurgical Review*, **13**, 155–159

4 Patton, G.W. and Parker, R.J. (1989) Rupture of the lateral head of gastrocnemius muscle at the musculotendinous junction mimicking a compartment syndrome. *Journal of Foot Surgery*, **28**, 433–437

5 Pedowitz, R.A., Hargens, A.R., Mubarak, S.J. *et al.* (1990) Modified criteria for the objective diagnosis of chronic compartment syndrome of the leg. *American Journal of Sports Medicine*, **18**, 35–40

6 Styf, J.R. and Korner, L.M. (1986) Chronic anterior-compartment syndrome of the leg. Results of treatment by fasciotomy. *Journal of Bone and Joint Surgery*, **68A**, 1338–1347

7 Amendola, A., Rorabeck, C.H., Vellett, D. *et al.* (1990) The use of magnetic resonance imaging in exertional compartment syndromes. *American Journal of Sports Medicine*, **18**, 29–34

8 Wiley, J.P., Short, W.B., Wiseman, D.A. *et al.* (1990) Ultrasound catheter placement for deep posterior compartment pressure measurements in chronic compartment syndrome. *American Journal of Sports Medicine*, **18**, 74–79

9 Rorabeck, C.H., Bourne, R.B., Fowler, P.J. *et al.* (1988) The role of tissue pressure measurement in diagnosing chronic anterior compartment syndrome. *American Journal of Sports Medicine*, **16**, 143–146

10 Allen, M.J., Stirling, A.J., Crawshaw, C.V. *et al.* (1985) Intracompartmental pressure monitoring the leg injuries. An aid to management. *Journal of Bone and Joint Surgery*, **67B**, 53–57

11 Mannarino, F. and Sexson, S. (1989) The significance of intracompartmental pressures in the diagnosis of chronic exertional compartment syndrome. *Orthopaedics*, **12**, 1415–1418

12 Egan, T.D. and Joyce, S.M. (1989) Acute compartment syndrome following a minor athletic injury. *Journal of Emergency Medicine*, **7**, 353–357

13 Martens, M.A. and Moeyersoons, J.P. (1990) Acute and recurrent effort-related compartment syndrome in sports. *Sports Medicine*, **9**, 62–68

14 Lutz, L.J., Goodenough, G.K. and Detmer, D.E. (1989) Chronic compartment syndrome. *American Family Physician*, **39**, 191–196

15 Styf, J. (1988) Diagnosis of exercise-induced pain in the anterior aspect of the lower leg. *American Journal of Sports Medicine*, **16**, 165–169

16 Allen, M.J. and Barnes, M.R. (1986) Exercise pain in the lower leg. Chronic compartment syndrome and medial tibial syndrome. *Journal of Bone and Joint Surgery*, **68B**, 818–823

17 Melbert, P.E. and Styf, J. (1989) Posteromedial pain in the lower leg. *American Journal of Sports Medicine*, **17**, 747–750

18 Bates, B.T., Osternig, L.R., Mason, M.S. *et al.* (1979) Foot orthotic devises to modify selected aspects of lower extremity mechanics. *American Journal of Sports Medicine*, **7**, 338–342

19 Burry, H.C. (1978) Pathogenesis of some traumatic and degenerative disorders of soft tissue. *Australian and New Zealand Journal of Medicine*, **8** (Suppl), 163–165

20 Leach, R.E., James, S., Wasilewski, S. (1981) Achilles tendinitis. *American Journal of Sports Medicine*, **9**, 93–98

21 Smart, G.W., Taunton, J.E., Clement, D.B. (1980) Achilles tendon disorders in runners: A review. *Medicine and Science in Sports and Exercise*, **12**, 231–243

22 Clement, D.B., Taunton, J.E. and Smart, G.W. (1984) Achilles tendinitis and peritendinitis: etiology and treatment. *American Journal of Sports Medicine*, **12**, 179–184

23 Williams, J.G.P. (1986) Achilles tendon lesions in sport. *Sports Medicine*, **3**, 114–135

24 Fornage, B.D. (1986) Achilles tendon: US examination. *Radiology*, **159**, 759–764

25 Maffulli, N., Regine, R., Angellillo, M. *et al.* (1987) Ultrasound diagnosis of Achilles tendon pathology in runners. *British Journal of Sports Medicine*, **21**, 158–162

26 Blei, C.L., Nirschl, R.P. and Grant, E.G. (1986) Achilles tendon: US diagnosis of pathologic conditions. *Radiology*, **159**, 765–776

27 Quinn, S.F., Murray, W.T., Clark, R.A. *et al.* (1987) Achilles tendon: MR imaging at 1.5 Tl. *Radiology*, **164**, 767–770

28 Bates, B.T., Osternig, L.R., Mason, M.S. *et al.* (1979) Foot orthotic devises to modify selected aspects of lower extremity mechanics. *American Journal of Sports Medicine*, **7**, 338–342

29 Lowdon, A., Bader, D.L. and Mowat, A.G. (1984) The effect of heel pads on the treatment of Achilles tendinitis: a double blind trial. *American Journal of Sports Medicine*, **12**, 431–435

30 Schepsis, A.A. and Leach, R.E. (1987) Surgical management of Achilles tendinitis. *American Journal of Sports Medicine*, **15**, 308–315

31 Kvist, M.H., Lehto, M.U.K., Jozsa, L. *et al.* (1988) Chronic Achilles paratenonitis. *American Journal of Sports Medicine*, **16**, 616–623

32 Inglis, A.E., Scott, W.N., Sculco, T.P. *et al.* (1976) Ruptures of the tendo achillis. *Journal of Bone and Joint Surgery*, **58A**, 990–993

33 Kuwada, G.T. and Schberth, J. (1984) Evaluation of Achilles tendon rupture. *Journal of Foot Surgery*, **23**, 340–343

34 Densted, T. Finn., and Doaas, A. (1979) Surgical treatment of partial Achilles tendon rupture. *American Journal of Sports Medicine*, **7**, 15–17

35 Canoso, J.J., Wohlgethan, J.R., Newberg, A.H. *et al.* (1984) Aspiration of the retrocalcaneal bursa. *Annals of Rheumatic Disease*, **43**, 308–312

36 Kernohan, J. and Hall, A.J. (1984) Treatment of a fractured ossified Achilles tendon. *Journal of Royal College of Surgeons of Edinburgh*, **29**, 263

12 Ankle joint

The ankle is a modified hinge joint. The lower end of the tibia with the medial and lateral malleoli are lined by articular cartilage to form a mortise into which the superior or trochlear surface of the talus fits (Figure 12.1). Two active movements, plantar and dorsiflexion, occur at the ankle. The axis of this movement runs through the body of the talus, passing from its medial surface distal to the medial malleolus to its lateral surface where it runs through the tip of the lateral malleolus. With the foot dorsiflexed, the broader anterior part of the body moves backwards into the mortise and the joint becomes more stable. When the foot is plantar flexed, the narrower posterior part of the body of the talus moves forwards into the mortise and the talus can be passively moved side to side between the malleoli.

The talus can also medially rotate a few degrees, accompanied by movement in the lateral malleolus, which also rotates internally and downwards [1].

Ankle stability is normally dependent on the integrity of the joint surfaces, as the talus is locked into the tibiofibular mortise with the malleoli on either side exerting a pincer-like effect. Its integrity also depends on the ligamentous support provided by the anterior tibiofibular ligament superiorly and the two collateral ligaments on either side of the ankle joint.

Examination

Examination of the ankle forms an integral part of foot examination and some abnormalities, such as deformities and gait disturbances, are discussed later. Examination includes the spine and the whole of the lower legs and feet. Measurements include leg length, muscle strength and torsional abnormalities. Examination of the ankle should be performed with the patient walking, standing and lying supine and then prone.

Ankle examination

1 Inspection.
   (a) Gait.
   (b) Deformities.
   (c) Swelling.
2 Movements.
   (a) Active.
   (b) Passive.
   (c) Accessory.
   (d) Isometric.

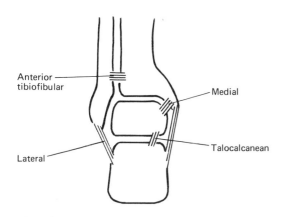

Figure 12.1 Ligaments stabilizing the ankle mortise

3 Palpation.
   (a) Warmth.
   (b) Synovial thickening.
   (c) Tenderness.
   (d) Arterial pulses.

Inspection

The ankle should be inspected both from the front and behind with the patient first standing, then walking, and finally lying down. The presence of an effusion in the ankle joint can best be appreciated by inspection of the ankle from the front and rear with the patient standing. Anteriorly, the effusion may be seen to bulge into the synovial space, which follows the line of synovial reflection proximally over the anterior surface of the tibia (Figure 12.2). Posteriorly, an effusion in the ankle joint may be seen bulging out behind the malleoli so that it fills in the normal gutter between the malleolus and the Achilles tendon. Effusions into the tendon sheaths crossing the ankle are readily visible. The tibialis posterior and peroneal tendons run behind their respective malleoli, and effusions in their tendon sheaths produce a crescent-shaped swelling along the line of the tendon.

These synovial swellings may need to be differentiated from oedema, which, because of the dependency of the leg or inflammatory changes in surrounding soft tissue, may complicate ankle

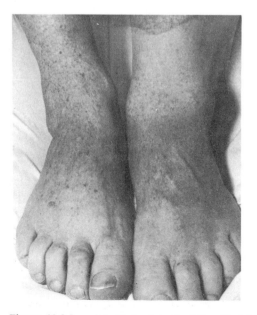

Figure 12.2 Synovial effusion into the left ankle joint

lesions. Bruising and swelling around the ankle may be evident after recent ligament sprains.

Movements

Active

Active movements at the ankle joint are dorsiflexion and plantar flexion. The active range is measured with the ankle in the neutral position, with the foot at 90 degrees to the leg. Movement in the midtarsal joints also contributes to the range of these movements which vary widely with age and physical training. The range may be restricted by arthritis, a sprained ligament or swelling around the ankle.

Passive

Dorsiflexion

Full passive ankle dorsiflexion is normally greater in range than active dorsiflexion.

METHOD
The patient lies supine with the ankle beyond the end of the couch. The subtalar joint must be in a neutral position (Chapter 13) as pronation here will also produce some dorsiflexion in the subtalar and midtarsal joints. The knee is kept extended. The foot is passively moved into dorsiflexion by holding the foot proximal to the midtarsal joint.

Clinical measurement of this range is important as it reflects the range of dorsiflexion available at the ankle during locomotion, and a minimum of 10 degrees of ankle dorsiflexion with the knee extended and the subtalar joint in neutral position is needed for locomotion. If decreased, compensation must occur in the knee or subtalar joint [2]. A decrease in dorsiflexion, equinus deformity, [3] may result from contracture of the gastrocnemius–soleus and Achilles tendon complex; bony lesions around the ankle; leg length discrepancy; muscle imbalance; or prolonged bed rest. It may be compensated for by excess pronation of the subtalar joint or by premature heel rise during ambulation.

Plantar flexion

The patient lies in the same position as for dorsiflexion. The passive range of plantar flexion is also normally greater than the active range. The range of passive movement may be found to be restricted and painless or restricted and painful. A painful restriction of this movement is most commonly from a sprain of the lateral ligament of the ankle joint.

Accessory movements

Accessory movements need to be tested first in the inferior tibiofibular joint and then in the ankle joint.

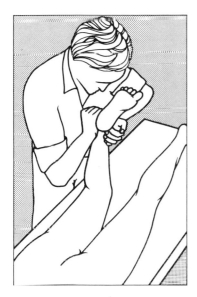

Figure 12.3 Posteroanterior accessory movement: inferior tibiofibular joint

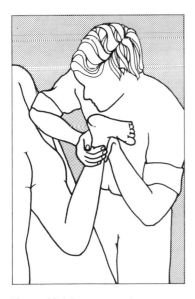

Figure 12.4 Anteroposterior accessory movement: inferior tibiofibular joint

Inferior tibiofibular joint

There are six accessory movements in the inferior tibiofibular joint:

1 Posteroanterior. An oscillatory pressure is produced by pressure against the posterior border of the lateral malleolus (Figure 12.3).
2 Anteroposterior, which is produced by pressure against the anterior border of the lateral malleolus (Figure 12.4).
3 Longitudinal caudad movement is produced by inversion of the calcaneus.
4 Longitudinal cephalad movement is produced by eversion of the calcaneus.
5 Separation of the fibula relative to the tibia occurs mainly on full dorsiflexion of the ankle.
6 Compression is produced by pressure over both malleoli (Figure 12.5).

Ankle joint

There are eight accessory movements at the ankle joint:

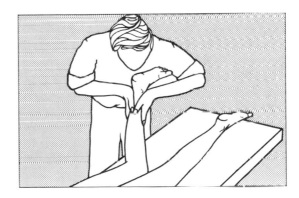

Figure 12.5 Inferior tibiofibular joint: compression

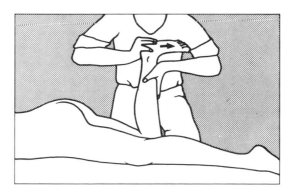

Figure 12.6 Posteroanterior accessory movement: ankle joint

1   Posteroanterior movement, which is produced by pushing the calcaneus forwards (Figure 12.6).
2   Anteroposterior movement is produced by gripping over the talus and pushing it posteriorly (Figure 12.7).
3   Longitudinal cephalad movement is produced by compression through the calcaneus (Figure 12.8).

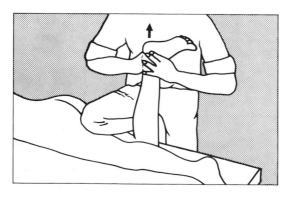

Figure 12.7 Anteroposterior accessory movement: ankle joint

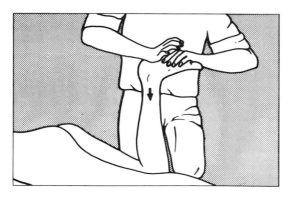

Figure 12.8 Longitudinal cephalad accessory movement: ankle joint

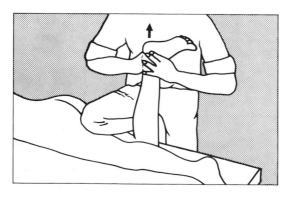

Figure 12.9 Longitudinal caudad accessory movement

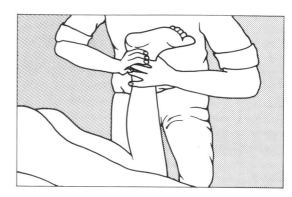

Figure 12.10 Ankle joint: medial rotation

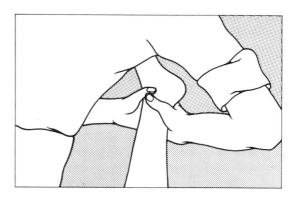

Figure 12.11 Ankle joint: lateral rotation

4   Longitudinal caudad movement is produced by distraction of the ankle (Figure 12.9).
5   Medial rotation is produced by movement of the talus and foot (Figure 12.10).
6   Lateral rotation is produced by an opposite movement of talus and foot (Figure 12.11).
7,8 Abduction and adduction (Figure 12.15).

Isometric tests

Dorsiflexion of the ankle is produced mainly by the anterior tibial muscle, which is inserted into the medial aspect of the first cuneiform and the base of the first metatarsus. It is tested with the foot fully inverted and the ankle fully dorsiflexed; the patient resists the examiner's attempt to force the foot into plantar flexion. The tendon may then be seen and palpated on the medial side of the ankle joint.

Pain and crepitus may result from either tendinitis of the muscle in the lower third of the leg, or to a tendinitis at its insertion. A painless weakness is associated with foot drop, which may be due to a lesion of the L5 nerve root or the lateral popliteal nerve.

Plantar flexion of the ankle is produced mainly by the gastrocnemius and soleus muscles. It is usually very difficult for the examiner to detect any weakness in these muscles by resisting plantar flexion of the foot. A better method of reproducing pain and weakness is to have the patient stand up and down ten times on the toes of one foot. Pain may be the result of a tear in the gastrocnemius or a lesion in the Achilles tendon. A painless weakness may be caused by an S1 nerve root lesion or a long-standing rupture of the Achilles tendon.

Palpation

The bony outlines of the malleoli and the anterior margin of the lower end of the tibia are subcutaneous and the anterior joint line is easily palpated. The joint line can also be palpated posteriorly behind the medial malleolus by having the patient actively dorsi-flex and plantar flex the ankle. The ankle is palpated for any increase in warmth by comparing it with the opposite ankle. Palpation should confirm the presence of synovitis in the ankle (Figure 12.12). The patient lies supine and the examiner holds the back of the ankle behind the malleoli with one hand to squeeze fluid into the more extensive anterior part of the joint. The anterior joint line is palpated using either the fingers or thumb of the other hand. Tenderness is sought especially over the joint line and attachments of the collateral ligaments.

Classification of ankle lesions

1   Soft tissue injuries.
    (a) Ligament sprains.
    (b) Ligament rupture and instability.
    (c) Recurrent instability of the ankle.
    (d) Tendon lesions.
2   Bone.
    (a) Talotibial exostoses.
    (b) Osteochondritis dissecans.

Soft tissue injuries

Ligament sprains

Ligament sprains are the most common injury in athletes [4].

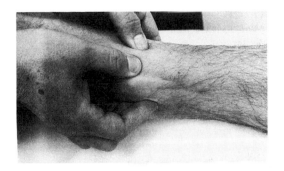

Figure 12.12 Palpation of the synovial swelling

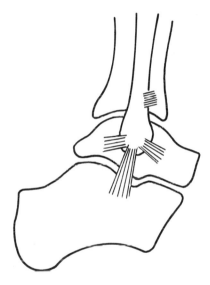

Figure 12.13 Lateral ligaments of the ankle joint

Lateral collateral ligament sprain

The three bands of fibres that make up the lateral ligament are injured by different mechanisms, determined by the function of the ligament and the direction in which the fibres run (Figure 12.13). They all run from the tip of the lateral malleolus.

1   The anterior talofibular ligament, the weakest of all ankle ligaments, runs to the neck of the talus and fuses with the anterior capsule of the ankle joint. It is taut throughout plantar flexion and so may be damaged by a sudden forced or excessive degree of inversion or plantar flexion. This is the position of the foot in which most injuries occur and the anterior ligament is the most commonly involved at either its upper or lower attachments,

more commonly the upper. The history is often one of having fallen while running, walking or jumping on a rough surface.

2   The fibulocalcaneal ligament runs vertically downwards to the lateral surface of the calcaneus and is taut with the ankle at a right angle.

3   The posterior talofibular ligament runs to the talus, strengthening the posterior aspect of the ankle capsule. Only rarely injured, it occurs, for example, in long jumpers who land on their feet with the ankle suddenly forcibly dorsiflexed.

Anterior tibiofibular ligament sprain

A sprain of the anterior tibiofibular ligament is common [5] and may follow the typical inversion strain or an eversion or a dorsiflexion injury. In an eversion injury the talus is forced against the medial malleolus, the ankle mortise is widened and fibres of the anterior tibiofibular ligament may be torn. Sprains may also follow forced dorsiflexion of the ankle in which the anterior part of the body of the talus is forced into the joint, disrupting ligament fibres. With severe degrees of injury this ligament may be ruptured and produce a diastasis of the inferior tibiofibular joint, with disruption of the normal ankle mortise. It may also produce a rupture of the Achilles tendon, or a malleolar fracture.

Medial ligament sprain

Sprains of the medial ligament are not common because the ligament is strong and eversion injuries are relatively uncommon.

Diagnosis of ligament sprains

The majority of ankle sprains are first degree, with pain and no instability, or second degree often with marked swelling, increased pain and only slight laxity. Third degree sprains with complete rupture produce instability but marked pain and swelling are uncommon [6].

Diagnosis depends on an accurate history of the mechanism of the injury, a history of previous sprains, the site of pain, and clinical examination and assessment of the degree of injury [4]. At the time of injury there may be an audible crack or snap, even in minor sprains. It is always useful to examine ankle movements as soon as possible after injury, before any swelling develops. The site of the sprain should be accurately localized and an assessment made of the degree of injury, which may require

examination over a few days. The normal leg is examined first to determine the normal range and degree of ligamentous laxity. The affected ankle is inspected for oedema, bruising, deformity or synovitis.

Pain is reproduced by stretching or compressing the injured ligament, by moving the foot into inversion, eversion, plantar and dorsiflexion. In a lateral ligament sprain, pain may be reproduced either on inversion of the foot or on full passive eversion of the foot, as the painful area in the ligament is compressed between the fibular malleolus and calcaneus. In sprains of the anterior tibiofibular ligament, pain may be reproduced on plantar or dorsiflexion of the ankle, but especially on plantar flexion with inversion of the foot. Tenderness is sought by palpation over the ligamentous attachments and surrounding soft tissues.

Routine radiographs are necessary in all but the mildest ankle sprains [6–10] and stress views are usually indicated [6] but may be unreliable [11]. Arthrography to detect leakage into surrounding soft tissues to indicate a capsular ligament tear is not often helpful [6,11].

Management

Ankle sprains are often poorly managed; if radiographs are taken or reported as normal, the patient is usually advised that it is 'only a sprain' and further treatment may not be undertaken. The common belief was that ankle sprains are a worse injury than a fracture, with prolonged disability. The management previously advocated with prolonged immobilization even for minor sprains, produced subsequent muscle weakness, joint stiffness and pain. Thus the popular concept of 'once a sprain, always a sprain': a negative outlook that should never have been allowed to prevent a patient's return to full activity.

Initial treatment

Treatment in the first 48 h after injury is designed to minimize pain and swelling by using rest, ice, compression and elevation. This prevents haemorrhage and oedema formation and so limits subsequent adhesion formation and stiffness. The lower leg is first shaved and Friar's Balsam is applied to the skin. A Gibney basketweave adhesive tape strapping [12] with a double heel-lock gives the most effective support [6,9] and when properly applied limits inversion, eversion and rotation of the ankle. The strapping is applied from the medial side of the leg, up the lateral side of the leg A piece of foam rubber may be incorporated over the ligament to prevent haematoma formation. After 2 days, the strapping is removed, bruising and oedematous swelling should be minimized, and the degree of ligament injury is reassessed.

Subsequent treatment

1 Most injuries are first degree or second degree sprains. The aim with these is to exercise and stretch the ankle within the limits of pain, to mobilize it as early and as rapidly as possible [5]. The patient is encouraged to start to walk as normally as possible with a heel-to-toe gait within the limits of pain [13]. The ligament needs to be protected by either taping or a cast-brace. The ankle may be strapped in maximum eversion and dorsiflexion. An alternative is a cast-brace with a lite-cast upper section work below the knee, into which a polyethylene plastic shoe insert is incorporated. This allows plantar and dorsiflexion but prevents inversion or eversion, with earlier exercise and ambulation [6,7,11,14–17].
2 Anti-inflammatory drugs given for pain relief [18].
3 Physical methods, heat or preferably ice are of benefit.
4 Isokinetic and active resisted exercises and postural re-education exercises with the use of a wobble board, tilt board or balance board are given daily. Ligament injury causes articular nerve fibres and their mechanoreceptors involved in reflex stabilization of the ankle joint to be disrupted [2]. Exercises to increase neuromuscular coordination by having the patient balance on a board that moves at first in one plane and then on one that moves in all planes leads to increased proprioceptive control [6,19].
5 Mobilization by passive movement to restore accessory and physiological movements to a full pain-free range is important for, without them, active exercises and the wobble board will not be able to restore muscle power and coordination.
6 Stretching techniques to the soft tissues around the ankle plus the Achilles tendon are essential.
7 Local injections and massage are contraindicated during this stage.

Treatment with complications

Using these methods, the ligament usually returns to its full function. In some patients, particularly those initially treated inadequately, the lateral ligament may remain tender and painful on movement, especially with full passive inversion of the foot. Pain is felt on running, often when changing direction suddenly. Tenderness is usually around the attachment of the lateral ligament to the malleolus. The pathological basis of this lesion has never been determined and has been assumed to result from adhesion formation. It is more likely to be an area of chronic granulation scar tissue as in tenoperiosteal lesions, e g lateral epicondylitis of the elbow. This ankle lesion may be treated by an injection of local anaesthetic and 1 ml of corticosteroid given into the tender area in the ligament on one or two occasions.

With sprains of the anterior tibiofibular ligament, pain occurs especially when running with sudden acceleration or deceleration. Tenderness is localized over the ligament and treated with local corticosteroid injection.

Manual therapy techniques are commenced using large-amplitude rocking movements, taking care not to produce any discomfort. Rotation, produced by holding around the patient's foot and rocking it, is the main technique. As pain decreases, this treatment is used at the limit of the range (Figure 12.10), so producing stretching and some discomfort. Distraction (Figure 12.14) with slow oscillatory stretching is also used. With pain and stiffness, the amount of treatment varies depending on the degree of joint irritability. Physiological movements, usually dorsiflexion of the ankle, are used first. Accessory movements are then added at the limit of the range of dorsiflexion, using posteroanterior movements (Figure 12.6), anteroposterior movements (Figure 12.7) and inversion of the heel (Figure 12.15).

If stiffness is predominant, dorsiflexion is again used, but is now taken further into the range (Figure 12.16). Additional physiological movements are used strongly in other directions and accessory movements are then added at the limit of each range. As the pain settles, active exercises are recommended.

Rehabilitation

As pain and tenderness resolve, exercises and stretching are increased, followed by walking, jogging in a straight line at about half pace, then running, followed by side-stepping and running in a figure of eight pattern and function activities until full activity is achieved [2]. The ankle should be strapped before each practice session and game for the rest of the season.

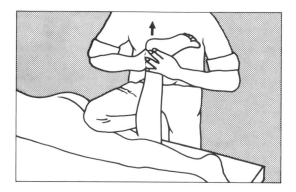

Figure 12.14 Distraction

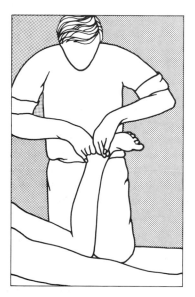

Figure 12.15 Inversion of the heel

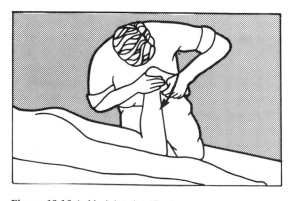

Figure 12.16 Ankle joint dorsiflexion

PREVENTION

This [20] includes care with shoes, especially cut-down shoes, care with training or playing surfaces, prophylactic ankle strapping, stretching, the use of bracing to prevent inversion [21], and proprioceptive training [21].

Ligament rupture and ankle instability

Lateral instability following rupture of the anterior talofibular and calcaneofibular ligaments [6,7,10,14] is often difficult to test for clinically [9]. It is tested with the ankle in plantar flexion and full passive inversion of the foot. A small range of movement is normally present, but a greater degree of inversion is possible if the ligament is ruptured and the talus rocks in the ankle mortise.

The diagnosis may be confirmed by radiography with stress inversion of the ankle to demonstrate the presence of any tilting of the talus (Figure 12.17). This first stresses the anterior talofibular ligament and the joint capsule. Should they be torn, the talus will tilt medially. Further inversion then stresses the calcaneofibular ligament so that gross tilting of the talus indicates a tear of this ligament also. The normal degree of talar tilt is from 0 to 5 degrees but varies with age and ligamentous laxity. If the significance of the tilt is uncertain, a similar view of the other ankle should be taken for comparison.

Anterior instability is caused by a rupture of the anterior talofibular ligament so that the talus becomes loose in its mortise (Figure 12.18). It is tested by the anterior drawer sign [6,8–10,15,22].

The patient sits over the edge of the couch with the legs hanging down and the foot in a slight plantarflexion. One hand is placed over the anterior aspect of the lower tibia to push the tibia posteriorly and the calcaneus is grasped with the other hand to pull it anteriorly. The talus may be felt to move anteriorly, often producing a 'clunking' noise. A lateral radiograph may show forward displacement of the talus greater than 3 mm.

Medial instability owing to a tear of the medial ligament is uncommon, and follows an injury with pronation and eversion of the foot with a tear of the anterior tibiofibular ligament and interosseous membrane [9] (Figure 12.19). It is tested clinically in a similar manner to a lateral ligament tear, but the examiner now everts the foot and the talus may be felt to tilt in the ankle mortise.

The diagnosis may be confirmed on radiographs, which show a widening of the space in the medial compartment of the ankle between the medial

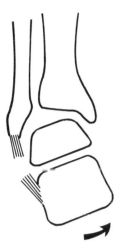

Figure 12.17 Talar tilt on inversion stress

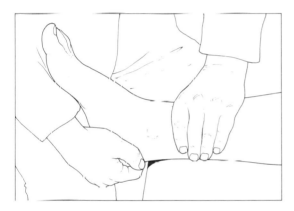

Figure 12.18 Testing for anterior instability

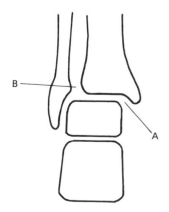

Figure 12.19 Rupture of the medial ligament. (A), Widening of the medial joint space; (B), diastasis of the inferior tibiofibular joint

malleolus and the talus, commonly associated with a diastasis of the inferior tibiofibular joint (Figure 12.19).

Management

Management of these injuries remains controversial. Surgical repair, cast immobilization and exercises have each been advocated [22]. In acute ruptures of ankle ligaments with talar instability, it might appear logical to attempt surgical repair of the disrupted ligament. Nevertheless, these injuries can be treated successfully by early mobilizing, active exercises and postural re-education of the ankle [6–9,11,13,15,16]. As pain resolves the patient and his ankle are managed (see above) with a graded return to full activity. Rupture of the medial and tibiofibular ligaments needs to have an internal screw fixation to approximate the separated joint surfaces.

Recurrent instability of the ankle

The patient with recurrent ankle instability may complain of recurrent ankle sprains, that the ankle turns over easily or that the ankle feels insecure and often lets him down. The ankle is often painful and stiff and there may be recurrent swelling. These symptoms may be present while walking or running, particularly over rough ground, and the patient usually can feel or hear a click in the ankle. Recurrent instability may be due to:

1 Function instability. This occurs after a ligament injury owing to loss of proprioception and postural control [21,23,24]. Ankle joint function is related to the ability to maintain equilibrium in single limb stance [24]. Sensory nerve fibres subserve a reflex arc that stabilizes the foot and ankle during locomotion and, when lost, reflex stabilization is lost and the foot tends to give way. Instability may be tested for by a modified Romberg's test [23]. Management is by intensive rehabilitation [25].
2 Ligament ruptures. Mechanical instability follows rupture of the capsular ligament structures of the lateral ligament, allowing the talus to become loose and subluxed in its mortise. Clinical tests and radiology, including arthrography, have been described above. With pain and instability, late reconstruction of the lateral ligaments may be indicated [8,26–28].

3   Inadequately treated sprains. These may lead to pain and a sudden giving way of the ankle, most likely when the patient is running and suddenly changes direction, swerving or turning quickly. The underlying pathological basis for this condition may be the formation of chronic granulation tissue at the ligament origin or the formation of adhesions. Examination of the foot and ankle will reveal pain on stretching this area, especially on adduction of the heel, inversion of the foot, or longitudinal caudad movement of the ankle. An area of marked tenderness can usually be palpated over the origin of the ligament from the lateral malleolus. Treatment is with mobilization techniques, deep friction massage or injection of local anaesthetic and corticosteroid.

Anterior capsule sprain leads to a loss of ankle movement. Pain may not be reproduced on testing active ankle plantar flexion but is present on testing passive movements. The range of full passive plantar flexion of the ankle is decreased and over-pressure reproduces pain. In football players this leads to considerable disability as the foot needs to be fully plantar flexed to kick a ball and sudden stretching of the capsule produces quite severe pain. Treatment consists of stretching the ankle under a general anaesthetic to restore the full passive range of plantar flexion.

4   Foot deformities. Foot deformities, especially a valgus deformity of the fore foot in which there is an alteration in peroneus longus function, are often associated with recurrent pain and disability in the lateral compartment of the ankle joint.

5   Undiagnosed causes. In a small proportion of patients, particularly females, no obvious cause can be demonstrated, although it has been attributed to wearing inadequate shoes, such as high heels or with heels that wear unevenly. Management may include orthotics, a float on the heel of the shoe and active rehabilitation and exercises.

Tenosynovitis of the ankle tendons

Tenosynovitis commonly involves either the peroneal tendons over the lateral compartment of the ankle or the tibialis posterior tendon over the medial compartment. It may follow trauma, such as a sprain of an ankle ligament; overuse; or inflammatory conditions such as rheumatoid arthritis or spondyloarthritis in which tenosynovitis may, at times, be the presenting symptom. The patient complains of pain, swelling and/or restricted movement, and

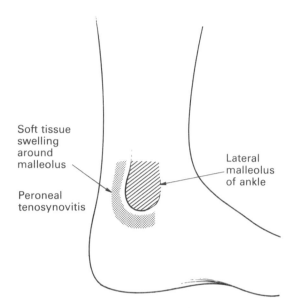

Figure 12.20 Peroneal tenosynovitis

examination reveals swelling that has a characteristic linear appearance as it bulges out from behind and below the malleolus.

Peroneal tendons

Peroneal tenosynovitis may occur along the course of the tendon from behind the fibular malleolus to the outer side of the foot (Figure 12.20).

MAJOR SIGN

Pain is reproduced by the examiner either fully resisting eversion of the foot, or stretching the peroneal tendons by fully passively inverting the foot. At the same time as these manoeuvres are being carried out, the examiner palpates for tenderness and crepitus over the peroneal tendons behind the lateral malleolus.

COMPLICATIONS

1   Subluxation of the peroneal tendons occurs after an ankle injury disrupts the peroneal retinaculum binding the peroneal tendons in their grooves behind the fibular malleolus. The tendons can then sublux over the fibular surface, usually during dorsiflexion of the foot, and are repositioned on plantar flexion of the foot. Treatment is surgical.

2 Tendovaginitis of the peroneal tendons [29,30] occurs as localized thickening of the common peroneal tendon sheath, similar to a de Quervain's syndrome at the wrist. It occurs as an overuse injury, particularly in athletes or ballet dancers. The patient presents with pain localized over the peroneal tendons, and a thickened, tender swelling may be palpated below the lateral malleolus. Treatment consists of rest and a local corticosteroid injection but, if pain persists, the peroneal sheath may be excised.
3 Rupture of the peroneal tendon is a rare complication that needs to be differentiated from weakness of ankle eversion as a result of a neurological lesion, such as an L5 nerve root lesion.
4 Weakness of these tendons may be associated with a recurrent sprain of the ankle.
5 A ganglion may be formed around the peroneal tendons.

Tibialis posterior tendon

Tenosynovitis involves the tibialis posterior tendon behind or just below the medial malleolus. Apart from the causes described above, tenosynovitis may also occur as a complication of a valgus deformity of the rear foot, producing strain on the medial compartment structures.

MAJOR SIGNS
Pain is reproduced by either resisting active inversion of the foot or stretching the tendon by fully passively everting the foot. At the same time, tenderness and crepitus are sought by palpating along the course of the tendon behind the medial malleolus.

COMPLICATIONS
1 A tarsal tunnel syndrome may develop (see Chapter 13).
2 Tendovaginitis occurs as localized thickening in the tendon sheath.
3 Rupture of the tibialis posterior tendon is associated with marked loss of foot function [31]. If untreated, progressive deformity may result which can only be adequately treated by rear foot arthrodesis [32,33].

Bone

Talotibial exostoses

This common sporting ankle lesion is characterized by the growth of bony exostoses on the surface of the

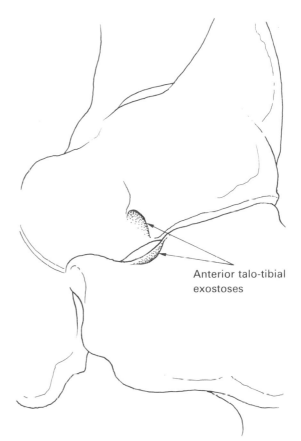

Figure 12.21 Anterior talotibial exostoses

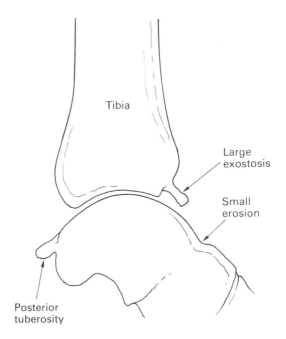

Figure 12.22 Talotibial exostoses and erosion

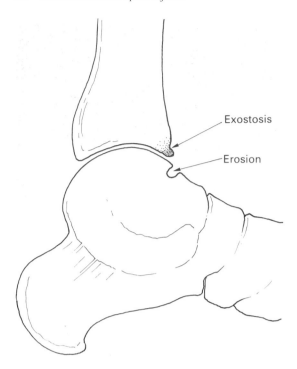

Figure 12.23 Tibial exostosis with a large erosion in the neck of the talus

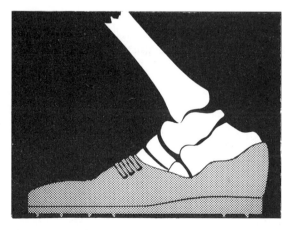

Figure 12.24 Diagrammatic representation of talotibial impingement on dorsiflexion of the ankle

talus and tibia around the ankle joint (Figure 12.21). On the anterior margins of the ankle joint exostoses develop on the upper surface of the neck of the talus and the lower end of the tibia just above the joint margin. They may reach large proportions and can develop anywhere along the anterior tibial margin (Figure 12.22). Similar bony changes also occur

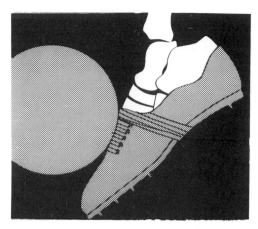

Figure 12.25 Diagrammatic representation of talotibial impingement on plantar flexion of the ankle

around the posterior margins of the tibia and talus. At times an exostosis develops only on the tibial surface and is associated with a large erosion in the neck of the talus (Figure 12.23). Occasionally the tibial exostosis may break off to form a loose bony body inside the joint (Figure 12.26).

In the push-off phase of running direct bony apposition results between the anterior border of the tibia and the talus (Figure 12.24). In full plantar flexion of the foot, as occurs on kicking, the posterior talus will hit the bony block of the lower posterior margin of the tibia (Figure 12.25). Anatomical considerations, such as a long posterior process of the talus or a separate os trigonum, make these lesions about the posterior aspect of the joint more likely. A long posterior process of the talus may be compressed more readily by the calcaneus against the tibia. Anterior and posterior exostoses are caused by the same fundamental mechanisms and often occur in the same ankle.

Clinical features

Pain, the usual presenting symptom, may be present on activity, especially running or going down stairs. A dull ache may be present after exercise. The ankle feels stiff and the athlete may complain of a loss of speed when pushing off to run. Locking of the ankle joint may occur if an exostosis is broken off to produce a loose bony foreign body. This needs to be differentiated from a meniscoid lesion by arthroscopy [34].

This condition usually produces more symptoms than signs, which may be difficult to elicit. On inspection some swelling or fullness over the anterior aspect of the ankle may be apparent. Active ankle movements may be of full range.

Major signs

Pain may be reproduced on either full passive plantar or dorsiflexion of the ankle. Anterior exostoses tend to be associated with pain and restriction at the limit of ankle dorsiflexion, and posterior exostoses with a painful restriction at the limit of plantar flexion. Over-pressure applied at the limit of either of these ranges usually reproduces pain.

Other signs

Anteriorly, tenderness is found over the anterior border of the tibia or the neck of the talus. Posteriorly, it is usually most marked just behind and above the medial malleolus; pressure over this site while the foot is fully plantar flexed should reproduce pain.

Management

1 Rest. The patient needs to rest from those activities, such as running, that cause pain.
2 Anti-inflammatory drugs are used to control pain.
3 Injections. The inflamed area around the anterior or posterior exostoses responds well to an injection of local anaesthetic and corticosteroid solution.
4 Physical methods. Ultrasound may be used to ease pain and localize the tender area. Exercises and massage are contraindicated.
5 Passive mobilization techniques are used when passive movements provoke pain to restore the maximal pain-free range of ankle movement.
6 Surgery is only rarely indicated; it should be used in those who fail to respond to conservative measures or have recurrent troubles on resuming full activity. Treatment by bevelling off the exostosis produces excellent results and the patient can usually resume normal activities. With joint locking, arthroscopic removal of the loose fragment is necessary (Figure 12.26).

Osteochondral fracture

An osteochondral fracture occurs at any age [35]. The usual site of involvement is the anterolateral surface of the articular dome of the talus [35]

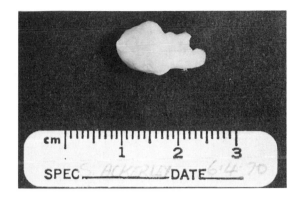

Figure 12.26 Loose osteochondral fragment from an anterior talotibial exostosis removed surgically

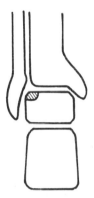

Figure 12.27 Usual site of osteochondral fracture of the talus

(Figure 12.27). It usually follows an inversion strain of the ankle, with the ankle dorsiflexed and so presents the broader posterior area of the talus in the ankle mortise, where it is more readily impinged against the fibular malleolus. It may also occur if the patient lands on the foot after having jumped into the air.

A second site, on the posteromedial surface, is caused by an inversion and plantar flexion injury, such as jumping into the air and coming down on the toes [35].

The patient presents usually as a sprained ankle or with pain, some intermittent swelling and a limp. There are no specific tests for this condition but compression of the joint surface may reproduce pain. While maintaining compression, the ankle is rocked through a full range of dorsi- and plantar flexion. Tenderness may be found over the superior surface of the talus.

Management

This lesion should be suspected in all patients with a 'sprained ankle' that fails to respond to treatment. Repeat radiography, nuclear bone scan, CT, MRI or arthroscopy [36] are then necessary. Occasionally symptoms are mild or intermittent, and treatment with rest and no weight-bearing for 6–12 months may suffice. If symptoms are persistent or there is locking of the joint, removal of the loose body with curetting of the cavity is indicated but can be a difficult operation if the fragment extends under the tibia. With degenerative changes, fusion of the ankle may be necessary.

References

1   Rasmussen, O. (1985) Stability of the ankle joint. *Acta Orthopaedica Scandinavica*, **56** (Suppl. 211), 13
2   Molnar, M.E. (1988) Rehabilitation of the injured ankle. *Clinics in Sports Medicine*, **7**, 193–204
3   Bouche, R.T. and Kuwada, G.T. (1984) Equinus deformity in the athlete. *Physician and Sports Medicine*, **12**, 81–91
4   Hergenroeder, A.C. (1990) Diagnosis and treatment of ankle sprains. A review. *American Journal of Diseases – Child*, **144**, 809–814
5   Smith, R.W. and Reischl, S.F. (1986) Treatment of ankle sprains in young athletes. *American Journal of Sports Medicine*, **14**, 465–471
6   Ryan, L.T.C., John, B., Hopkinson, L.T.D. *et al.* (1989) Office management of the acute ankle sprain. *Clinics in Sports Medicine*, **8**, 477–495
7   Nemeth, V.A. and Thrasher, E. (1983) Ankle sprains in athletes. *Clinics in Sports Medicine*, **2**, 217–224
8   Lightowler, C.D.R. (1984) Injuries to the lateral ligament of the ankle. *British Medical Journal*, **289**, 1247
9   Cox, J.S. (1985) Surgical and non-surgical treatment of acute ankle sprains. *Clinical Orthopaedics and Related Research*, **198**, 118–126
10 Rijke, A.M., Jones, B. and Vierhout, P.A.M. (1986) Stress examination of traumatized lateral ligaments of the ankle. *Clinical Orthopaedics and Related Research*, **210**, 143–151
11 Jackson, J.P. and Hutson, M.A. (1986) Cast-brace treatment of ankle sprains. *Injury*, **17**, 251–255
12 Capasso, G., Maffulii, N. and Testa, V. (1989) Ankle taping: Support given by different materials. *British Journal of Sports Medicine*, **23**, 239–240
13 Linde, F. and Hvass, I. (1986) Early mobilizing treatment in lateral ankle sprains. *Scandinavian Journal of Rehabilitation*, **18**, 17–21
14 Hughes, I.L.T., Lauren, Y., Stetts, I.L.T. *et al.* (1983) A comparison of ankle taping and a semirigid support. *Physician and Sports Medicine*, **11**, 99–103
15 Cass, J.R. and Morrey, B.F. (1984) Ankle instability: current concepts, diagnosis, and treatment. *Mayo Clinic Proceedings*, **59**, 165–170
16 Cetti, R., Christensen, S.E. and Corfitzen, M.T. (1984) Ruptured fibular ankle ligament: plaster or Pliton brace? *British Journal of Sports Medicine*, **18**, 104–199
17 Carne, P. (1989) Non-surgical treatment of ankle sprains using the modified Sarmiento brace. *American Journal of Sports Medicine*, **17**, 253–257
18 Sloan, J.P., Hain, R. and Pownall, R. (1989) Benefits of early anti-inflammatory medication following acute ankle injury. *Injury*, **20**, 81–83
19 Tropp, H., Askling, C. (1988) Effects of ankle disk training on muscular strength and postural control. *Clinical Biomechanics*, **3**, 88–91
20 McCluskey, G.M., Blackburn, T.A. and Lewis, T. (1976) Prevention of ankle sprains. *American Journal of Sports Medicine*, **4**, 151–157
21 Tropp, H., Askling, C. and Gillquist, J. (1985) Prevention of ankle sprains. *American Journal of Sports Medicine*, **13**, 259–262
22 Muwanga, C.L., Hellier, M., Quinton, D.N. *et al.* (1986) Grade III injuries of the lateral ligaments of the ankle: the incidence and a simple stress test. *Archives of Emergency Medicine*, **3**, 247–251
23 Tropp, H. and Askling, C. (1988) Effects of ankle disk training on muscular strength and postural control. *Clinical Biomechanics*, **3**, 88–91
24 Tropp, H. and Odenrick, P. (1988) Postural control in single limb stance. *Journal of Orthopaedic Research*, **6**, 833–839
25 Lightowler, C.D.R. (1984) Injuries to the lateral ligament of the ankle. *British Medical Journal*, **289**, 1247
26 *Lancet* (1989) Editorial, p. 1056
27 Karlsson, J., Bergsten, T., Lansinger, O. *et al.* (1989) Surgical treatment of chronic lateral instability of the ankle joint. *American Journal of Sports Medicine*, **17**, 268–274
28 Ahlgren, O. and Larsson, S. (1989) Reconstruction for lateral ligament injuries of the ankle. *Journal of Bone and Joint Surgery (Br)*, **71B**, 300–303
29 Andersen, E. (1987) Stenosing peroneal tenosynovitis symptomatically simulating ankle instability. *American Journal of Sports Medicine*, **15**, 258–259
30 Zivot, M.L., Pearl, S.H., Pupp, G.R. *et al.* (1989) Stenosing peroneal tenosynovitis. *Journal of Foot Surgery*, **28**, 220–224
31 Alexander, I.J., Johnson, K.A. and Berquist, T.H. (1987) Magnetic resonance imaging in the diagnosis of disruption of the posterior tibial tendon. *Foot Ankle*, **8**, 144–147
32 Jahss, M.H. (1982) Spontaneous rupture of the tibialis posterior tendon: clinical findings, tenographic studies and a new technique of repair. *Foot Ankle*, **3**, 158–166
33 Johnson, K.A. (1983) Tibialis posterior tendon rupture. *Clinical Orthopaedics*, **177**, 140–147
34 McCarroll, J.R., Schrader, J.W., Shelbourne, K.D. *et al.* (1987) Meniscoid lesions of the ankle in soccer players. *American Journal of Sports Medicine*, **15**, 255–257
35 Savastano, A.A. (1982) Articular fractures of the dome of the talus. *Physician and Sportsmedicine*, **10**, 113–119
36 Lundeen, R.O. (1989) Arthroscopic evaluation of traumatic injuries to the ankle and foot. Part I: Acute injuries. *Journal of Foot Surgery*, **28**, 499–511

13 Foot

The foot may conveniently be divided into three areas: the hind foot, the midtarsal region and the fore foot. The hind foot comprises two bones: the talus and calcaneus. The midtarsal region is made up of five bones: the navicular, cuboid and three cuneiform bones. The fore foot comprises five metatarsal bones and their corresponding toes (Figures 13.1 and 13.2).

Subtalar joint

The talus articulates with the calcaneus at two separate sites, one anterior and the other posterior, to form the synovial talocalcaneal joints which form a functional unit, the subtalar joint (Figure 13.3) [1,2]. The anterior talocalcaneal joint is also continuous with the talonavicular joint which also forms

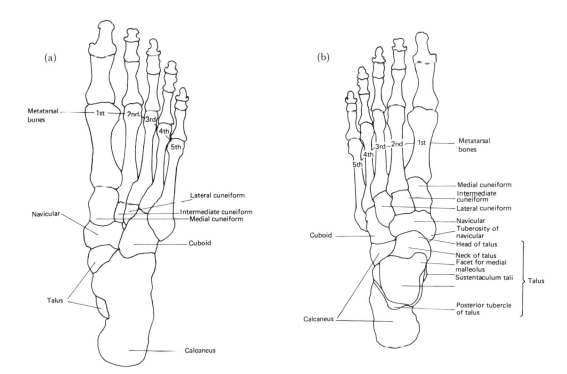

Figure 13.1 Bones of the left foot. (a), Plantar aspect; (b), dorsal aspect

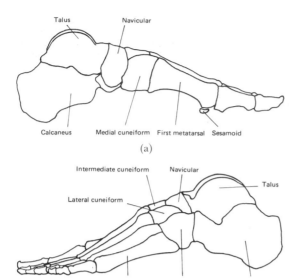

Figure 13.2 Bones of the left foot. (a), Medial aspect; (b), lateral aspect

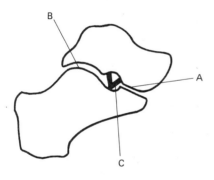

Figure 13.3 (A), Anterior talocalcanean joint; (B), posterior talocalcanean joint; (C), tarsal tunnel, with V-shaped interosseous ligament

part of a functional unit, the transverse tarsal joint, which comprises the talonavicular and calcaneocuboid joints.

The anterior and posterior talocalcaneal joints are separated by a tunnel, the sinus tarsi, formed by two grooves (sulci) on the reciprocal surfaces of the talus and calcaneus [1]. This tunnel contains the powerful interosseous ligament, important for stability and dynamic function of the subtalar joint [3,4]. It is lax on pronation (Figure 13.4) and is tense on supination, when it produces increased stability of the foot.

The axis of movement for the subtalar joint, the subtalar or Henkes axis, runs at an angle of 42 degrees to the transverse plane and 16 degrees to the frontal plane (Figure 13.5). Movement in the subtalar joint can take place in three separate body planes around this axis so producing supination and pronation. Supination produces inversion, adduction and plantar flexion; pronation eversion, abduction and dorsiflexion [5].

The subtalar joint forms the major key to normal and abnormal foot function [4–6]. Its triplanar action allows the normal foot to adapt to alterations in ground contours and to be maintained flat on the ground with the leg in varying angular positions, e.g. when turning while running at speed. It can also compensate for foot deformities, as described later.

With the foot non-weight bearing, the talus is fixed in the ankle mortise and the calcaneus moves under it. With the foot firmly planted and the calcaneus fixed, movements are imparted to the talus so producing rotary movements of the lower leg [4].

The total range of pronation–supination in the subtalar joint is approximately 30 degrees. The minimum range necessary for locomotion is considered to be 8–12 degrees.

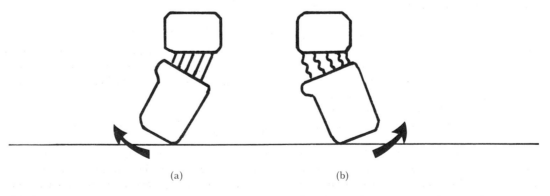

Figure 13.4 (a), On supination the interosseous ligament is tense and increases stability in the foot; (b), on pronation it is lax

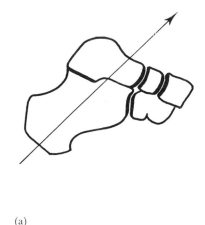

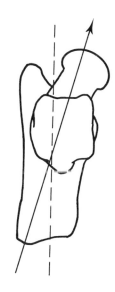

(a)

(b)

Figure 13.5 Subtalar axis of Henke (arrow): (a) from the side; (b) from above. It runs at an angle to the long axis of the foot (dotted line)

Transverse (or mid) tarsal joint

The lateral aspect of this joint lies between the calcaneus and cuboid; its medial aspect lies between the talus and the navicular. The cuneiforms and cuboid can rotate on the navicula and calcaneus especially in supination.

The transverse tarsal joint [1] has two axes of motion, one longitudinal and one oblique, that allow the gliding talonavicular and calcaneocuboid joints to function together to produce supination and pronation. With the subtalar joint in the neutral position, the axis of the calcaneocuboid joint lies parallel with the ground and the axis of the talonavicular joint lies slightly oblique to it (Figure 13.6).

With pronation, the axes of the talonavicular and calcaneocuboid joints lie parallel to each other so that free movement at the midtarsal level is possible (Figure 13.7a). This unlocking of the midtarsal joint allows the hind foot to adapt to the underlying surface during weight-bearing and brings the fore foot flat onto the ground [4].

During supination, the axes of the talonavicular and calcaneocuboid joints lie at an increased angle to each other (Figure 13.7b). Movement in the midtarsal region is restricted or locked and the foot is converted into a rigid support to form an efficient lever for propulsion [4].

Supination is controlled by the tibialis anterior and posterior muscles, which are attached medial to the subtalar axis. Pronation is controlled by the peroneal muscles attached lateral to the subtalar axis.

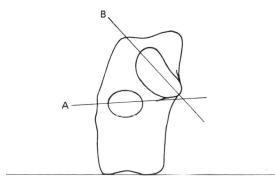

Figure 13.6 Transverse tarsal joint In the neutral position, the axis of the calcaneocuboid joint (A) is parallel with the ground. The axis of the talonavicular joint (B) crosses it at an oblique angle

Intercuneiform movements

These are small and gliding: (1) in a plantar and a dorsal direction during plantar flexion and dorsiflexion, and (2) in a rotary direction during supination and pronation.

Tarsometatarsal joints

These form part of the transverse arch of the foot, with the second cuneiform bone as its keystone, supported by the peroneus longus tendon. The metatarsal bone with its corresponding toe and tarsometatarsal joint form a functional unit, or ray.

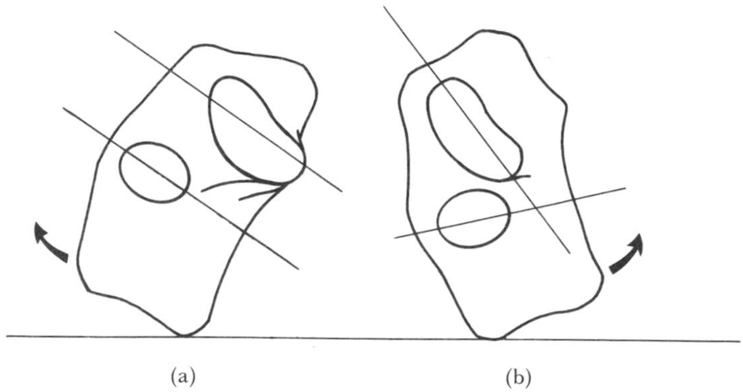

(a)   (b)

Figure 13.7 (a), With pronation of the subtalar joint the axes of the talonavicular and calcaneocuboid joints are parallel and the transverse tarsal joint is unlocked; (b), with supination of the subtalar joint the transverse tarsal joint is locked

Foot function

The normal foot is ideally adapted to its function of weight-bearing and locomotion [7]. The lateral border of the foot is buttressed by bone and the inner border is formed into a longitudinal arch that functions as an ideal elastic shock absorber but can also become a rigid weight-bearing system for forward propulsion of the foot. The joints of the foot need to be flexible to allow this function and at the same time allow the foot to adapt to irregularities in the ground. The foot must be correctly presented to the ground and the position it needs to adopt varies according to the angle or position of the leg and alterations in the slope of the ground.

Running gait

Running consists of alternating stance (or support), and swing (or air-borne) phases [8]. One full gait cycle is described from heel strike in one leg to the next heel strike of the same leg. The support phase goes through three well-defined stages: heel strike (contact), midstance and propulsion. Running is accompanied by considerable rotation in the pelvis and leg which aids in lengthening the stride. Just before heel strike the leg is in lateral rotation.

On initial contact, heel strike, the foot and subtalar joint are slightly supinated, the tibia in lateral rotation and the calcaneus hits the ground in an inverted position.

As the foot moves into its stance phase, the tibia immediately rotates medially with concomitant pronation of the subtalar joint. This allows absorption of the initial contact force and adaptation to the running surface. The transverse tarsal joint is unlocked and the foot becomes more flexible and mobile.

At midstance, the swing leg passes over the stance leg, the centre of gravity moves in front of the stance foot and the ankle dorsiflexes. The subtalar joint now supinates stabilizing and locking the midtarsal joint and medial, longitudinal arch, thus allowing the foot to become a rigid lever for propulsion.

Toe off occurs as the first ray is stabilized for active propulsion of the hallux. This begins with heel lift and the body weight shifts from the lateral to the medial side of the foot.

Examination

Examination of the foot and ankle follows examination of the back and lower leg. Muscle function, full neurological evaluation and the arterial supply, by palpating dorsalis pedis and tibialis posterior arteries, are assessed [9]. The ankle is then tested with the patient standing, walking, sitting and lying down.

Examination of the foot

1   Inspection.
    (a) Deformities.
    (b) Skin changes.
    (c) Swelling.
    (d) Muscle wasting.
    (e) Shoes.
    (f) Gait.
2   Movements.
    (a) Active and passive.
    (b) Accessory.
    (c) Isometric.
3   Palpation.

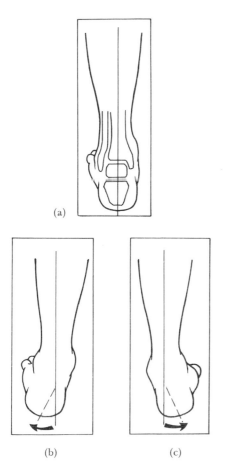

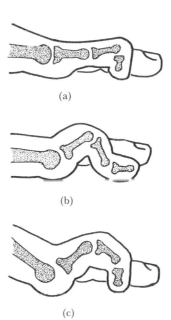

Figure 13.9 (a), Mallet toe; (b), claw toe; (c), hammer toe

Figure 13.8 (a), Normal alignment of the talus and calcaneus; (b), valgus deformity of the left hind foot; (c), varus deformity of the left hind foot

Inspection

The foot is examined with the patient standing, walking, sitting with the feet over the edge of the couch, lying supine and then prone. The patient stands looking straight ahead and the foot is inspected from the front, side, and from behind. It should also be inspected with the patient first adopting as natural a posture as possible, and then standing with the feet together. The normal posture of the foot with the patient standing should reveal that the calcaneus lies vertical to the floor, the subtalar joint is in a neutral position, and the five metatarsal heads lie in contact with the ground. The general conformation of the foot is noted, including the relative length of the toes.

Deformities

The hind foot may show either a valgus or a varus deformity. A valgus deformity is manifested by an eversion of the calcaneus relative to the weight-bearing surface. A varus deformity is manifested by an inversion of the calcaneus relative to the weight-bearing surface (Figure 13.8).

In the midtarsal region the medial longitudinal arch may be either depressed (pes planus) or elevated (pes cavus). A deformity of the fore foot relative to the hind foot may be in either varus or valgus.

Fore foot

The toes may be laterally deviated into valgus deformity, which most commonly involves the great toe (hallux valgus). Other toe deformities include:

1 Mallet toe, in which there is a flexion deformity of the terminal interphalangeal joint.
2 A cock-up deformity, or claw toe, in which the proximal phalanx is subluxed dorsally onto the metatarsal head, which is depressed into the sole of the foot. The proximal interphalangeal joint develops a flexion deformity and the terminal interphalangeal joint is hyperextended (Figure 13.9).

3   Hammer toe, in which a hyperextension deformity of the metatarsophalangeal joint is associated with a flexion deformity of the interphalangeal joints.

Skin changes

The skin is inspected for any rashes, colour changes,
nodules, ulcers or nail changes. A callus is an area of
thickened skin in the sole of the foot that results from
abnormal friction or pressure. They are commonly
found under the metatarsal heads or in the heel and
are produced by abnormal foot mechanics. Hard corns
are areas of hyperkeratosis developing in the thin skin
over deformed toes as the result of abnormal pressure
from the shoe. They normally have a painful central
core, which is evident when the outer layers of skin are
removed. Soft corns occur in the moistened surfaces
between the toes, especially in the fourth interdigital
cleft, and also result from abnormal pressure.

Swelling

Soft tissue swelling is usually evident on inspection.
Synovitis of the subtalar joint usually causes a bulge
laterally through the sinus tarsi, and synovitis of the
midtarsal joint bulges onto the dorsum of the foot.
Tendon sheath swelling usually occurs either in the
retromalleolar areas as a linear swelling or over the
dorsum of the foot. Swelling in the bursa over the
first or fifth metatarsophalangeal joint may be
evident on inspection. A generalized swelling of the
toes in patients with spondyloarthritis produces a
typical 'sausage-shape' deformity.

Muscle wasting

Wasting of the small muscles is not easily detected
in the foot although wasting of the extensor digitorum brevis may be evident over the sinus tarsi in
patients with L5 nerve root compression.

Shoes

These are inspected to see their type and whether
they conform to the shape of the foot [9,10]. Unequal
wearing of a part of the shoe may correspond to the
presence of any foot deformity. For example, with an
equinus deformity of the ankle [11] the tips of the
soles are excessively worn; with a valgus deformity of

the rear foot the inner side of the heel is worn and
the medial counter is broken; prominent displaced
metatarsal heads will indent the anterior part of the
sole. In a toe-out gait, excessive shoe wear is
produced on the lateral aspect of the heel and the
medial part of the forefoot. With a toe-in gait, wear
is most prominent on the medial aspect of the heel
and the lateral part of the fore foot.

Gait

Abnormalities of gait have been described in
Chapter 9. In the foot, gait can also be disturbed by
pain and restriction in its joints, ligaments or
tendons. The foot is examined on walking, then on
heels and toes towards, away from and then across
in front of the examiner.

The angle of gait is the position adopted by the
feet during locomotion. Normally the foot forms an
angle of 7–10 degrees of abduction, i.e. toe-out,
relative to the line of progression. However, the
position of the foot varies from person to person and
even in the same person from step to step. The angle
tends to increase with age but should not exceed 15
degrees. It may be altered by structural changes in
the foot, especially in the subtalar joint, or in the
lower limb so that the angle is decreased (toe-in
gait) or increased (toe-out gait).

Movements

Active and passive movements

Those active and passive movements tested routinely
include:

1   Subtalar joint movements.
2   Intertarsal joints: adduction and abduction.
3   Tarsometatarsal joints: adduction and abduction.
4   First tarsometatarsal joint: plantar flexion, dorsiflexion and rotation.
5   Metatarsophalangeal joints: flexion and extension.
6   Proximal interphalangeal joints: flexion and
extension.
7   Terminal interphalangeal joints: flexion and
extension.
8   Intermetatarsal joints.

Subtalar joint

The subtalar joint needs to be examined first in its
neutral position. With the patient lying supine, the
head of the talus is palpated between the index finger

and thumb. The foot is then passively moved through an arc of pronation and supination. On pronation, the head of the talus becomes prominent medially and will then disappear on supination. During this arc of motion there is a point at which the talar head is found to be prominent on either side of the navicular. This position, neither supinated nor pronated, is taken as the neutral position.

It is difficult to measure the range of pronation–supination in this joint accurately because of its triplanar nature, but it can be assessed by two methods. (1) The patient lies supine and the calcaneus is grasped from behind and moved passively into full eversion and inversion. (2) Supination–pronation is tested by a combination of active and passive movements. The patient lies supine with the knee flexed to 90 degrees and the ankle fully dorsiflexed to fix the talus in its mortise. The heel is moved inwards and then outwards (Figure 13.10) and the patient cooperates in this movement by simultaneously turning the heel inwards and outwards. The normal range is approximately 20 degrees of inversion and 10 degrees of eversion.

Intertarsal joints

Passive movements of supination–pronation and abduction–adduction are tested with the subtalar joint in neutral position. These are tested passively with the patient lying prone and knee flexed to a right angle.

Abduction of the forefoot on the hind foot is tested by holding the heel with the right hand with the thumb over the lateral border of the calcaneus (Figure 13.11). The left hand holds over the lateral border of the foot with the thumb over the cuboid. Movement is produced through the examiner's arms by approximating the elbows, not by pressure from the thumbs. The normal range is up to 10 degrees.

Adduction is tested by holding the medial border of the foot with both hands, the left thumb over the talus and the right thumb over the navicular (Figure 13.12). Movement is produced by the arms. The normal range is up to 20 degrees.

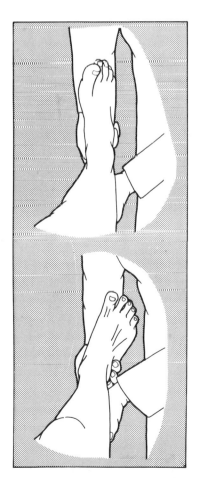

Figure 13.10 Test for movement in the subtalar joint

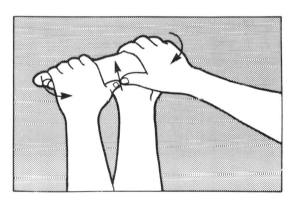

Figure 13.11 Abduction of the forefoot on the hind foot

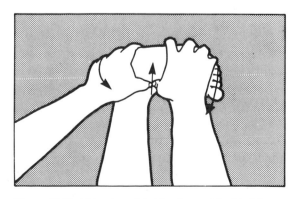

Figure 13.12 Adduction of the forefoot on the hind foot

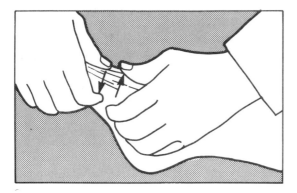

Figure 13.13 Test for passive movement at the first tarsometatarsal joint

Tarsometatarsal joints

Abduction and adduction of the tarsometatarsal joints are tested in a similar manner. For abduction the thumbs are placed over the cuboid and the tuberosity of the fifth metatarsal bone, respectively. For adduction the thumbs are placed over the medial cuneiform and the base of the first metatarsal bone, respectively.

First tarsometatarsal joint

This is tested by the examiner fixing the patient's first cuneiform bone with his left hand and holding the head of the first metatarsal with his other (Figure 13.13). The first metatarsal is then moved in a plantar and then in a dorsal direction. The normal range is about 10 degrees in each direction. Rotation can also be tested in this joint by holding the cuneiform with one hand and rotating the metatarsal by gripping the phalanx.

Metatarsophalangeal joints

The range of metatarsophalangeal joint movement is best tested passively. The metatarsophalangeal joint of the great toe normally passively extends to approximately 90 degress and flexes to about 35 degrees. In the lateral four joints, the range is approximately 40 degrees flexion and 40 degrees extension.

Proximal interphalangeal joints

These joints can be actively flexed to about 50 degrees but there is no active extension of these joints.

Terminal interphalangeal joints

These joints are tested passively. They can normally be flexed to about 60 degrees and extended by about 30 degrees.

Accessory movements

Subtalar joint

There are ten accessory movements in the subtalar joint:

1 Medial gliding of the calcaneus under the talus.
2 Lateral gliding of the calcaneus under the talus.
3 Adduction of the calcaneus under the talus.
4 Abduction of the calcaneus under the talus.
5 Anteroposterior gliding of the calcaneus.
6 Posteroanterior gliding of the calcaneus.
7 Medial rotation.
8 Lateral rotation.
9 Longitudinal caudad.
10 Longitudinal cephalad.

Transverse tarsal joint

There are ten accessory movements in this joint. Similar types of movements take place in the talonavicular, navicular–cuneiform, and calcaneocuboid joints, which are tested separately.

Talonavicular joint

The ten accessory movements in this joint are:

1 Superoinferior gliding movement of the navicular in a plantar direction on the talus.
2 Inferosuperior gliding movement of the navicular in a dorsal direction on the talus.
3 Medial gliding of the navicular on the talus.
4 Lateral gliding of the navicular on the talus.
5 Supination around the axis of the foot.
6 Pronation around the axis of the foot.
7 Longitudinal caudad.
8 Longitudinal cephalad.
9 Adduction.
10 Abduction.

Calcaneocuboid joint

The ten accessory movements in this joint are similar to those in the talonavicular joint except that the cuboid is moved relative to the calcaneus.

Cuneiform–navicular joint

Ten accessory movements are similar to those in the transverse tarsal joint.

Intercuneiform joints

There are four accessory movements in these joints:

1 Superoinferior gliding.
2 Inferosuperior gliding.
3 Supination.
4 Pronation.

Tarsometatarsal joint

Five accessory movements are:

1 Posteroanterior movement.
2 Anteroposterior movement.
3 Gliding is produced by holding a metatarsal in one hand and the corresponding tarsal bone in the other and moving adjacent bones in opposite directions.
4 Rotation. The examiner passively flexes the toe at its metatarsophalangeal and interphalangeal joints and rotates the appropriate metatarsal bone.
5 Small medial and lateral gliding movements are produced by applying pressure with the thumbs against the anterolateral or anteromedial surfaces of the bases of the metatarsal to push it either medially or laterally

Intermetatarsal joints

Four accessory movements tested routinely are anteroposterior and posteroanterior gliding movements, and horizontal flexion and extension.

Isometric tests

Five isometric movements are tested routinely:

1 Supination.
2 Pronation.
3 Dorsiflexion of the great toe.
4 Dorsiflexion of the toes.
5 Flexion of the great toe.

Supination of the foot

This is tested by first fully passively pronating the foot and then fully resisting an attempt to move the foot back into supination. This movement is controlled by the tibialis anterior and the tibialis posterior whose tendons are palpated during the test. A painful weakness usually indicates tendinitis or tenosynovitis of the tibialis posterior. A painful weakness occurs with rupture of this tendon, with L4 nerve root compression or an entrapment of the deep peroneal nerve.

Pronation of the foot

This is tested by first fully passively supinating the foot and then fully resisting an attempt to move the foot back into pronation. This movement is controlled mainly by the peroneus longus muscle and its tendon is palpated behind the lateral malleolus. A painful weakness usually indicates a lesion of the peroneus longus. A painless weakness occurs either with rupture of the tendon, with an L5 nerve root compression or entrapment of the lateral popliteal nerve at the fibular head.

The extensor hallucis longus muscle

This is tested by fully resisting an attempt actively to dorsiflex the great toe. A painful weakness occurs with tenosynovitis of the tendon. A painless weakness usually indicates the presence of an L5 nerve root compression.

The extensors of the toes

These are tested by fully resisting an attempt to dorsiflex the toes. A painful weakness of this movement indicates tenosynovitis of the extensor digitorum longus and a painless weakness occurs in an L5 nerve root lesion.

The flexor hallucis longus

This is tested by resisting attempts to flex the great toe. A painful weakness indicates tenosynovitis of this tendon and a painless weakness may occur with rupture of the tendon or in patients with a tarsal tunnel syndrome.

Palpation

Many of the foot structures lie subcutaneously and are identifiable on palpation. On the lateral side of the foot the lateral malleolus of the fibula is easily identified and the peroneal tendons as they run at first behind and then below it. The opening of the sinus tarsi may be palpated one fingerbreadth in front and below the anterior border of the lateral malleolus. It is covered by the fleshy belly of the extensor hallucis brevis, which is the only intrinsic muscle on the dorsum of the foot. The sinus tarsi may be felt to open up when the foot is inverted. The peroneal tubercle can be felt a finger-breadth below as a bony swelling on the lateral aspect of the calcaneus. It separates the two peroneal tendons and the peroneus longus tendon passes under it. Three finger-breadths anteriorly lies the styloid process at the base of the fifth metatarsal bone into which the peroneus brevis is inserted. The calcaneocuboid joint may be felt to open and close halfway between the lateral malleolus and the styloid process during inversion and eversion of the foot. The shaft of the fifth metatarsal runs distally from the styloid process and ends in the rather prominent metatarsal head of the fifth metatarsophalangeal joint.

On the medial side of the foot, the medial malleolus is easily palpable, as is the tibialis posterior which runs behind and then under it. A thumb's breadth anteriorly lies the sustentaculum tali, which supports the head of the talus. A further two fingerbreadths anteriorly lies the tuberosity of the navicular, which becomes more prominent on the inversion of the foot. The line of the talonavicular joint lies between these two bony prominences, and the movement of the joint is easily appreciated during inversion and eversion of the foot. The head and neck of the talus can easily be grasped between the fingers and thumb just below the ankle joint and the head can be brought into prominence by extension of the foot. A fingerbreadth distal to the tuberosity of the navicular, the base of the first metatarsal bone can be palpated where it flares out slightly. The first metatarso–cuneiform joint lies at this level. The first metatarsal can be palpated along its length to the first metatarsophalangeal joint.

To palpate the dorsum of the foot, the medial and lateral malleoli are again identified. Three tendons cross the front of the ankle joint. The most medial and easily recognized is the tibialis anterior tendon as it passes to its insertion into the medial cuneiform and base of the first metatarsal bone. The tendon of the extensor hallucis longus and the dorsalis pedis artery may be palpable between this tendon and the tendons of the extensor digitorum longus. In the heel, the tuberosity of the calcaneus is subcutaneous and the Achilles tendon may be felt at its insertion. The medial tubercle of the calcaneus can be palpated on the plantar surface of the hind foot.

The interphalangeal joints are palpated by placing the thumb and forefinger between the toes and feeling over the joints for any swelling or tenderness.

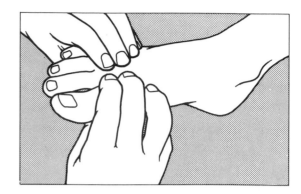

Figure 13.14 Palpation of the second metatarsophalangeal joint

The metatarsophalangeal joints should always be examined carefully as they are a common source of disability. Accurate assessment requires considerable experience but will often provide a clue to the clinical diagnosis. There are two methods of palpation:

1 By placing both thumbs under the plantar surface of the joint and palpating with the index finger of both hands over the dorsal surface of the joint and then between adjacent metatarsal heads to detect the presence of any synovitis, soft tissue swelling or thickening (Figure 13.14).
2 By placing the thumb over the dorsal aspect of the joint and the index finger under its plantar aspect. The finger on the plantar surface is placed a few millimetres more distally as the plantar surface of this joint extends slightly more distally than the dorsal surface. The joint is then moved up and down between the examiner's finger and thumb.

The alignment of the joint can also be palpated and plantar deviation of the metatarsal head or dorsal displacement of the proximal phalanx may be palpable. In Freiberg's disease the enlarged metatarsal head is usually easily palpable. Stress fracture of the metatarsal can usually be accurately localized over the site of involvement in the shaft of the bone. Palpation between the metatarsal heads may reveal a digital entrapment neuropathy (Morton's metatarsalgia). Any painful condition in this region may be exacerbated by squeezing the metatarsal heads together.

Midtarsal region

Swelling is usually visible on the dorsum of the foot here and tenderness, swelling or warmth may also be palpated. Localized bony tenderness over the navicular is present in patients with Kohler's disease or a stress fracture.

Heel

In the heel, the tuberosity of the calcaneus and the retrocalcaneal areas are palpated for any soft tissue or bony tenderness.

Classification of foot disorders

Foot pain and disability caused by musculoskeletal disorders are divided into: (1) generalized, and (2) localized conditions. Neurological, vascular, metabolic and skin disorders need to be differentiated but will not be considered here.

1 Generalized conditions.
   (a) Deformities.
   (b) Sudeck's atrophy.
   (c) Entrapment neuropathics.
   (d) Arthritis.
2 Localized regional conditions.
   (a) Pain in the toes.
   (b) Pain in the anterior metatarsal region.
   (c) Pain in the midtarsal region.
   (d) Pain in the heel.
   (e) Pain in the plantar region.

Generalized conditions

Foot deformities include:
1 Pes planus.
2 Pes cavus.
3 Varus deformity of the hind foot.
4 Varus deformity of the fore foot.
5 Valgus deformity of the fore foot.

Pes planus

Pes planus, flat feet or pronated feet should be regarded as a clinical finding, the cause of which needs to be determined and which may not be the cause of the patient's symptoms. A normal arch is important, especially in runners when pain and instability may be experienced with this deformity. It can occur as the result of excessive subtalar joint pronation which is associated with a valgus deformity of the rear foot, the most common cause being as a compensation for a fore foot varus to allow the fore foot to reach the ground [12]. Other causes include: genu varum, tibia varum, unequal leg lengths, tight Achilles tendons, and hypermobility syndromes [12].

Symptoms do not correlate with the degree of these structural alterations and symptoms may be absent while the foot remains supple. Even when this deformity is present it is not necessarily the cause of pain and pain may indicate that the compensatory mechanisms that maintain stability are beginning to fail. In symptomatic cases pain in the midtarsal or anterior metatarsal regions is usually the presenting symptom. Pain is usually exacerbated by activity and becomes worse as the day goes on. The patient may also complain of aching legs or cramps. Symptoms often commence during adolescence, often after sporting activities or starting a new occupation or possibly owing to growth. In adults, symptoms may also be brought on or exacerbated by pregnancy, increasing weight, trauma, after a period of prolonged bed rest or by plantar fasciitis.

MANAGEMENT
This condition requires treatment only if it is painful. Arch supports have been traditionally prescribed but should no longer be used as they do not form a system with the foot to provide sufficient biomechanical control.

1 Orthotic supports [12,13]. The valgus deformity of the hind foot may be controlled by orthotic supports, with a supinator wedge placed under the inner side of the calcaneus to return it to its vertical position. A thinner pronator wedge may be placed under the base of the fifth metatarsal bone to lift the lateral border of the foot, combined with a support under the navicular if pain is severe.
2 The shoe should be made with a reinforced heel counter to stabilize the hind foot and the waist made tight over the instep. Running shoes should have an extended medial flare.
3 Mobilization techniques. These should be used to improve joint stiffness or pain and allow exercises and postural control to be more effective.
4 Exercises designed to strengthen the intrinsic muscles of the foot to restore the medial arch. An exercise for the plantar flexors of the toes include picking up objects such as marbles or a piece of cloth. Stretching exercises to correct a tightened Achilles tendon are usually necessary, combined with exercises to increase the range of internal

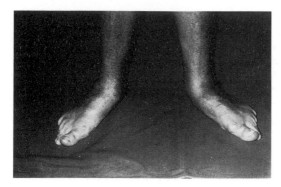

Figure 13.15 Rigid flat feet

rotation of the lower leg. Heel to toe walking with the weight on the outer border of the foot is encouraged.

RIGID DEFORMITY

A rigid flat foot may follow arthritis, such as rheumatoid arthritis, involving the subtalar joint [14] or as a late change in flat feet (Figure 13.15). Degenerative changes appear in joints around the navicular, evident on radiographs. Strong mobilizing techniques may dramatically relieve the pain and improve function even if only a small improvement in range is achieved.

SPASTIC FLAT FOOT

This condition, also known as peroneal spastic flat foot, is not uncommon. It is associated with a marked spasm mainly of the peroneal muscles but also of the long extensors of the toes; the underlying cause appears to be synovitis of the subtalar joint. It may be associated with congenital tarsal bars, which alter the normal foot mechanics and render the subtalar joint liable to trauma or overuse, so producing a synovitis. Synovitis may also occur after trauma or in the early stages of degenerative arthritis of the subtalar joint. This condition occurs most commonly in adolescent boys and is usually unilateral. There is often a history of recent sprain or overuse of the ankle or of having recently started work that entails prolonged standing or walking (apprentice's foot). Pain is usually severe and felt over most of the foot, especially midtarsal. It is worse as the day goes on, is exacerbated by weight-bearing, is eased to some extent by rest and may cause a limp.

Signs include a flattening of the medial longitudinal arch and marked muscle spasm in the peroneal and long extensors of the toes, and the foot is everted. The outer toes may be hyperextended at the metatarsophalangeal joints with a flexion deformity of the interphalangeal joints produced by the spasm in the long extensor muscles. Tenosynovitis may occur in the peroneal tendon sheath. Passive inversion of the foot is markedly restricted by pain and produces an increase in the degree of muscle spasm. Ankle movements are usually normal.

Radiographs are necessary to determine the presence of a bony synostosis and oblique views, tomograms or CT scans may also be necessary.

MANAGEMENT

1   Rest to the foot is essential and weight-bearing may need to be avoided. If pain is severe the foot and ankle are immobilized in the neutral position in a cast. A general anaesthetic may first be required to overcome the spasm and the foot is manipulated into the neutral position. The cast is worn for 6–8 weeks, after which symptoms usually subside.

2   Analgesics and anti-inflammatory drugs are given as required.

3   Injection of the subtalar joint. The patient lies supine with the foot fully inverted to open up the site of injection through the lateral opening of the tarsal canal. This can be easily palpated one fingerbreadth below and one fingerbreadth anterior to the tip of the lateral malleolus and can be felt to gap open as the foot is passively inverted. A 23-gauge needle inserted into the canal opening is directed slightly anteriorly for approximately 4 cm. It normally meets no resistance and 1 ml of corticosteroid and 2 ml of local anaesthetic are injected.

4   Manipulation or mobilization of the painful joints does much to relieve pain and muscle spasm.

5   Surgery may be required in patients with a congenital bony bar who do not respond to conservative therapy.

Pes cavus

This deformity is associated with an increased elevation of the medial longitudinal arch, so that the fore foot lies at a lower level than the hind foot. It typically has a rigid deformity of the fore foot which is in valgus. The toes become clawed, the foot is foreshortened, the subtalar joint is supinated and the heel goes into varus. Claw toes follow muscle imbalance between long toe extensors and weak intrinsic muscles of the foot. Muscle imbalances may result from neurological disorders such as peroneal muscular atrophy, Freidrich's ataxia, spina bifida or poliomyelitis. In most patients no underlying neurological disease is evident and it is classified as idiopathic. In some cases the deformity may not be marked and may be asymptomatic. Pain is usually caused by the excessive pressure under the second and third metatarsal, where painful callosities develop. Pain may also result from pressure effects over the dorsal surface of the clawed toes. Hind foot pain may result from ankle instability and recurrent sprains which may be a cause of falls in the elderly.

MANAGEMENT

Treatment is required if the foot is symptomatic. Management then consists of:

1 Orthotic supports [13] are designed to distribute pressure more evenly and relieve pain under the metatarsal head. A varus or valgus deformity of the hind foot is corrected by a pronator or a supinator wedge.
2 Shoes need to be made with sufficient room to accommodate the orthosis and the clawed toes. They should also have a low heel and stout leather soles.
3 Mobilization techniques are used to relieve pain and improve movements.
4 Exercises are mainly designed to strengthen the intrinsic muscles of the foot. Faradic foot baths may also be used for this purpose.
5 Operations are rarely indicated. Soft tissue release and tendon transfers, either tenotomies of the extensor tendons or transfer of the flexor tendons into the extensor tendons, may be combined with arthrodesis of the interphalangeal joints of the toes. Surgery to elevate the first ray above the level of the outer four metatarsals may be indicated. An osteotomy of the calcaneus may be necessary to correct a varus deformity of the hind foot.

Varus deformity of the hind foot

This is a common deformity [6] in which the posterior surface of the calcaneus is inverted relative to the ground, with the subtalar joint in neutral position. It is not considered to be of functional significance unless the deformity is greater than 5 degrees in the adult or 8 degrees in children. It may be produced by a varus deformity of the tibia or any congenital or acquired lesions of the subtalar joint, with decreased range of movement. As a result of the hind foot varus deformity, the plantar surface of the foot becomes inverted and the patient tends to walk

on the lateral surface of the foot. To compensate and maintain the foot on the ground during walking, pronation occurs in the subtalar joint. This in turn leads to hypermobility of the fore foot, with pain and callus under the metatarsal heads (especially the second) and a shearing strain is imposed on the soft tissue under the metatarsal heads on walking. Posterior heel pain may result from plantar fasciitis or a retrocalcaneal exostosis that develops as a reactive hyperostosis to abnormal pressure at heel strike and Achilles tendinitis. Excess pronation produces abnormal movement in the knee and may result in anterior knee pain.

MANAGEMENT

An orthotic device is used with a rear foot post to hold the rear foot inverted by the same number of degrees as the deformity. Pain may be relieved by mobilization of the subtalar joint, using strong techniques at the limit of range and large amplitude movements up to the limit of range. Surgery for the varus deformity is rarely indicated.

Varus deformity of the fore foot

This common deformity [6], in which the fore foot is inverted relative to the hind foot with the subtalar joint in neutral position, is also known as metatarsus adductus or varus (Figure 13.16). The basic abnormality lies in the development of the talus, as the normal varus torsion of the talar head and neck is retained [6]. Until the age of 2 years varus deformity of up to 5 degrees is common and requires no treatment. Deviation of the fore foot greater than 5 degrees will ultimately lead to foot pain and needs to be treated. The first metatarsal may become hypermobile owing to ligamentous stretching and

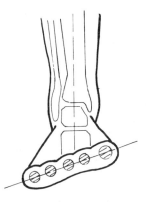

Figure 13.16 Varus deformity of the right forefoot relative to the hind foot

pain results as excessive weight is taken by the second metatarsal head. To compensate and allow the fore foot to bear weight during walking,the subtalar and midtarsal joints must pronate.

Examination of the compensated adult foot while standing shows the fore foot inverted relative to the hind foot and the medial metatarsal heads are raised relative to the outer ones. There is a convexity of the lateral border of the foot so that the base of the fifth metatarsal appears unduly prominent. The medial border of the boot is concave, with an increased medial angulation at the first metatarsotarsal joint and increased space between the first and second toe. The hind foot is usually in valgus. This condition needs to be differentiated from pes planus in which the fore foot is abducted. Measurement of the degree of fore foot varus is made with the patient lying prone and comparing the line of the metatarsal heads to an imaginary line drawn to bisect the calcaneus. This angle may also be measured on radiographs by drawing a line to bisect the calcaneus and the line of the fore foot.

MANAGEMENT

In children, this deformity may be corrected by a series of plaster casts applied while the foot is manipulated into a position of varus at the hind foot with the fore foot in abduction. In adults, a rigid type of orthotic device is made to accommodate the deformity with the subtalar joint in neutral. Numerous operations, including soft tissue releases and osteotomy of the metatarsals or the first cuneiform, have been described.

Valgus deformity of the fore foot

This condition, which occurs when the plane of the fore foot is everted relative to the calcaneus (Figure 13.17) with the subtalar joint in neutral position, is caused by an increased valgus torsion in the head and neck of the talus during development. It may involve all of the metatarsals or only the first metatarsal, which is plantar flexed. Compensatory mechanisms to overcome this valgus fore foot deformity take place by supination in the midtarsal joints and then in the subtalar joints.

The patient may present with fore foot pain, usually below the second or fifth metatarsal heads, with callus formation. The midtarsal joint is unable to develop full pronation during the push-off phase of walking, so excessive strain is placed on the first metatarsal ray, which becomes unstable. Pain is also experienced in the lateral compartment of the ankle and the patient may present with recurrent ankle sprains.

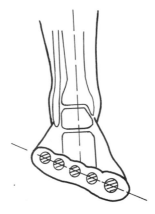

Figure 13.17 Valgus deformity of the forefoot relative to the hind foot

PLANTAR FLEXED FIRST RAY

In this the head of the first metatarsal lies below the transverse plane of the other metatarsal heads. It may be a congenital deformity or more commonly is associated with a valgus forefoot deformity. A fixed flexion deformity of the first metatarsal develops so that it is impossible to push its head up to the plane of the lateral metatarsals. On walking, the rigid first metatarsal strikes the ground first. The foot must then supinate quickly to bring the foot level with the floor and so the fifth metatarsal hits the ground forcibly. Pain and callus formation develop under the first and fifth metatarsal heads.

MANAGEMENT

1 An orthotic device to control the biomechanics of this deformity should be made.
2 In severe cases operation may be required to elevate the head of the first metatarsal. The peroneus longus tendon may be lengthened, or a vertical osteotomy through the base of the first metatarsal may be necessary.

Sudeck's atrophy

This form of reflex sympathetic dystrophy causes severe pain, swelling and disability in the foot. Its aetiology is unknown but the neurovascular disorder leads to an intense hyperaemia and osteoporosis. It may be idiopathic or follow prolonged immobilization but commonly follows trauma, which may be trivial. The natural history is one of prolonged pain and disability lasting up to 2 years; the condition then resolves, usually without any joint deformity. At times it may resolve in the affected foot only to appear later in the other foot.

The patient, usually middle-aged, presents with foot pain which may be of sudden onset. The pain becomes progressively worse, so that the patient is unable to walk on the foot, and may be present at night. The foot is swollen, often markedly, and the skin red and hot. Stiffness and swelling in the ankle and foot joints are common. Any area in the foot may be involved, not necessarily the site of the original trauma.

Radiographs are necessary to confirm the diagnosis, but changes appear after a variable length of time. Osteoporosis may be severe but joint spaces always remain well preserved, an important point in differentiation from arthritis. A CT scan or radionuclide bone scan (which may show similar changes in the unaffected leg) are positive earlier than radiographic changes. Laboratory tests are usually normal.

MANAGEMENT

1   The patient needs to be reassured that the ultimate prognosis is good, although the course of the disease may be prolonged and painful.
2   Analgesic and anti-inflammatory drugs are given to control pain.
3   Mobilization of individual joints in the foot should be used to relieve pain, thus assisting active movement and exercises [14a].
4   Encourage walking as much as possible even though pain is a problem because prolonged rest makes it worse.
5   Physical methods used in an attempt to control pain and swelling include alternate applications of heat and cold, TENS, interferential therapy, and active exercises which may be performed in a warm bath.
6   A translumbar sympathetic nerve block may be given and repeated if it succeeds in relieving pain.

Entrapment neuropathies

Tarsal tunnel syndrome

This is an entrapment neuropathy of the posterior tibial nerve as it passes in its neurovascular bundle behind and then below the medial malleolus to gain access into the foot [14b]. The nerve runs in a fibro-osseous tarsal tunnel, roofed over by the flexor retinaculum which runs from the medial malleolus to the calcaneus. The tunnel also contains the tibialis posterior, flexor digitorum longus and flexor hallucis longus tendons, each surrounded by a synovial sheath [3,15]. As the posterior tibial nerve passes through the tarsal tunnel it divides into the medial and lateral plantar nerves. The medial plantar nerve supplies sensation to the skin of the heel and the medial three and a half toes; the lateral plantar nerve supplies the lateral one and a half toes through its superficial division.

The syndrome may be caused by a tenosynovitis, especially of the posterior tibial tendon, which follows trauma, overuse or inflammatory conditions. It may follow sprain of the medial ligament or a fall onto the feet, and cause bilateral tarsal tunnel compression. Postural abnormalities of the foot, particularly pronation, may be associated with this condition. Overuse often follows sporting activity or occupations involving excessive use of the ankles, e.g. by climbing ladders. Tarsal tunnel syndrome may complicate rheumatoid arthritis or even more rarely may be its presenting symptom.

The patient presents with pain, described as burning or throbbing and often severe, in the plantar aspect of the foot and toes. At first it may be brought on by prolonged standing or ankle movements but subsequently it may be present at rest or radiate up the leg. Pins and needles or numbness in the plantar distribution of the nerve may also be present.

Examination reveals tenderness over the tarsal tunnel just posterior and distal to the tip of the medial malleolus. Pressure over this area for a few minutes should reproduce the patient's symptoms and a positive Tinel's signs may also be elicited. In the foot, sensory disturbances may be found in the distribution of the nerve and occasionally there is weakness of flexion of the interphalangeal joints. Evidence of tibialis tenosynovitis or of foot deformities may be present. Confirmatory evidence is obtained by nerve conduction studies to demonstrate sensory or motor disturbances in the branches of the plantar nerves.

MANAGEMENT

1   Any foot deformity should be corrected with the use of orthotic devices.
2   Local injection of 1 ml of corticosteroid into the tarsal tunnel is often most successful. A 25-gauge needle is used directed from above downwards into the hollow directly behind the medial malleolus to slide under the retinaculum.
3   If these methods fail exploration and surgical decompression of the tarsal tunnel will be necessary.

Medial plantar nerve

The medial plantar nerve is a branch of the posterior tibial nerve and may be entrapped in an opening in the abductor hallucis muscle. It may follow a foot deformity or trauma, either direct or secondary to wearing an ill-fitting arch support. Symptoms are similar to those of a tarsal tunnel syndrome but tenderness is located in the sole of the foot over the anterior portion of the calcaneus. Pressure localized here should reproduce the patient's symptoms.

Deep peroneal nerve

The deep peroneal nerve crosses the dorsum of the ankle covered by the extensor retinaculum. It then lies superficial to the tarsal bones and ends by supplying sensation to the lateral half of the great toe and medial half of the second toe. The nerve may be entrapped in front of the ankle as it lies beneath the extensor retinaculum and, because of its exposed position, it may be damaged by direct trauma, such as wearing poorly designed lace up shoes. The patient complains of sensory disturbances in the first interdigital cleft.

Localized regional conditions

Pain in the toes

Painful conditions of the toes may be due to:

1 Hallux valgus.
2 Hallux rigidus.
3 Hammer toes.
4 Mallet toes.
5 Varus deformity of the fifth toe.
6 A bunion of the fifth metatarsal head.
7 Arthritis.

Hallux valgus

Hallux valgus, a lateral deviation of the proximal phalanx of the great toe on the first metatarsal, is easy to recognize clinically but its aetiology is much more complex. It becomes symptomatic most often in middle-aged women but symptoms may develop during the teens. Hereditary factors play a part in its aetiology but it may also complicate conditions with ligament laxity and bony abnormalities such as metatarsus primus varus, a congenital shortening of the first metatarsal, varus deformity of the forefoot, pes planus and inflammatory arthritis. The wearing of tight or fashion shoes remains a controversial cause, although they can be implicated in the production and aggravation of symptoms. It is not uncommon in athletes and follows excessive pronation of the foot [16].

Other components of this deformity include:

1 Rotation of the great toe around its longitudinal axis, which causes the plantar surface of the great toe to face the second toe.
2 The extensor tendon comes to lie on the lateral side of the metatarsophalangeal joint, which increases the lateral deviation.
3 A bony exostosis develops on the medial side of the metatarsal head, covered by an adventitious bursa (bunion) which may become inflamed.
4 The sesamoid bones in the flexor tendons move laterally.
5 The great toe crowds out the second toe, which is forced to lie either over or under the great toe. At times the second metatarsophalangeal joint may dislocate.
6 Degenerative changes may develop in the first metatarsophalangeal joint.
7 Corns develop at pressure sites, usually over the dorsal and plantar aspects of the toes.
8 There may be a valgus deformity of the interphalangeal joint of the great toe.

CLINICAL FEATURES
The patient may present with pain related to the first metatarsophalangeal joint or to any of the above changes. Pain may be due to an inflamed bunion, which may become infected and break down forming a fistula. At times the only complaint may be painless deformity or swelling of the metatarsophalangeal joint. Pain under the outer metatarsal heads may follow either unequal weight distribution or an entrapment neuropathy of a plantar digital nerve. The diagnosis is readily made on inspection and the remainder of the foot is examined for any associated abnormalities. Radiography may be performed to record the degree of deformity and the degree of metatarsus primus varus.

MANAGEMENT
Conservative measures cannot correct this deformity but pain may be eased by wearing a moulded, roomy shoe with special protective pads. Mobilization of the metatarsophalangeal joint, with oscillatory movements in flexion–extension, abduction, adduction and rotation and compression, may provide pain relief.

Surgery is indicated for pain and needs to be carefully planned for satisfactory results:

1 Soft tissue operations include simple bunionectomy, which is not often of lasting value and McBride's operation to transfer the adductor hallucis tendon to the first metatarsal.
2 Arthroplasty of the metatarsophalangeal joint is the most common procedure and three operations have been described. Keller removes the proximal third of the proximal phalanx and the prominent medial part of the metatarsal head. Mayo excises the metatarsal head but results in shortening of the first metatarsus with extra weight being taken under the other metatarsal heads. A Swanson arthroplasty uses a silicone implant.
3 Osteotomy of the first metatarsal either through its neck or near its base.
4 Arthrodesis of the first metatarsophalangeal joint relieves pain but may give rise to subsequent degenerative changes in the interphalangeal joint.

Aftercare. The use of functional orthotics is essential to avoid recurrences.

Hallux rigidus

This descriptive title for osteoarthritis of the first metatarsophalangeal joint is not particularly apt, because restricted joint movement rarely produces complete rigidity. It occurs most often in middle-aged men and is often bilateral, and may occur in long distance runners. Dorsiflexion of the great toe is restricted because of restriction of plantar flexion of the first ray and symptoms arise because in the push-off phase of walking or running the joint becomes traumatized. Prominent osteophytes develop on the dorsal aspect of the joint, which becomes palpably thickened.

The patient usually presents with a gradual onset of pain and stiffness in the metatarsophalangeal joint. Pain may become quite severe and persistent, especially after standing or walking for any length of time. The interphalangeal joint compensates by becoming hyperextended and may develop a painful callosity on its plantar surface. Pressure from the shoe may then result in pressure effects on the toenail, which becomes thickened. Pain under the outer metatarsal heads may sometimes be the main complaint owing to rolling the foot to attain extension for propulsion.

The metatarsophalangeal joint becomes enlarged by osteophytes and an adventitious bursa over the dorsal surface of the joint. The normal passive range of metatarsophalangeal movement is lost, most markedly in extension. In younger patients or athletes degenerative changes may be much less prominent and symptoms are related to synovitis, often of sudden onset and palpable on the dorsum of the toe.

Diagnosis is confirmed by radiography. In older patients it may be asymptomatic and a chance radiological finding but in younger patients or athletes symptoms may be in excess of the radiological changes.

MANAGEMENT
1 Shoes and supports. Shoes need to be roomy to avoid friction against the hyperextended interphalangeal joint. A thick pad may be made to fit under the sole with a gap cut in it to fit under the metatarsophalangeal joint of the great toe and allow some freedom of movement. A rocker bar placed under the first metatarsophalangeal joint may also allow pain-free gait.
2 An injection of corticosteroid is useful to relieve symptoms of acute painful episodes. It is given on the dorsal surface directly into the synovium of the joint by directing a 25-gauge needle under the extensor tendon.
3 Firm mobilization techniques can often assist in relieving pain.
4 Surgery for the relief of pain is often necessary. Swanson arthroplasty is a satisfactory procedure. Arthrodesis is also advocated to relieve pain and does not cause any major functional disability as the patient is accustomed to having a stiff joint.

Hammer toes

This common deformity is due to a fixed flexion contraction of the PIP joint, which may be congenital or acquired. One or more of the outer four toes may be involved but most commonly the second. In time the extensor hood, which extends from the metatarsophalangeal joint to the distal third of the proximal phalanx, may develop a contracture. The proximal phalanx becomes hyperextended and the head of the metatarsal migrates plantarwards, with the formation of a painful callosity under the metatarsal head.

Pain results because of pressure from the shoe, which produces a painful callosity over the dorsum of the involved proximal interphalangeal joint.

Palliative treatment, strapping, pads, removal of the painful corns or wearing roomier shoes is rarely successful. Surgical treatment includes resection of the head of the proximal phalanx, with release of the extensor hood, or removal of the proximal end of the middle phalanx. Arthrodesis of the proximal interphalangeal joint is a satisfactory alternative.

Mallet toe

A mallet toe is a flexion deformity of the terminal interphalangeal joint of one or more toes. Pain is caused by a callosity that develops under the pulp of the toe or over the dorsum of the joint. Treatment is surgical and may entail amputation of the terminal joint.

Varus deformity of the little toe

This is a congenital deformity in which the little toe comes to lie across the base of the fourth toe. In adulthood pressure effects may become an increasing problem with a hard corn on the dorsal surface of the little toe and a soft corn between the fourth and fifth toes. Surgery may be necessary.

Bunion of the fifth metatarsal head

Inflammation in an adventitious bursa overlying the lateral aspect of the fifth metatarsal head may occur in rheumatoid arthritis, but is more commonly caused by an exostosis in the underlying bone. It has been named 'tailor's bunion' because tailors sit cross-legged. If surgery is indicated either the bony exostosis or the head of the fifth metatarsal may need to be resected.

Arthritis

In the spondyloarthritis of psoriasis or Reiter's disease, inflammatory changes in the interphalangeal joints and tendons on the dorsum of the toe lead to a reddened swelling of the digit, aptly named 'sausage-shaped'. Examination may also reveal the presence of associated nail changes and radiographs may show joint changes and/or periostitis.

Anterior metatarsalgia

Pain in the fore foot is a common symptom, and pain arising in the musculoskeletal system is given the descriptive title of anterior metatarsalgia. It needs to be differentiated from other causes of pain in this region that may result from diabetes or vascular, neurological or skin diseases. The anterior transverse arch, described as spanning the heads of the first and the fifth metatarsal bones and as having the second metatarsal as its keystone, is only an anatomical concept in the non-weight-bearing foot. The arch flattens out in the standing position and on walking so that body-weight is taken by all five metatarsal heads. The amount of weight transmitted to each metatarsal head varies according to the different positions adopted by the leg and foot, and most is borne by the first and fifth metatarsals.

It was previously considered that anterior metatarsalgia was caused by a dropped anterior arch, often from ligamentous weakness. As the forepart of the foot does not function as an arch this concept must be incorrect. Clinically, it may be found that the line of the metatarsal heads may become convex and weight distribution is abnormal, but the causes for this and for pain must be investigated further. The common musculoskeletal causes of anterior metatarsalgia are:

1 Foot deformities.
2 Trauma.
3 Entrapment neuropathy.
4 Freiberg's disease.
5 Morton's syndrome.
6 Hypermobility of the first metatarsal.
7 Arthritis of the metatarsophalangeal joints.

Foot deformities

Most of the foot deformities may be the underlying cause of anterior metatarsalgia. Symptoms usually arise from unequal distribution of body-weight so that excess weight is carried under the metatarsal heads with pain and callus formation under the metatarsophalangeal joints. In pes planus the fore foot is abducted and the peroneus longus tendon functions poorly in controlling first metatarsal movement, allowing excess weight to be taken on the more lateral metatarsal heads. The extensor tendons have an increased angle of pull on the phalanges, extending the toes and producing plantar deviation of the metatarsal heads. Pes cavus, with claw toe formation, leads to excessive weight being borne under the metatarsal heads and eventual plantar subluxation of the metatarsophalangeal joints.

Trauma

Traumatic conditions include stress fracture, traumatic synovitis of metatarsophalangeal joint and sesamoiditis.

STRESS FRACTURE

A stress fracture may occur in any of the metatarsals. The second is most commonly involved because it is the longest and most fixed of the metatarsals. It usually occurs as an overuse phenomenon in runners but may also develop in middle-aged people, especially women, owing to conditions producing overloading of the second metatarsal, such as a short first metatarsal or hypermobility of the first ray. It may also occur as a complication of other foot disorders. The condition was first described in army recruits involved in unaccustomed heavy activity (march fracture). Any part of the bone may be involved but most commonly in the neck, followed by the middle third, and rarely at the base.

The patient presents with an aching pain, usually of sudden onset and made worse by activity. If exercise is continued pain becomes quite severe. There may be some oedema over the dorsum of the foot and tenderness can be accurately localized over the bone. As the fracture heals, excess periosteal new bone is formed and may be palpable as a tender lump.

The diagnosis should be confirmed by radiography, although changes can take some time to develop. Periosteal new bone is seen around the shaft and the fracture line may be visible.

Treatment first consists of rest from weight-bearing combined with strapping around the foot. The patient can usually walk without producing an exacerbation of pain after a few days and can resume full activity in approximately 6 weeks.

TRAUMATIC SYNOVITIS OF THE METATARSOPHALANGEAL JOINT

Traumatic synovitis comes about when the second metatarsal functions under increased stress if the first metatarsal is not accepting its normal weight-bearing. It is usually brought on by running which may result in hypertrophy or stress fracture of the second metatarsal, synovitis of, or callus formation under, the second metatarsophalangeal joint. Active and passive flexion and extension of the metatarsophalangeal joint may be restricted and painful with tenderness localized over the joint. Synovial swelling may be visible or palpable. It needs to be differentiated from a stress fracture or Freiberg's disease by radiography.

Treatment consists of rest, a metatarsal pad behind the metatarsophalangeal joint and injection of corticosteroid into the dorsal aspect of the joint. Passive mobilization, gently at first but progressing as pain recedes, is valuable.

SESAMOIDITIS

Pain arising from a lesion of the two sesamoid bones in the flexor tendon of the great toe is usually from trauma. A fracture may result from direct trauma, or a stress fracture from overuse. The separated parts of the ossicle are evident on radiographs but must be distinguished from a developmental bipartide sesamoid, which should also be present on radiographs of the other foot. Pain may also occur owing to degenerative changes produced by osteochondral damage.

TREATMENT

This consists of support with a sponge rubber pad, placed behind the sesamoid bone. An injection of corticosteroid can be given using a 25-gauge needle around the flexor tendon. A fracture of the sesamoid is immobilized in a plaster cast. Occasionally, surgical excision of the sesamoid may become necessary if osteoarthritis produces recurrent symptoms.

Entrapment neuropathy of digital nerve

An entrapment neuropathy of the digital nerve between the metatarsal heads most commonly involves the third plantar digital nerve, which supplies sensation to adjacent surfaces of the third and fourth toes. The second interdigital space is the next most common site of involvement. The plantar nerves travel deep to the level of the metatarsal heads in a narrow fibrous tunnel, then angulate dorsally through the intermetatarsal ligament. Entrapment may follow excessive dorsal angulation of the nerve owing to overuse of the foot or alterations in the normal anatomical relationship. Overuse may occur in walking, running or with excessive extension of the toes, e.g. in occupations which involve squatting, such as carpet layers, or wearing high-heel or tight shoes.

It occurs most commonly in middle-aged females, may be bilateral and has characteristic symptoms. Pain usually described as severe, burning or throbbing is sited at first in the region of the metatarsal heads, shooting up into the toes. Pain may at times be localized to the opposing surfaces of the involved toes and may radiate proximally into the foot. It is usually related to walking but may be persistent. A most characteristic symptom is that the patient has to stop walking, sit down, remove his shoe and massage the foot to try to obtain relief. The patient may also complain of paraesthesiae in the toes.

An extremely tender area in the soft tissues between, not over, the metatarsal heads can be palpated and sustained pressure here should reproduce pain. It may also be reproduced by squeezing the metatarsal heads together for some minutes. Sensory disturbances may be elicited in the corresponding toes. Occasionally the swelling around the nerve may be palpable. The whole of the foot should be examined for the presence of any predisposing deformities.

MANAGEMENT

Conservative treatment should be instituted first because it often provides relief.

1 The patient should avoid the use of high-heeled or tight shoes and try to avoid stress, hyperextension of the metatarsophalangeal joints or excessive walking.
2 It is not usually possible to design a support to alter the anatomical relationships of the nerve but a metatarsal support may occasionally provide some pain relief.
3 Injections of local anaesthetic and corticosteroid into the affected area are easy to perform and produce pain relief for varying lengths of time.
4 Mobilization of the intermetatarsal area may be valuable for the relief of pain.
5 Surgery to divide the intermetatarsal ligament and remove the area of swollen nerve is indicated if symptoms are sufficiently severe.

Freiberg's disease

Freiberg's disease involves the head of the second, or rarely the third, metatarsal during adolescence. Usually classified as an osteochondritis, owing to an avascular necrosis of the bone, it has also been considered as an osteochondritis dissecans or an osteochondral fracture. At times a loose bony fragment may be found within the involved metatarsophalangeal joint.

It may be asymptomatic or present with pain, swelling and localized tenderness made worse on weight-bearing. Enlargement of the metatarsal head may be palpable. Radiographs after a few weeks show typical deformity with broadening of the head and sometimes the neck of the metatarsal and the articular surface has an S-shaped deformity. The bone in the centre of the head is sclerotic and the joint space is widened. Pain resolves slowly over weeks or months but radiographic appearances remain unaltered. In later years degenerative joint changes develop.

MANAGEMENT

In its early stages management consists of a suitably placed metatarsal pad and rest to the foot. Surgery to increase blood supply to the metatarsal head before the bone ends separate may be successful. Later the metatarsal head may be resected but symptoms may persist. More relief may be obtained from excision of the base of the proximal phalanx and remodelling the metatarsal head or by removing loose bony fragments.

Morton's syndrome

The configuration of the foot in this syndrome was though to be similar to that of prehistoric man. There is congenital shortening of the first metatarsal with hypermobility of the first tarsometatarsal joint, which is also abducted (metatarsus primus varus). The second metatarsal is longer than the others, takes excessive weight and becomes hypertrophied with callus formation under its metatarsal head. A similar clinical picture may result from an acquired deformity of the first metatarsal after surgical correction for hallux valgus. Athletes with this condition may develop a stress fracture of the second metatarsal.

Orthotics or a platform built under the head of the first metatarsal to redistribute the weight should relieve pressure on the second metatarsal.

Hypermobility of the first metatarsal

The fundamental cause of this condition is ligamentous laxity of the first tarsometatarsal joint [6] leading to hypermobility of the first ray and it may develop as a complication of a varus fore foot. It becomes symptomatic on weight-bearing as the first metatarsal does not take its share of the load, and the second metatarsophalangeal joint receives excessive weight causing pain and callus formation under the second metatarsal head.

Hypermobility may be tested for by placing one thumb under the plantar surface of the first metatarsophalangeal joint and the other thumb under the plantar surface of the second metatarsophalangeal joint. These two joints are then forced into passive dorsiflexion and the examiner notes whether an increased range is present in the first ray.

Midtarsal pain

Midtarsal pain is commonly the result of:

1 Foot deformities.
2 Joint disorders.
    (a) Hypomobility, cuboid syndrome.
    (b) Arthritis.
3 Bone lesions.
    (a) Stress fracture of the navicular.
    (b) Osteochondritis of the navicular.
    (c) Dorsal exostosis.
4 Soft tissue lesions.
    (a) Peroneal brevis tendinitis.
    (b) Sinus tarsi syndrome: instability of the subtalar joint.

Foot deformities

Patients with either a pes planus or a pes cavus may present with midtarsal pain. Preliminary examination usually reveals that supination or pronation is painful and restricted in the subtalar and the midtarsal joints. Additional tests are then necessary to find the appropriate joint.

Joint disorders

Hypomobility lesions of the midtarsal joints, also called the cuboid syndrome [17] are relatively common and may follow trauma with sprain of these joints. Pain may be felt diffusely in the midtarsal region but is most common on the plantar aspect of the foot under the cuboid. Pain is often made worse on walking. Accessory movements in the transverse tarsal joint are lost and these movements reproduce the pain. Radiographs are normal.

Hypomobility in the midtarsal joints is treated by passive mobilization, usually with rapid improvement. Mobilizations use small-amplitude movements into the painful range at the limit of the restricted range. If dorsiflexion is painful and limited, treatment consists of small-amplitude dorsiflexion movements localized to this area by the thumbs (Figure 13.18). Otherwise, treatment by manipulation may be necessary. The patient lies prone with legs over the edge of the couch. Two thumbs are placed over the plantar surface of the cuboid and the fore foot grasped with the hands. A quick downwards thrust with the thumbs moves the cuboid dorsally and laterally over the calcaneus.

Bone lesions

1 Stress fractures of the navicular are becoming more common [18,19]. They occur in athletes, usually sprinters, and involve the middle third of the navicular bone. Radiographs may not always be diagnostic at first and technetium bone scans may be more useful. The diagnosis should then be subsequently confirmed by radiography or CT scan. Treatment, by a non-weight-bearing cast, is often sufficient but in cases of non-union surgery is indicated [20].
2 Osteochondritis of the navicular (Kohler's disease) is rare. The patient is usually a child with pain in the midtarsal area and a limp. There may be some localized swelling and tenderness, and radiographs show a small squashed sclerotic navicular; this will revert to normal over approximately 2 years but degenerative changes in the talonavicular joint may develop in later life.

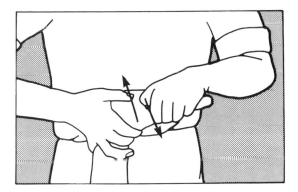

Figure 13.18 Intertarsal dorsiflexion

3 Dorsal exostosis is an osteocartilaginous swelling over the dorsum of the first tarsometatarsal joint. It is often painless, and may represent a response to pressure, as from lacing shoes too tightly, and an adventitious bursa may sometimes develop over it. Radiographs usually show surprisingly little change. Treatment is by preventing pressure from the shoe.

Soft tissue lesions

PERONEAL BREVIS TENDINITIS
An overuse lesion of the peroneus brevis tendon inserted into the base of the fifth metatarsal is not uncommon. Pain around the base of the fifth metatarsal bone is made worse by running. Isometric contraction of the muscle, by resisting eversion of the foot, reproduces pain.

Treatment consists of rest, anti-inflammatory drugs, mobilization and injection of the locally tender area around the styloid process with 1 ml of local anaesthetic and 1 ml of corticosteroid.

This injury needs to be differentiated from an avulsion or stress fracture of the styloid process of the fifth metatarsal bone, which will be evident on radiographs.

Heel pain

Causes include:

1 Soft tissue lesions.
   (a) Plantar fasciitis.
   (b) Bruised heel.
   (c) Lesions of the Achilles tendon (see p. 181).

2   Bone.
   (a) Exostosis of the superior tuberosity of the calcaneus.
   (b) Osteochondritis of the calcaneus.
   (c) Stress fracture of the calcaneus.
3   Joints.
   (a) Hypomobility of the subtalar joint.
   (b) Synovitis of the subtalar joint.

Soft tissue lesions

PLANTAR FASCIITIS

The plantar fascia originates from the tuberosity of the calcaneus and extends distally, covering the intrinsic foot muscles. Its bowstring effect plays an important role in maintaining the integrity of the medial longitudinal arch and stabilizing the foot during toe-off [2]. It becomes stretched either when the medial arch is flattened or on take-off when extension of the toes pulls the fascia more distally. Stretching produces traction on its calcaneal attachment and tension may increase to twice body-weight. Forces are obviously increased during running, especially on a hard surface [2]. Inflammation of the plantar fascia occurs at its attachment into the periosteum.

Plantar fasciitis is common in either sex, usually over the age of 40 years, except in active sportsmen when the patient, usually a male, may be in his twenties [21]. It is common in occupations involving prolonged standing or walking, or in some foot deformities, hallux rigidus, or may be associated with restricted movement in the subtalar joint.

Pain is localized over the medial tuberosity of the calcaneus, but may radiate along the sole of the foot. It may be severe and then usually interferes with function. Pain is made worse by activity, such as walking or climbing stairs, may be present at night, is often present when first getting out of bed and tends to be relieved by rest. Pain may begin suddenly during activity, when it may be caused by a tearing of some of the fibres, or may follow direct trauma.

Examination usually localizes the site of pain and tenderness accurately to the fascial attachment. Pain may be reproduced by stretching the fascia, e.g. on full dorsiflexion of the ankle. Entrapment of the posterior tibial or medial calcaneal nerves may also cause pain.

Radiographs may be normal or show a calcaneal spur, which represents the process of repair as hypertrophic bones grow out along the lines of stress in the fascia. The spur should not be regarded as the source of pain and it may be asymptomatic or a chance finding on radiographs. Radiography in inflammatory arthritis may reveal erosive or periosteal changes. A bursa commonly found under the attachment of the fascia may be inflamed in rheumatoid arthritis. Subcutaneous nodules here become painful and tender on walking. Gout does not often involve this area but should it do so the patient usually has long-standing clinical gout.

MANAGEMENT

1   Rest. The patient is advised to rest from running until pain settles, which unfortunately often takes a considerable time and other activities such as swimming, bicycling or flotation exercises may be substituted.
2   Orthotics are designed to relieve some of the stress on the plantar fascia and will vary according to the presence of any underlying foot deformity [21].
3   Supports. A sponge or Sorbo rubber pad with a piece removed to correspond with the painful heel area is placed under the heel to raise it approximately 1 cm and lessen the strain on the fascial attachments. It is worn at all times in shoes or slippers, but rarely provides much relief. In patients with a varus or valgus deformity of the hind foot, a suitable wedge may be inserted into the shoe or a spring-loaded heel used in the shoe.
4   Anti-inflammatory drugs may be given for pain relief.
5   Mobilization techniques may relieve pain by stretching the plantar fascia or mobilizing the hind foot and subtalar joint.
6   Corticosteroid injections into the painful area in the heel are quite effective. The tender area over the tuberosity of the calcaneus is found by palpation and a 21-gauge needle directed through the heel pad to the periosteum. It is usually quite a painful injection and 3 ml of local anaesthetic should be added to 1 ml of corticosteroid. The area around the bone and the plantar fascial attachments must be widely infiltrated. The patient is advised to rest from weight-bearing for a day after the injection and warned that the pain may be severe. The injection may be repeated several times at intervals of 2 weeks.
7   Physical methods are not usually very successful although daily application of ultrasound may lessen pain and help to localize the tender area.
8   Surgery is rarely indicated. Stripping of the plantar fascia from its origin on the calcaneus is only moderately successful. The spur is removed at the same time, but removal of a spur without stripping the fascia is not advisable. Release of an entrapped nerve may be successful [8].

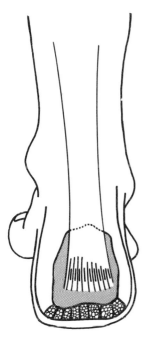

Figure 13.19 Structure of the fibro-fatty pad of the heel

BRUISED HEEL

The normal structure of the fibro-fatty pad of the heel is shown in Figure 13.19. With age or repeated trauma in running or jogging the fibrous septa of this pad may be disrupted and the fat pad may be dispersed. The heel is painful and swollen and may feel tender and thickened on palpation.

Treatment is often difficult and may require prolonged rest. Heel pads are of little value and more relief can be obtained from a moulded cup to compress the sides of the calcaneus to prevent the fat pad from being dispersed. Prevention by use of well-padded shock-absorbing heels is necessary.

Bone

EXOSTOSIS OF THE SUPERIOR TUBEROSITY OF THE CALCANEUS

This bony exostosis on the posterolateral surface of the calcaneus is usually found in young adults often associated with a varus deformity of the hind foot. In young females it may be caused by wearing high-heel shoes. The patient may present with an unsightly swelling, pain made worse by wearing shoes, or with an Achilles bursitis.

Treatment Varus deformity of the heel is corrected by use of suitable orthotics. Shoes are worn with a high heel and pliable uppers with a sponge-rubber pad to cushion the back of the heel. Surgical removal of the exostosis is very successful if conservative measures fail.

OSTEOCHONDRITIS OF THE CALCANEUS

This condition occurs mainly in young males, aged 7 to 14 years, owing to traction by the Achilles tendon on the un-united calcaneal apophysis. Radiographs reveal fragmentation and sclerosis of the calcaneal apophysis, although these findings are often non-specific. The child is nearly always engaged in sports involving running, and usually presents during the middle of the athletics or football season with heel pain and stiffness. Pain, at first related to activity and relieved by rest, usually increases and he is unable to continue running.

Examination localizes the lesion to the Achilles tendon insertion into the posterior aspect of the calcaneus, where there may be some degree of swelling, thickening or tenderness. It is often associated with a varus hind-foot deformity with an inefficient action of the Achilles tendon and loss of passive ankle dorsiflexion.

Osteochondritis dissecans may rarely occur in older age groups [22].

Management This consists of rest from running and a pad to elevate the heel. Physical methods usually produce only temporary relief.

Joints

HYPOMOBILITY OF THE SUBTALAR JOINT

Restriction of movement in the subtalar joint may develop in patients who have had an ankle sprain, have spent a prolonged period of time in bed, or had a leg immobilized in plaster. Mobilization techniques are the treatment of choice.

SYNOVITIS OF THE SUBTALAR JOINT

Synovitis may follow trauma to the foot or a sprain of the ankle joint. Pain, usually felt in the heel or the midtarsal region, persists after the original trauma has settled. Movement in the subtalar joints is restricted and painful and a valgus hind foot deformity may be found. Degenerative changes in the posterior talocalcaneal joint increase pain and stiffness and progressive valgus deformity of the hind foot.

SINUS TARSI SYNDROME

This relatively ill-defined syndrome comprises pain related to the opening of the sinus tarsi on the lateral side of the hind foot (Figure 13.3). It may follow trauma with resultant stiffness of the subtalar joint.

Investigations may include arthrography [23]. Preferred treatment is with joint mobilization and injection of corticosteroid into the sinus tarsi itself.

This disorder may ultimately lead to subtalar instability [24].

Management

1 The patient needs extra rest from weight bearing and the joint may be supported by a posterior slab worn at night.
2 Anti-inflammatory drugs are prescribed.
3 Injection of local anaesthetic and corticosteriod may be given into the lateral opening of the tarsal canal.
4 Mobilization techniques are used to ease joint pain and stiffness.
5 A triple arthrodesis may be necessary for persistent pain owing to osteoarthritis.

Plantar pain

Pain in the plantar aspect of the foot involving the heel and fore foot or from a tarsal tunnel syndrome has been discussed above. Other causes include:

1 Soft tissue lesions.
   (a) Tendinitis of the flexor hallucis longus.
   (b) Ledderhose's disease.
2 Foot deformities.
3 Joint disorders.
   (a) Arthritis.
   (b) Hypomobility lesions.
   (c) Acute strain of the medial longitudinal arch.

Soft tissue lesions

TENDINITIS OF THE FLEXUS HALLUCIS LONGUS TENDON

This is not uncommon, especially as a sporting injury from running on an unaccustomed surface, or running barefoot in sand. Pain is usually reproduced by the examiner fully resisting plantar flexion of the great toe or by stretching the flexor tendon. An area of tenderness may be found along the course of the tendon, usually proximal to the head of the first metatarsal.

Treatment consists of rest from running, ultrasound, mobilization, and injection around the tendon sheath with 1 ml corticosteroid.

LEDDERHOSE'S DISEASE

This is a fibromatous swelling in the plantar fascia, most often in the medial aspect of the middle portion, and may be present in both feet. It is related to Dupuytren's contracture in the hand and Peyronie's disease of the penis, either or both of which may be present. It can be asymptomatic but may produce pain especially on weight bearing and may cause a compression neuropathy of the medial plantar nerve.

A sponge rubber cushion or an insole in which a hole is cut to accommodate the tender nodule may help. If not a wide excision of the fascia may be necessary.

Foot deformities

Plantar pain may be the presenting symptom in patients with pes planus or pes cavus.

Joint disorders

Plantar pain may occur in:
1 Inflammatory arthritis.
2 A hypomobility lesion of the transverse tarsal joint, which most commonly involves the talonavicular joint with pain related to the spring ligament. It responds well to mobilization techniques.
3 Acute strain of the medial longitudinal arch occurs mainly as a result of running with repetitive depression of the medial arch. This overuse injury involves the tibialis posterior tendon, the spring ligament or the flexor hallux longus tendon. Pain felt under the medial side of the foot is made worse by activity.

References

1 Riegger, C.L. (1988) Anatomy of the ankle and foot. *Physical Therapy*, **68**, 1802–1804
2 Perry, J. (1983) Anatomy and biomechanics of the hindfoot. *Clinical Orthopaedics and Related Research*, **177**, 9–15
3 Ericksson, S.J., Quinn, S.F., Kneeland, J.B. *et al.* (1990) MR imaging of the tarsal tunnel and related spaces: Normal and abnormal findings with anatomic correlation. *American Journal of Roentgenology*, **155**, 323–328
4 Evans, P. (1990) Clinical biomechanics of the subtalar joint. *Physiotherapy*, **76**, 47–51
5 Oatis, C.A. (1988) Biomechanics of the foot and ankle under static conditions. *Physical Therapy*, **68**, 1815–1821
6 Tiberio, D. (1988) Pathomechanics of structural foot deformities. *Physical Therapy*, **69**, 1840–1849

7 Maitland, G.D. (1982) *Gait.* Videotape no. 24. Postgraduate Study Centre Medizinische Abteilung, Bad Ragaz, Switzerland, CH-7310

8 Rodgers, M.M. (1988) Dynamic biomechanics of the normal foot and ankle during walking and running. *Physical Therapy,* **68**, 1822–1830

9 Giallonardo, L.M. (1988) Clinical evaluation of foot and ankle dysfunction. *Physical Therapy,* **68**, 1850–1856

10 McPoil, T.G. Jr. (1988) Footwear. *Physical Therapy,* **68**, 1857–1865

11 Bouche, R.T. and Kuwada, G.T. (1984) Equinus deformity in the athlete. *Physician and Sports Medicine,* **12**, 81–91

12 Subotnick, S.I. (1981) The flat foot. *Physician and Sports Medicine,* **9**, 85–91

13 Lockard, M.A. (1988) Foot orthoses. *Physical Therapy,* **68**, 1866–73

14a Rolf, G. (1988) The treatment of patients with Sudeck's atrophy syndrome including the use of passive mobilization techniques. *International Federation of Orthopaedic Manipulative Therapists,* 50–51

14b Schon, L.C. and Baxter, D.E. (1990) Neuropathies of the foot and ankle in athletes. *Clinics in Sports Medicine,* **9**, 489–509

15 Zeiss, J., Fenton, P., Ebraheim, N. *et al.* (1990) Normal magnetic resonance anatomy of the tarsal tunnel. *Foot and Ankle,* **10**, 214–218

16 Berman, D.L. (1982) Etiology and management of hallux valgus in athletes. *Physician and Sports Medicine,* **10**, 103–108

17 Newell, S.G. and Woodle, A. (1981) Cuboid syndrome. *Physician and Sports Medicine,* **9**, 71–76

18 Keene, J.S. and Lange, R.H. (1986) Diagnostic dilemmas in foot and ankle injuries. *Journal of the American Medical Association,* **256**, 247–251

19 Torg, J.S., Pavlov, H., Cooley, L.H. *et al.* (1982) Stress fracture of the tarsal navicular – a retrospective review of twenty-one cases. *Journal of Bone and Joint Surgery,* **64A**, 700–712

20 O'Connor, K., Quirk, R., Fricker, P. *et al.* (1990) Stress fracture of the tarsal navicular bone treated by bone grafting and internal fixation: Three case studies and a literature review. *Excel,* **6**, 16–22

21 Roy, S. and Eugene, O.R. (1983) How I manage plantar fasciitis. *Physician and Sports Medicine,* **11**, 127–131

22 Taylor, P.M. (1982) Osteochondritis dissecans as a cause of posterior heel pain. *Physician and Sports Medicine,* **10**, 53–59

23 Goosens, M., de Stoop, N., Claessens, H. *et al.* (1989) A useful tool in the diagnosis of hindfoot disorders. Posterior subtalar joint arthrography. *Clinical Orthopaedics and Related Research,* **249**, 248–255

24 Heilman, A.E., Braly, W.G., Bishop, J.O. *et al.* (1990) An anatomic study of subtalar instability. *Foot and Ankle,* **10**, 224–228

14 Temporomandibular joint

This synovial joint is formed between the condyle of the mandible and the saddle-shaped mandibular fossa and articular eminence of the temporal bone (Figure 14.1). This joint has several unique features: it is a bilateral articulation in which two joints function as a unit; it is lined by fibrous not hyaline cartilage; and it contains an intra-articular disc or meniscus that divides each joint into two separate synovial cavities, an inferior and a larger superior space which do not normally communicate. The disc has thickened anterior and posterior bands. The posterior band connects to the bilaminar zone of vascular elastic connective tissue (Figure 14.2). The smaller anterior band attaches to the condyle, the articular eminence and the capsule. On its medial and lateral sides, the disc is attached to the neck of the condyle. The joint is surrounded by a loose capsule, strengthened by ligaments on its medial and lateral surfaces. The muscles of mastication, including the temporal, masseter and pterygoids, produce movement and also stability in the temporomandibular joint.

Synchronous movements of the temporomandibular joint produce opening and closing of the mouth, protraction and retraction of the mandible, and a lateral side to side movement of the chin. On opening the mouth, the inferior portion of the joint acts as a hinge joint and the disc and condyle rotate forwards together to be placed under the articular eminence. In the superior joint the condyle translates anteriorly under the eminence. On further opening, the posterior band of the disc abuts against the posterior surface of the condyle.

On closing the mouth these movements are reversed [1,2] and the meniscus is withdrawn to its resting position by elastic fibres in the bilaminar zone. In the upper compartment, a gliding movement in an anteroposterior direction allows for protraction and retraction of the jaw and a lateral side to side movement [3,4].

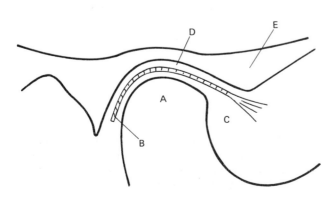

Figure 14.1 Temporomandibular joint. (A), Condyle of mandible; (B), intra-articular meniscus, with attachment to (C) lateral pterygoid muscle; (D), mandibular fossa; (E), articular eminence of the temporal bone

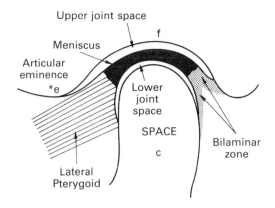

Figure 14.2 Normal anatomy of the temporomandibular joint. c, Mandibular condyle; e, articular eminence of temporal bone; f, articular fossa of temporal bone. (Courtesy of *Medical Journal of Australia*)

Temporomandibular pain

Pain in the jaw is a common complaint and needs to be differentiated from numerous other causes of facial pain. It may be referred from an unerupted molar or from carcinoma of the mouth or pharynx, from upper cervical spine trauma or degeneration. Confusion may arise when the neck and jaw have been simultaneously injured. Pain in the jaw may also occur in cranial arteritis when pain brought on by eating is the result of an intermittent claudication of the jaw muscles. Other features of this disease are usually present and the erythrocyte sedimentation rate (ESR) is invariably elevated. Diagnosis may be confirmed by a temporal artery biopsy. Jaw pain of psychogenic origin is not common, but should be suspected if a patient complains of a diffuse facial or head pain, usually of sudden onset and associated with inability or difficulty in opening the mouth. The patient will often describe this pain by placing one hand over all of the side of the face.

Pain and disability arising from the temporomandibular joint [5] have long been a controversial subject since the original description of dysfunction by Costen in 1934. Recently new forms of investigations, including arthroscopy, CT scans and MRI, have resulted in more accurate definitions and diagnoses [6].

Local causes of pain in the temporomandibular joint are most commonly the result of dysfunction of the temporomandibular joint in the younger age group and to osteoarthritis in the elderly but in all age groups these may need to be differentiated from an inflammatory synovitis.

Temporomandibular joint dysfunction refers to an internal derangement of the joint owing mainly to anterior displacement of the disc [1,4,7,8]. Myofascial pain and dysfunction is a separate, distinct, less common entity with no demonstrable evidence of organic disease [1,4].

Clinical examination

1 Inspection.
   (a) Symmetry.
   (b) Swelling.
   (c) Deformities.
   (d) Teeth.
2 Movements.
   (a) Active.
   (b) Passive.
   (c) Accessory.
3 Palpation.
   (a) Warmth.
   (b) Tenderness.
   (c) Swelling.
   (d) Clicks and crepitus.

Inspection

Inspection first notes facial symmetry at rest and on facial movements. The face is then inspected to detect the presence of any swelling, asymmetrical development, deviation of the chin, and underdevelopment (micrognathia) or enlargement (prognathism) of the jaw. In patients with condylar hyperplasia, excessive growth in the mandibular condyle results in deviation of the chin to the opposite side, with bowing of the mandible and a posterior open bite. Synovial swelling, which has to be marked before it becomes clinically obvious, presents just anterior to the external auditory meatus. Teeth and their occlusion are noted.

Movements

Active

The patient is asked to open and close the mouth, move the mandible to left and right and then to protrude it forwards while noting any deviation of the joint to one or other side.

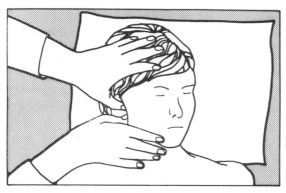

Figure 14.3 Transverse medial accessory movement

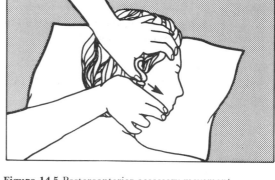

Figure 14.5 Posteroanterior accessory movement

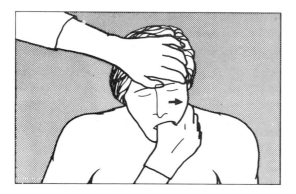

Figure 14.4 Transverse lateral accessory movements

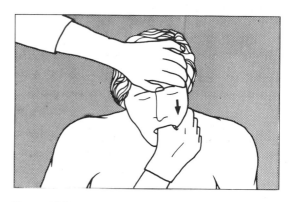

Figure 14.6 Longitudinal caudad movement

The range of vertical motion is tested with the jaw open maximally and slightly protruded. The distance between the upper and lower incisor teeth is usually between 4 and 6 cm [3]. The range of lateral motion is tested with the mouth partially open, the lower jaw protruded and wriggled from side to side. The range is approximately 2 cm.

Passive

These movements are then carried out passively. Over-pressure is applied at the limit of each available range and is best performed by taking a firm grasp of the mandible with the thumb inside the patient's mouth to assess end-feel and any muscle spasm.

Accessory

There are five accessory movements to be tested in the temperomandibular joint: transverse medial,

transverse lateral, posteroanterior, longitudinal caudad and longitudinal cephalad movements.

Transverse medial

Starting position The patient lies supine with the head turned to the left and resting on a pillow. The pads of the thumbs are placed together over the head of the mandible, fingers apart (Figure 14.3).

Method A transverse medial movement of the mandible head is produced by a movement through the examiner's arms and thumbs. If only one thumb is used to produce movement, the other hand can be used to palpate transverse lateral movement in the opposite joint.

Transverse lateral

Starting position The patient lies supine looking straight ahead. The examiner stands on the left side and stabilizes the forehead with the right hand. The pad of the left thumb is placed in the mouth near the head of the mandible. The pad of the left index finger is placed over the temporomandibular joint to feel the range of movement (Figure 14.4).

Method Lateral movement of the head of the mandible is produced by movement of the examiner's arm.

Posteroanterior

Starting position The patient lies supine with the head turned to the left and resting on a pillow. The examiner stands by the right shoulder with the pads of both thumbs against the posterior surface of the head of the mandible behind the lobe of the ear (Figure 14.5).

Method Posteroanterior movement is produced with the patient's mouth slightly opened.

Longitudinal caudad

Starting position The patient lies supine with the examiner on the left side with his left thumb over the right lower molars and his index finger over the lateral surface of the temporomandibular joint. The right hand is placed over the forehead to stabilize the head (Figure 14.6).

Method Distraction of the joint surfaces is produced by pressure with the thumb against the right lower molars. The range of movement may be felt by placing the index finger over the temporomandibular joint.

Longitudinal cephalad

Starting position The patient lies supine and the examiner stands on the left side; the heel of the left hand is placed on the inferior margin of the right mandibular angle and the right hand stabilizes the head.

Method Compression of the joint surfaces is produced by pushing upwards with the left hand.

Palpation

The temporomandibular joint is palpated at rest to determine the relationship between the head of the mandible and the articular eminence of the temporal bone, and then the muscles around the jaw are palpated. Both joints are palpated at rest and on movement for any warmth, local tenderness, clicks, crepitus, and soft tissue swelling or thickening. Capsular thickening is palpable in the chronic joint disorders and is more readily appreciated by comparing the normal side. The joint is also palpated by placing one finger in front of the external auditory meatus and next just inside the meatus to assess temporomandibular joint movement or any clicks or crepitus.

Lesions of the temporomandibular joint

1. Dysfunction and pain.
   (a) Temporomandibular joint dysfunction.
   (b) Myofascial pain syndrome.
2. Arthritis.
   (a) Inflammatory.
       (i) Rheumatoid arthritis.
       (ii) Spondyloarthritis.
       (iii) Juvenile chronic arthritis.
       (iv) Crystal synovitis.
   (b) Osteoarthritis.
   (c) Ankylosis.

Dysfunction and pain

Temporomandibular joint dysfunction

This is the best term to describe this common disorder, characterized by pain and internal derangement of the disc in the temporomandibular joint. The problem arises when the mouth is closed and the disc is displaced anteriorly to impinge against the condyle. Then, on opening the mouth, the condylar head, instead of rotating under the thin central zone, impinges on the posterior band of the disc (Figure 14.7) [4]. As the disc is crushed, clicks or crepitus may be heard on either opening or closing the mouth, especially opening (Figure 14.8). Movement is usually restricted. Subsequently, the disc is unable to return to its normal position and so remains anteriorly displaced even when opening the mouth, called 'closed lock'. Finally, the disc displacement may lead to a perforated disc, usually in the bilaminar layer [1]. This ultimately can lead to degenerative changes and osteoarthritis. It occurs much more commonly in females than males, is usually unilateral and any age group may be affected, although it tends to present in the early twenties. Some patients

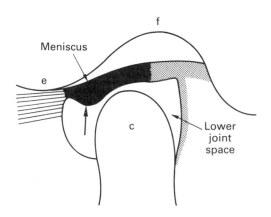

Figure 14.7 Anterior dislocation of the meniscus. The mouth is opened to a position just before a click occurs. The meniscus forms an impression on the anterosuperior aspect of the contrast-filled lower joint space (arrow). e, c and f, see Figure 14.2. (Courtesy of *Medical Journal of Australia*)

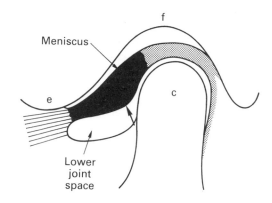

Figure 14.9 Anterior dislocation of the meniscus in a locked jaw. The meniscus forms an impression on the superior aspect of the lower joint space (arrow), as it is wedged between the head of the mandible (c) and articular eminence of the temporal bone (e). (Courtesy of *Medical Journal of Australia*)

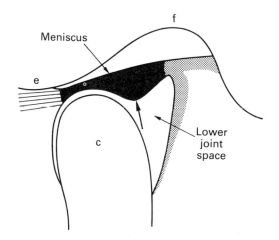

Figure 14.8 On opening the mouth a little further a click has occurred. The condyle (c) has moved forward under the articular eminence (e). The meniscal bulge (arrow) has now moved behind the condyle, and forms an impression on the lower joint space contrast there. The rapid movement of this meniscal bulge over the condyle causes the 'click'. (Courtesy of *Medical Journal of Australia*)

may have generalized joint hypermobility [4]. Symptoms may be intermittent, can be severe and widespread or chronic.

The presenting complaint is usually pain either in the jaw or the ear, but it often radiates widely into the face, head or even neck. Pain is often described as an aching, with a history of clicking in the jaw.

The patient is often conscious of a sensation of stiffness in the jaw which may interfere with eating or be worse in the early morning. Locking of the jaw is a rare and usually late complication.

MAJOR SIGNS

Abnormal joint movement may be either a restriction of movement or, on opening the mouth, a deviation of the jaw towards the painful side which returns to the midline at maximal opening. Clicking during jaw movement may be audible or palpable. Tenderness and thickening may be felt on palpation over the joint with the mouth both closed and open.

INVESTIGATIONS

Plain radiographs are usually non-contributory but arthrotomography, CT scans, MRI and arthroscopy have delineated the pathology [1,6,7,8,9,10–12]. The disc may be displaced anteriorly, perforated, buckled or torn from its attachments [13].

MANAGEMENT

Acute episodes are best managed with avoidance of exacerbating factors, heat and a soft diet. Surgery, and recently arthroscopic surgery, with either disc repair, if possible, or disc removal [6] may be indicated [1,12].

For a locked jaw a firm grasp of the mandible is taken with the thumb inside the patient's mouth and the head of the mandible is distracted away from its opposing joint surface (Figure 14.9).

Myofascial pain dysfunction

This separate entity in which there is no demonstrable evidence of organic disease or of internal joint derangement [4] is also a common cause of temporomandibular joint pain.

Pain is dull and aching, aggravated by chewing or other use of the jaw and usually becomes diffuse. It is unilateral and may be continuous or intermittent. It usually does not prevent sleep but may be present on awakening. It is often associated with headache and, less commonly, neck pain. Symptoms are often diffuse and include tinnitus, vertigo, hypersensitivity to sound and fullness in the ears. Jaw restriction and stiffness may be present. The muscles of mastication are tender to palpate, more so than the temporomandibular joint [3]. Routine investigations and radiographs are normal.

The aetiology is unknown [14] and several theories, that may be interrelated, have been proposed to explain the disability in the joint and surrounding muscles. There may be hypomobility of the temporomandibular joint following trauma or a primary muscle disorder with spasm or postural imbalance [3]. It has been ascribed to a psychosomatic disorder [6] with emotional stress causing tension and spasm in the muscles of mastication which may then lead to incoordination of movement. Such muscle tension may also be the underlying cause of habitual jaw clenching (bruxism) and teeth grinding. Joint pain may be associated with malocclusion, or abnormal dental occlusion, which may displace the condyle when the teeth are biting. This is often the result of loss of molar support and abnormal or compulsive chewing habits, such as clenching or grinding the teeth, or excessive use of chewing gum. These dental findings are rarely primary [3].

MANAGEMENT

1 It is most important to treat the patient and not just the temporomandibular joint itself. The patient needs to be reassured about the benign nature of his condition and the mechanism of pain production should be explained. Diazepam may be prescribed if muscle tension appears to be a major factor.
2 Physical methods of treatment, such as heat or ice, have little role to play in this condition.
3 Exercises to stretch the tightened muscles and restore coordinated movement have been advocated [3,15,16].
4 Relaxation exercises reinforced with biofeedback and behavioural therapy are of more value,

especially as tension appears to play a large role in this condition.
5 Mobilization techniques play a role in restoration of pain-free movement.
   (a) Accessory movements applied externally to the head of the mandible are used for pain.
   (b) With joint stiffness mobilization techniques to stretch the physiological movements and accessory movements at the limit of physiological range are used. Active exercises are given to retain the increased range.
6 In most cases, management should include a dental consultation to assess the degree of any malocclusion present. A temporary bite-raising appliance may be used at night to modify the position of the condyle of the mandible in its glenoid to lessen joint loading and so allow for muscle relaxation. Occlusal grinding to alter the shape and grinding surfaces of the teeth to achieve contact of the teeth when the jaw is clenched is rarely successful.

Arthritis

Inflammatory lesions

An inflammatory arthropathy may involve the temporomandibular joint. It is usually bilateral and may be due to juvenile chronic arthritis or rheumatoid arthritis and spondyloarthritis in older age groups. Juvenile chronic arthritis [17] commonly results in a disturbance of the bone growth with an underslung lower jaw with receding chin (micrognathia) and with bilateral temporomandibular joint involvement, the mandible remains small, but is symmetrical. In unilateral temporomandibular joint involvement there is maldevelopment of the mandible as the affected side is smaller than the other normal side so the face appears skewed. Pain is not very common and the condition may first become apparent when the second teeth erupt and the underdeveloped mandible is then too small to accommodate them.

In rheumatoid arthritis, the incidence of temporomandibular involvement varies in reported series, but some degree of clinical involvement is common [3]. Changes on radiography or CT are usually bilateral and can occur in up to 60% of cases [17]. Erosions in the anterior margins of the condyles and fossa are followed by destructive changes, subluxation or resorption. Patients have pain and swelling and subsequent changes may include progressive separation in the upper teeth and change in the bite.

Synovitis occurs in seronegative spondyloarthritis and may give similar types of changes [17]. Acute pseudogout has been reported [18].

Osteoarthritis

Degenerative changes also involve the temporomandibular joint [3] and may follow trauma, such as an intracapsular fracture of the condylar head. It affects women more commonly than men, usually in the fifth decade. It may be asymptomatic and symptoms include pain, stiffness and crepitus. Pain is present at rest or during movement such as shaving or yawning, and is frequently described as deep-seated, dull and aching in the preauricular region. Stiffness is often worse in the morning, making cleaning the teeth or eating difficult. Crepitus, tenderness and thickening are commonly present over the joint.

Radiographic changes are necessary to confirm the diagnosis but standard views usually do not provide sufficient detail and special views are needed. Early changes usually involve flattening of the condylar head and subsequently osteophytes develop on the anterosuperior aspect of the joint.

MANAGEMENT

Treatment should consist at first of conservative measures with anti-inflammatory drugs, the use of mobilization techniques, correction of dental faults and intra-articular injections of corticosteroids. If symptoms persist, condylectomy may be undertaken.

Ankylosis

Ankylosis of the joint may follow trauma, inflammatory arthritis, or septic arthritis [19]. In a child, ankylosis of the joint leads to micrognathia and the appearance of the bird-like face. The diagnosis is confirmed by CT scan.

Treatment is by temporomandibular joint arthroplasty. Teflon implants have been used [16] but may be complicated by an erosive arthritis [20] and their use has diminished [6].

References

1 Kaplan, P.A. and Helms, C.A. (1988) Current status of temporomandibular joint imaging for the diagnosis of internal derangements. *American Journal of Roentgenology*, **152**, 697–705

2 Gorman, E.S. and Warfield, C.A. (1987) The temporomandibular joint syndrome. *Hospital Practice*, **22**, 134–142

3 Hall, L.J. (1984) Physical therapy treatment results for 178 patients with temporomandibular joint syndrome. *American Journal of Otology*, **5**, 183

4 Harinstein, D., Buckingham, R.B., Braun, T. *et al.* (1988) Systemic joint laxity (the hypermobile joint syndrome) is associated with temporomandibular joint dysfunction. *Arthritis and Rheumatism*, **31**, 1259–1264

5 Gorman, E.S. and Warfield, C.A. (1987) The temporomandibular joint syndrome. *Hospital Practice*, **22**, 134–142

6 Solberg, W.K. (1988) Temporomandibular joint syndrome. *Seminars in Neurology*, **8**, 291–297

7 Schellhas, K.P., Wilkes, C.H., Fritts, H.M. *et al.* (1988) Temporomandibular joint: MR imaging of internal derangements and postoperative changes. *American Journal of Roentgenology*, **150**, 381–389

8 Westesson, P., Katzberg, R.W., Tallents, R.H. *et al.* (1987) CT and MR of the temporomandibular joint: comparison with autopsy specimens. *American Journal of Roentgenology*, **148**, 1165–1171

9 Burnett, K.R., Davis, C.L. and Read, J. (1987) Dynamic display of the temporomandibular joint meniscus by using 'fast scan' MR imaging. *American Journal of Roentgenology*, **149**, 959–962

10 Bare, V.L. (1987) Temporomandibular joint arthroscopy: a new treatment alternative. *AORN Journal*, **45**, 1368–1373

11 Rudy, T.E., Turk, D.C., Zaki, H.S. *et al.* (1989) An empirical taxometric alternative to traditional classification of temporomandibular disorders. *Pain*, **36**, 311–320

12 Schellhas, K.P., Wilkes, C.H., Omlie, M.R. *et al.* (1988) The diagnosis of temporomandibular joint disease: two-compartment arthrography and MR. *American Journal of Roentgenology*, **151**, 341–350

13 Gerschman, J.A. and Reade, P.C. (1988) Disorders of the temporomandibular joint and related structures. *Australian Family Physician*, **14**, 239–244

14 Passero, P.L., Wyman, B.S., Bell, J.W. *et al.* (1985) Temporomandibular joint dysfunction syndrome: A clinical report. *Physical Therapy*, **65**, 1203

15 Santiesteban, A.J. (1989) Isometric exercises and a simple appliance of temporomandibular joint dysfunction: a case report. *Physical Therapy*, **69**, 463–466

16 Talaat, A.M., El-Dibany, M.M. and El-Garf, A. (1986) Physical therapy in the management of myofacial pain dysfunction syndrome. *Annals of Otology, Rhinology and Laryngology*, **95**, 225–228

17 Avrahami, E., Segal, R., Solomon, A. *et al.* (1989) Direct coronal high resolution computed tomography of the temporomandibular joints in patients with rheumatoid arthritis. *Journal of Rheumatology*, **16**, 298–301

18 Hutton, C.S., Doherty, M. and Dieppe, P.A. (1986) Acute pseudogout of the temporomandibular joint: a report of three cases and review of the literature. *British Journal of Rheumatology*, **26**, 51–52

19 Sawhney, C.P. (1986) Bony ankylosis of the temporomandibular joint: follow-up of 70 patients treated with arthroplasty and acrylic spacer interposition, **77**, 29–38

20 Kaplan, P.A., Ruskin, J.A., Tu, H.K. *et al.* (1988) Erosive arthritis of the temporomandibular joint caused by Teflon-proplast implants: plain film features. *American Journal of Roentgenology*, **151**, 337–339

Index